Highly Infectious Diseases in Critical Care

Jorge Hidalgo • Laila Woc-Colburn
Editors

Highly Infectious Diseases in Critical Care

A Comprehensive Clinical Guide

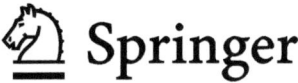 Springer

Editors
Jorge Hidalgo, MD, MACP, MCCM, FCCP
Division of Critical Care
Karl Heusner Memorial Hospital
Belize City
Belize

Laila Woc-Colburn, MD, DTM&H, FACP,
FIDSA
National School of Tropical Medicine
Baylor College of Medicine
Houston, TX
USA

ISBN 978-3-030-33805-3   ISBN 978-3-030-33803-9   (eBook)
https://doi.org/10.1007/978-3-030-33803-9

This Springer imprint is published by the registered company Springer Nature Switzerland AG
The registered company address is: Gewerbestrasse 11, 6330 Cham, Switzerland

To our families who have been able to cope with our time constraints and frustrations, always supporting us, making everything worthwhile.

Preface

We are delighted to introduce the book on highly infectious diseases, providing the physician with a guide to both the approach to the patient and the treatment.

Highly infectious disease (HID) is transmissible from person to person, carries a high rate of mortality, and represents a serious hazard in the healthcare setting and the community, which requires specific control measures. In the twenty-first century, due to our ability to move from one country to another, environmental factors, changes in lifestyle, and many other factors, we often have seen and experience the emergence of this disease, like SARS and more recently Ebola. With this book, we plan to present a description of the more common and highly infectious diseases to the healthcare practitioners, as well as to the institution, so they can prepare and plan for the potential outbreaks of emerging or resurgent HID. This book will help the critical care physician to define their role in defining the logistics, leading a team, and proving care for these patients. Also, it will help in identifying the barriers to conventional ICU practices when managing a patient with a particular pathogen and ways to circumvent these barriers. We hope the medical community will find it refreshing, exciting, and useful in daily practice.

Belize City, Belize   Jorge Hidalgo, MD, MACP, MCCM, FCCP
Houston, TX, USA   Laila Woc-Colburn, MD, DTM&H, FACP, FIDSA

Acknowledgments

The preparation of this book required the efforts of many individual. We particularly wish to thank each of the authors; their contributions, prepared in the midst of extremely busy schedules, are responsible for the value of this book. We are deeply appreciative of the help to make this book a reality.

We sincerely appreciate the talents and accomplishments of the Springer professionals, in particular Mr. Andy Kwan, who partner with us all along and took our manuscript and produced it into this book. We welcome all comments, pros and cons, as well as suggested revisions.

Contents

Contributors

Azka Afzal, MD Department of Internal Medicine, University of Chicago, Chicago, Illinois, USA

Adel Mohamed Yasin Alsisi, MD Prime Healthcare Group, LLC, Dubai, UAE

Pedro Arriaga, MD St Michaels Hospital, Toronto, ON, Canada

Catherine M. Berjohn, MD, MPH Division of Infectious Diseases, Naval Medical Center, San Diego, CA, USA

Uniformed Services University, Bethesda, MD, USA

Sarah Bezek, MD Department of Emergency Medicine, Baylor College of Medicine, Houston, TX, USA

Stephen Brannan, MD Department of Anesthesiology, University of Nebraska Medical Center, Omaha, NE, USA

Alex Loarca Chávez, MD Adult Intensive Care, Hospital Regional de Occidente, San Juan de Dios, Quetzaltenango, Guatemala

Daniel S. Chertow, MD, MPH, FCCM Critical Care Medicine Department, National Institutes of Health Clinical Center and Laboratory of Immunoregulation, National Institute of Allergy and Infectious Diseases, Bethesda, MD, USA

Bruno Alvarez Concejo, MD University of Texas Southwestern, Dallas, TX, USA

Denise Marie A. Francisco, MD Infectious Diseases, Baylor College of Medicine, Houston, TX, USA

Daniel Godinez, MD Department of Internal Medicine, Belize Healthcare Partners Limited, Belize City, Belize

Jorge Hidalgo, MD, MACP, MCCM, FCCP Division of Critical Care, Karl Heusner Memorial Hospital, Belize City, Belize

Ajay Hotchandani, MD General Medicine, Belize Healthcare Partners Limited, Belize City, Belize

Michael Jaung, MD Department of Emergency Medicine, Baylor College of Medicine, Houston, TX, USA

Holland Kaplan, MD Department of Internal Medicine, Baylor College of Medicine, Houston, TX, USA

Department of Infectious Diseases, Baylor College of Medicine, Houston, TX, USA

Jason Kindrachuk, MD Laboratory of Emerging and Re-Emerging Viruses, Department of Medical Microbiology, University of Manitoba, Winnipeg, MB, Canada

Joy Mackey, MD Department of Emergency Medicine, Baylor College of Medicine, Houston, TX, USA

Gerald Marín-García, MD VA Caribbean Healthcare System, Pulmonary Critical Care Section, San Juan, PR, USA

Ryan C. Maves, MD, FCCP, FIDSA Division of Infectious Diseases, Naval Medical Center, San Diego, CA, USA

Uniformed Services University, Bethesda, MD, USA

Tina Motazedi, MD Massachusetts General Hospital, Boston, Massachusetts, USA

Javier Pérez-Fernández, MD, FCCM, FCCP Critical Care Section, Baptyist Hospital of Miami, Florida International University, Miami, FL, USA

Michael J. Plotkowski, MPAS, PA-C Department of State, Foreign Service Medical Provider, U.S. Embassy Belmopan, Belmopan, Belize

Ignacio J. Previgliano, MD Hospital General de Agudos J. A. Fernández, Buenos Aires, Argentina

Universidad Maimonides, Buenos Aires, Argentina

Talha Qureshi, MD Department of Internal Medicine, Baylor College of Medicine, Houston, TX, USA

Department of Infectious Diseases, Baylor College of Medicine, Houston, TX, USA

Juan Ignacio Silesky-Jiménez, MD, FCCM, MSc University of Costa Rica, San José, Costa Rica

James Sullivan, MD Department of Anesthesiology, University of Nebraska Medical Center, Omaha, NE, USA

Ahmed Reda Taha, MD, FRCP, FCCP, FCCM Sheikh Khalifa Medical City, Critical Care Department, Abu Dhabi, United Arab Emirates

Gloria Rodríguez-Vega, MD HIMA-San Pablo, Caguas, PR, USA

Laila Woc-Colburn, MD, DTM&H, FACP, FIDSA Section Infectious Diseases, Department of Medicine, National School of Tropical Medicine, Baylor College of Medicine, Houston, TX, USA

Chapter 1
How Infectious Diseases Have Influenced Our Culture

Laila Woc-Colburn and Ajay Hotchandani

The history of mankind may be viewed and analyzed through the lens of infectious disease [1]. The history of the world has been influenced by the impact infectious diseases have had on the population. To grasp the correlation between infectious disease and culture, we must first look at what each is. Infectious diseases are disorders caused by organisms – such as bacteria, viruses, fungi, and parasites [2]. Culture is viewed as the customary beliefs, social forms, material traits, and characteristic features of everyday existence shared by people of the same group, religion, or ethnicity. So how does an organism invisible to the naked eye change the course of humanity? Its impact is so profound that, long after the disease is not a threat, the changes and effects continue.

In 1991, the Institute of Medicine of the National Research Council appointed multidisciplinary experts to study the emergence of microbial threats. In their report, they concluded that six categories of factors could explain the emergence/reemergence of infectious diseases [3]. These factors are as follows:

(a) Human demographics and behavior
(b) Breakdown of public health measures
(c) Economic development and land use
(d) International travel and commerce
(e) Microbial adaptation and change
(f) Technology and industry

L. Woc-Colburn
Section Infectious Diseases, Department of Medicine, National School of Tropical Medicine, Baylor College of Medicine, Houston, TX, USA

A. Hotchandani (✉)
General Medicine, Belize Healthcare Partners Limited, Belize City, Belize

© Springer Nature Switzerland AG 2020
J. Hidalgo, L. Woc-Colburn (eds.), *Highly Infectious Diseases in Critical Care*,
https://doi.org/10.1007/978-3-030-33803-9_1

Human Demographics and Behavior

The demographics of the human population and distribution history have, on numerous occasions, demonstrated the detrimental impact infectious diseases have had on the demographics of a nation. The European bubonic plague ("Black Death") occurred between 1348 and 1350. During a span of 2 years, it killed 20 million people, 2/3 of the European population at the time. The citizens made the correlation between close contact and crowded settings with being affected by the Black Death. It resulted in a decreased rate of urbanization, industrial development, and economic growth as people left cities and returned to a rural and agricultural lifestyle [4].

In 1875, measles was introduced to Fiji by travelers from the West. It resulted in a substantial number of deaths reducing the population by 25% within a few months. The deaths included those who governed the island leading to political unrest and resulted in colonization. Despite losing 25% of their population to measles, the Fijians fared better than the people of Hispaniola, who became virtually extinct after the arrival of Columbus and the pathogens brought over from Europe.

While those events saw the accidental introduction of pathogens into particular demographics, it did highlight the destructive power of infectious diseases on such populations. The strategic introduction of an infectious disease into a particular demographic for the purposes of causing harm is known as "germ warfare." It has been used several times throughout history with the threat of being it used during modern times through "bioterrorism". One such possible concern is that the virus which results in smallpox is being stored in a Russian laboratory. Since being eradicated in 1980, there has been less of an effort to immunize against smallpox thereby making the impact of a bioterrorism attack catastrophic.

With the improvement of infrastructure and delivery of medical care, the threat of living in an urban setting has declined. Human migration has been shifting toward cities and urban centers. The urban population jumped from 29% in 1950 to 50.5% in 2005 [4]. Working backward from the United Nation's prediction that the world will be 51.3% urban by 2010, Dr. Ron Wimberley, Dr. Libby Morris, and Dr. Gregory Fulkerson estimated 23 May 2007 to be the first time the urban population outnumbered the rural population in history [5].

Another event that affected the world's population, in a positive manner, was the introduction of antibiotics. In 1943, allied WW2 soldiers begin receiving supplies of antibiotics, saving thousands of lives [6]. As noted in Table 1.1, the general trend was an approximately 23% increase in population during a 50-year period. In 1950, there was a spike in the percentage of population increase by 137%. While there are multiple factors that may have contributed to the population growth, the widespread availability of antibiotics help saved lives that may have been lost to a respiratory or urinary tract infection, thereby having arguably the greatest impact on population growth.

Culture We are taught from childhood that it is important to socialize and be part of a group. If a child lacks social interaction, there is the possibility that they might be evaluated as to why they chose not to belong. Living in dense urban areas allows people to more easily interact and socialize with those they share the same beliefs and values allowing them to engage in activities representing these beliefs. Migration

Table 1.1 World population [7]

Year	Million
1500	458
1600	580
1700	682
1750	791
1800	978
1850	1262
1900	1650
1950	**2521**
1999	**5978**
2008	6707
2011	7000
2015	7350
2018	7600

patterns reflect ethnic populations, hence why you hear of an area within a city referred to as "Little _____" or "_____town," i.e., Little Italy or Chinatown. The sense and want of belonging helps drive urbanization, but also places a larger population at risk.

While difficult to prove, different forms of greeting may have contributed to a possible reduction in the spread of an infectious disease. Among males, it is now common to greet someone with bumping fists rather than shaking hands, thereby reducing the possibility of spreading a possible infection via contact. There are cultural greetings that avoid contact which can possibly reduce the spread of infectious diseeases i.e. Namaste (praying hand in India), Ojigi (bowing in Japan).

Breakdown of Public Health Measures

Public health measures are non-medical interventions used to reduce the spread of disease. They include, but are not limited to, providing public education, conducting case and contact management, closing schools, limiting public gatherings, issuing travel restrictions, and screening travelers. The type of public health measures used and the timing depend on the epidemiology of the microbe [8]. When implemented appropriately, these measures will help decrease the number of individuals exposed to the infectious disease, reduce illness and death, and slow the spread of disease in order to provide more time to implement medical measures to combat the infectious microbes.

A breakdown in any or all of these measures may result in epidemics becoming pandemics with detrimental consequences. A review of these measures, what they entail, and possible consequences as a result of a breakdown of that measure are laid out in Table 1.2 [8].

Culture The mindset of a country and its people are what can make or break the effectiveness of public health measures or occur as a result of a breakdown in public health measures. In August 2014, an Ebola quarantine center was raided and looted by men claiming that Ebola is a fictitious disease. During times of pandemics, the faster the public education is done and proper measures put in place, the less the citizens have to fear. We have become a society of instant gratification. We want to know and we want to know now. We turn to search engines such as Google and online social media such as Facebook to get any update from any source. Any delay in getting information out by the proper authorities leaves room for a mischief maker to publish "fake news".

Economic Development and Land Use

Health disasters such as the Ebola virus disease epidemic in West Africa, the Middle East respiratory syndrome (MERS) outbreak in the Republic of Korea, and the rise of antimicrobial-resistant pathogens have catalyzed investments in global health security. As the public health community works to strengthen national systems to avoid international spread of disease, governing bodies increasingly recognize that biological threats have not only global health impacts but also wide-ranging socio-economic disruptions [9].

Land-use change is rapidly converting forests and savannas into "anthro-habitat": land whose primary focus is the production of agriculture, shopping or sports facilities, or housing estates, all of which provide some direct benefit to the human economy. But how do these changes modify habitats in ways that change the probability of infectious disease outbreaks? Habitat conversion significantly alters the interactions between the environment and populations of humans and domestic livestock. The resulting changes in the infection dynamics of many vector- and waterborne disease systems could create new opportunities for pathogen infections, or could modify the dynamics toward pathogen reduction or eradication [10].

Culture In 2009, Mexico City came to an almost standstill during the H1N1 outbreak. The president started to shut down government offices and urged the private sector to close down also, stating being at home was the safest thing to do. Some private entities defied this request noting that they had to stay open as they cannot afford to lose any business. Some even thought they would capitalize on it seeing that their competitors were closed. The news of the H1N1 caused the stock market to slide down and a drop in the value of the Mexican peso. The World Bank has stated that a severe flu pandemic which triggers a clampdown on trade could cost the global economy trillions of dollars.

International Travel and Commerce

The terrifying scenario that something we cannot see with our naked eye can travel half way across the world and spark a global pandemic is a storyline all too familiar in Hollywood. Unfortunately, it is a scenario that has some roots in history. As men-

Table 1.2 Public health measure

Public health measure	Activities to implement measure	Timeframe and duration	Result of breakdown
Public education	Public education regarding infection prevention and control, social quarantine, and accessing medical care	This should occur as early as possible and remain throughout the event Trigger: First lab confirmation in country or region	With the advent of social media, (mis)-information can spread within minutes. A lack of public education will result in inaccurate information being circulated leading to confusion, mistrust, and loss of valuable time. It is crucial that the proper authorities are first in getting information; otherwise they will have to dedicate as much resources to public education as they will to combat false information
Travel restrictions	Foreign travel advisories, voluntary foreign travel restrictions, closing borders, and reducing transit time in places where public transportation is used	This is usually implemented once mode of spreading is determined to be droplet or airborne and an epidemic in a country or region has been declared. It remains as long as public health is at risk Trigger: Evidence of a pandemic strain	There is oftentimes a lag between medical diagnoses and when the data becomes available for analysis. Making a decision to restrict travel has economic consequences for any country, and therefore, they may be hesitant to make a decision too early thereby allowing the disease to enter their borders. Governments often weight multiple factors when deciding to restrict travel, and the delay in obtaining those factors can prove fatal
Case management	Voluntary isolation, self-care, medication, and public health follow-up	Often used in the early stages when there are fewer cases and the main goal being confirmation of the strain Trigger: Cluster of cases	A critical part of case management is providing information and strategies to infected individuals on how to reduce transmission to others. Improper case management can result in greater number of infected family members, drain on limited resources, and harder time trying to contain the infectious disease
Contact management	Education, voluntary and modified quarantine, and public health follow-up	Often used in the early stages when there is a chance to contain the spread and confirm the diagnosis is the same Trigger: Cluster of cases	If an individual who became infected and is not contacted may then become the carrier and spread the disease, one flight and the chances of proper contact management become virtually impossible

(continued)

Table 1.2 (continued)

Public health measure	Activities to implement measure	Timeframe and duration	Result of breakdown
School closing	Infection prevention and control measures, social distancing and school and day care closures	This has to be implemented at the beginning of a suspected outbreak Trigger: Cluster of cases within ministry of education region	Schools and day cares can be breeding grounds for infectious diseases. Failure to close schools will result in the introduction of the microbe into a very dense population in a very short period of time. They further propagate the infection when they come in contact with their family, which can include elderly people whom are housebound
Social distancing in the community	Workplace infection prevention and control for non-healthcare settings, restrict public gatherings, educate public on limiting private events	This is implemented during the early stages and maintained until the all clear is given Trigger: Cluster of cases within/nearby a local public health unit	If not implemented or implemented too late, it will result in greater than warranted close contacts which increases the chances of being infected and/or spreading the infectious disease. Mainly for economic reasons, some companies may be hesitant to implement any protocol that will limit their productivity and reduce financial gains

tioned earlier, those who traveled to the island of Hispaniola almost wiped out the population with infectious diseases.

Infectious diseases are spreading around the world faster than ever, says the World Health Organization, and new diseases are emerging at the unprecedented rate of 1 a year. Several factors have helped accelerate the spread of diseases around the world, namely, the increasing ease of international travel (each year airlines carry more than 2 billion passengers), population growth, resistance to drugs, under-resourced healthcare systems, intensive farming practices, and degradation of the environment [11]. Three important consequences of global transport network expansion are infectious disease pandemics, vector invasion events, and vector-borne pathogen importation.

Humans travel in numbers and at speeds like never before. Travelers visit remote areas as well as major population centers. With almost no limitations to traveling, it means that humans can reach almost anywhere within the incubation period for most microbes that cause disease in humans. Travel is also discontinuous, often including many stops and layovers along the way [12]. This situation creates the perfect scenario to infect numerous people without ever being able to track back "patient zero" when conducting Case and Contact Management.

Global travel has increased from 200 million international travelers in 1970 to 1.4 billion in 2018 [13]. In addition to the marked increase in the overall number, there has also been a shift in areas visited by travelers, especially to areas in Asia.

The 2006 figures from the World Tourism Organization showed the most rapid relative increase was to sub-Saharan Africa. Travel between regions was increasing faster than travel within regions, and air transport was growing at a faster pace than ground and water transport with air travel accounting for 46% of transport.

Political instability and disease outbreaks can also influence travel destinations, sometimes abruptly.

The biomass of humans constitutes only a fraction of the matter moved about the earth. Humans carry and send a huge volume of plants, animals, and other materials all over the face of the globe. Much of this movement results from the planned transport of goods from one place to another, but some is an unintended consequence of shipping and travel. All has an impact on the juxtaposition of various species in different ecosystems. "Hitchhikers" include all manner of biologic life, both microscopic and macroscopic. Animals can carry potential human pathogens and vectors. The globalization of markets brings fresh fruits and vegetables to dinner tables thousands of miles from where they were grown, fertilized, and picked. Tunnels, bridges, and ferries form means to traverse natural barriers to species spread. The roads built to transport people often speed the movement of diseases from one area to another. Mass processing and wide distribution networks allow for the amplification and wide dissemination of potential human microbes [14].

Culture With the advent of the Internet and online booking, it is becoming easier and cheaper to travel to foreign destinations than ever before. With a smartphone, one can literally book their transportation (flight, cruise, ground transportation) and accommodations (hotel or private housing such as AirBnb) and purchase goods and services at their destination without ever having to step into a travel agency or bank to get foreign currency. While at those locations, travelers often try local cuisines and drinks sometimes leading to the infamous "traveler's diarrhea."

Microbial Adaptation and Change

The time may come when penicillin can be bought by anyone in the shops. Then there is the danger that the ignorant man may easily underdose himself and by exposing his microbes to non-lethal quantities of the drug make them resistant. – Sir Alexander Fleming

The rapid emergence of resistant bacteria is occurring worldwide, endangering the efficacy of antibiotics, which have transformed medicine and saved millions of lives. Many decades after the first patients were treated with antibiotics, bacterial infections have again become a threat. The antibiotic resistance crisis has been attributed to the overuse and misuse of these medications, as well as a lack of new drug development by the pharmaceutical industry due to reduced economic incentives and challenging regulatory requirements [15].

The overuse of antibiotics clearly drives the evolution of resistance. Epidemiological studies have demonstrated a direct relationship between antibiotic consumption and the emergence and dissemination of resistant bacteria strains. In bacteria, genes can be inherited from relatives or can be acquired from nonrelatives on mobile genetic elements such as plasmids [15]. Resistance can also occur spontaneously through mutation. Antibiotics remove drug-sensitive competitors, leaving resistant bacteria behind to reproduce as a result of natural selection. Despite warnings regarding overuse, antibiotics are overprescribed worldwide. In many other countries, antibiotics are unregulated and available over the counter without a prescription. This lack of regulation results in antibiotics that are easily accessible, plentiful, and cheap, which promotes overuse [16]. An estimated 80% of antibiotics globally are purchased outside of hospitals [17]. Although many of these antibiotics are purchased without prescriptions, increased regulation to restrict sales may not be an appropriate solution for communities that lack access to antibiotics. Interventions that target incentives linked to consumers, prescribers, and retailers and that educate the public and healthcare providers will be required to change consumption patterns in communities.

Incorrectly prescribed antibiotics also contribute to the promotion of resistant bacteria. Studies have shown that treatment indication, choice of agent, or duration of antibiotic therapy is incorrect in 30–50% of cases [18].

In both the developed and developing world, antibiotics are widely used as growth supplements in livestock. An estimated 80% of antibiotics sold in the USA are used in animals, primarily to promote growth and to prevent infection [19]. The antibiotics used in livestock are ingested by humans when they consume food [20]. The transfer of resistant bacteria to humans by farm animals was first noted more than 35 years ago, when high rates of antibiotic resistance were found in the intestinal flora of both farm animals and farmers. More recently, molecular detection methods have demonstrated that resistant bacteria in farm animals reach consumers through meat products [19].

Antibacterial products sold for hygienic or cleaning purposes may also contribute to this problem, since they may limit the development of immunities to environmental antigens in both children and adults. Consequently, immune system versatility may be compromised, possibly increasing morbidity and mortality due to infections that would not normally be virulent [21].

The development of new antibiotics by the pharmaceutical industry, a strategy that had been effective at combating resistant bacteria in the past, had essentially stalled due to economics. Of the 18 largest pharmaceutical companies, 15 abandoned the antibiotic field. Antibiotic research conducted in academia has been scaled back as a result of funding cuts due to the economic crisis. Antibiotic development is no longer considered to be an economically wise investment for the pharmaceutical industry. Because antibiotics are used for relatively short periods and are often curative, antibiotics are not as profitable as drugs that treat chronic conditions, such as diabetes, psychiatric disorders, asthma, or gastroesophageal reflux [19].

Estimates regarding the medical cost per patient with an antibiotic-resistant infection range from $18,588 to $29,069. The total economic burden placed on the US economy by antibiotic-resistant infections has been estimated to be as high as $20 billion in healthcare costs and $35 billion a year in lost productivity [20].

Antibiotic-resistant infections also burden families and communities due to lost wages and healthcare costs [19].

Culture In developing nations where some areas lack medical facilities, patients with respiratory, urinary, or gastrointestinal infection often time seek medical advice from anyone and anywhere, like pharmacies. Often times they would describe their symptoms to the person behind the counter who would dispense what they believe to be the appropriate treatment. Another common practice is sharing leftover antibiotics. Leftover antibiotics signal that the initial patient did not complete the recommended course of treatment and the possibility of the antibiotics being expired or spoilt.

Technology and Industry

Infodemiology (i.e., information epidemiology) refers to "the set of methods, which study the data specifically, health data on the internet for the purpose of public health studies and policies." Infoveillance (i.e., information surveillance) can be defined as a syndromic surveillance that analyzes online data to detect disease outbreaks at a shorter time than traditional surveillance. Social media has been used in various health applications. Many researchers have built prediction models of disease spread outbreak using health-related data extracted from the Internet. The utilization of Google Search queries has introduced a Web-based tool for real-time surveillance of disease outbreaks [22].

Online social network ("OSN") communication is a revolutionary trend that utilizes Web 2.0, which introduces a new feature that enables users to become active. Users can freely express what they feel and share their health condition. By contrast, users only passively read the content in websites based on Web 1.0. The popularity and the proliferation of OSNs have created an extensive social interaction among users and generated a large amount of social data. They offer a unique opportunity to study and understand social interaction and communication among far larger populations now more than before [23]. OSNs have received considerable attention as a possible tool for tracking a pandemic. The increasing attention on using OSN as a surveillance system to track a pandemic is due to the real-time user-generated data provided by social media. OSNs are a perfect source for early-stage pandemic detection because of their real-time nature. This characteristic also enables for fast communication between health agencies and the public in the early stage of pandemic outbreak detection [22].

Traditional pandemic surveillance such as influenza pandemic is entirely manual, and thus it causes 1 to 2 weeks of time lag between the time of medical diagnosis and the time when the data become available [24]. OSNs have the potential to eliminate the time lag in traditional surveillance by enabling the extraction of millions of real-time text data, which include geographical location and information regarding one's personal well-being. However, the accuracy of OSN surveillance systems depends on the quality of the algorithms used to distinguish between pandemic-related data and other social media communication data. OSN-based surveillance systems are limited to public data only.

One particular research [25] was aimed in detecting the Ebola virus in the early stage by tracking tweets related to Ebola (#Ebola). Analysis of the tweets captured the early stage of Ebola outbreak. Ebola-related tweets in Nigeria were chosen 3 to 7 days before the official declaration of the first probable Ebola case.

In 2008, an experiment in digital epidemiology occurred at Google, where engineers launched the disease-forecasting tool Google Flu Trends. The company planned to analyze Google search data for keywords relating to symptoms of the flu. The hope was it would analyze the data to accurately determine the likelihood of a flu or dengue outbreak 2 weeks earlier than the CDC could. A visit to the site reveals that as of 2014 they are no longer publishing data; however, no reason was given as to why.

Culture There is a saying found on t-shirts and coffee mugs stating "Don't confuse your Google search with my medical degree". Doctors are finding themselves increasingly having to correct an individual's wrong self-diagnosis made using Google (or other search engines).

The Internet and software applications that are now available place humanity at the cusp of change against the fight of infectious diseases. Throughout history, infectious diseases have caused humanity to make certain changes to lifestyle and habitation. This was due to the time it took to confirm there was a pandemic, signal the alarm, get information out, and arrange testing and treatment. With data being transmitted at breakneck speeds, a population is no longer dependent on their government or an NGO to tell them something is going wrong around them. As noted above, using OSN, outbreak trends can be detected up to 2 weeks earlier than traditional methods thereby notifying a population earlier allowing them to take precautionary measures, which would result in fewer contacts and a decrease in the spread of an infectious disease. I would hypothesize that there will be an inverse correlation between the number of mobile phones connected to the Internet and the number of people affected by an infectious disease during an epidemic/pandemic.

Foodborne Illness

There are many indicators that point to the fact that the incidence of foodborne disease is increasing globally and is a substantial cause of morbidity and mortality worldwide. For industrialized countries in general, it has been estimated that up to one-third of the population suffer a foodborne illness each year [26]. Although the vast majority of cases are mild, a significant number of deaths do occur, and the high levels of acute infections and chronic sequelae lead to billions of dollars in medical costs and lost productivity [27].

Although foodborne disease data collection systems often miss the mass of home-based outbreaks of sporadic infection, it is now widely accepted that many cases of foodborne illness occur as a result of improper food handling and preparation by consumers in their own kitchens, as shown in a review of studies from both Europe and North America [28]. In addition, a study of *Escherichia coli* O157 outbreaks in the USA [29] found that 80% of suspect hamburgers were prepared and eaten at home. In Australia, approximately 90% of *Salmonella* species infections are generally thought to be associated with non-manufactured foods and the home [30]. Data available from Canada covering 1996 and 1997 has identified the home as the most common exposure setting for cases of *Salmonella* species, *Campylobacter* species, and pathogenic *E. coli* infection [31].

The four most common mistakes in handling and preparing food at home are the inappropriate storage of food (including inadequate refrigeration), the failure to attain a required cooking and/or reheating temperature, any actions that result in cross-contamination, and the presence of an infected food handler.

There are also a number of global factors that have an impact on food safety inside the twenty-first century home. In particular, the globalization of the food supply impacts homes all over the world. World meat consumption is expected to double between 1983 and 2020, to 300 million metric tons, and most of this increase will occur in developing countries [32]. The impact on food safety for homes in these countries may be significant, considering that meat processing may not be well regulated and home kitchens may not be equipped for storage and preparation of raw meats. Import statistics indicate that more than 50% of fresh vegetables in the developed world marketplace are imported from developing countries [33], prompting food safety experts to quip that consumers only have to travel as far as the local food market and home again to experience "traveler's diarrhea."

Culture The origins of many food taboos appear to be linked to infectious diseases. These include prohibitions on drinking raw animal blood, on sharing cooking and eating utensils and plates between meat and other foods, and on eating pork in Judaism and Islam (most likely concerned about dangerous pig tapeworms) [34].

Recent examples of these food exclusions that are still the norm today include the following:

- Consumption of raw milk being illegal in many countries, to prevent spread of bovine (cow) tuberculosis
- Not eating soft cheeses when pregnant to avoid contracting listeria, which can cause miscarriages and stillbirths
- Trying to stop people licking the cake bowl because of the risk of eggborne *Salmonella* bacteria

When traveling to any developing nation, the advice given, in order to avoid getting sick, is stay away from the street food. When speaking with the locals, their advice as to where to find the best food is often times the street food. For those seeking an authentic experience, they will, most often times than not, eat street food and document it with a post on social media.

Conclusion

Forever engaged in a battle of dominance, we fight something we cannot even see with our naked eye. We travel faster, but take the bug with us. We develop stronger antibiotics only to provide bacteria with the selective pressure to mutate. Our history and culture have been forged by the deadly hands of plagues and pandemics. With prevention being better than cure, we now have a tool that can help us turn the tide on infectious diseases. The Internet has afforded us the ability to increase public education without depending on governments or NGOs; the Internet has allowed faster reporting, leading to people in certain areas to self-imposed quarantining; the Internet has allowed people to reach out for help and alert the world when a disease rears its ugly head.

I would hypothesize that there will be an inverse correlation between the number of mobile phones connected to the Internet and the number of people affected by an infectious disease during an epidemic/pandemic. We may even see an overall decrease in the number of epidemics/pandemics declared and the duration of each.

References

1. Cunha BA. Historical aspects of infectious diseases, part 1. Infect Dis Clin North Am. 2004;18:xi–v.
2. Infectious Diseases – Mayo Clinic. https://www.mayoclinic.org/diseases-conditions/infectious-diseases/symptoms-causes/syc-20351173.
3. Brachman P. Infectious disease – past, present and future. Int J Epidemiol. 2003;32:684–6.
4. CIA.gov. World factbook – world statistics archived 1 February 2010 at WebCite.
5. World Population Becomes More Urban That Rural. https://newatlas.com/go/7334/.
6. https://www.ukri.org/research/themes-and-programmes/tackling-antimicrobial-resistance/.
7. "The World at Six Billion". UN Population Division. Archived from the original on March 5: Elsevier; 2016, Table 2 https://web.archive.org/web/20160305042439/http://www.un.org/esa/population/publications/sixbillion/sixbilpart1.pdf.
8. Peterborough County-City Health Unit. Pandemic influenza plan section 6: public health measures. December 2007 https://www.longwoods.com/articles/images/PIP-6-public-health-measures.pdf.
9. Regional Bureau For Africa, Undp. (2015). Socio-economic impact of Ebola virus disease in West African Countries A call for national and regional containment, recovery and prevention. https://doi.org/10.13140/RG.2.2.29620.04481.
10. Land Use Change and Infectious Disease. https://www.nceas.ucsb.edu/featured/dobson.

11. O'Dowd A. Infectious diseases are spreading more rapidly than ever before, WHO warns. BMJ. 2007;335(7617):418.
12. Infectious disease movement in a borderless world: workshop summary. Institute of Medicine (US) Forum on Microbial Threats. Washington, DC: National Academies Press (US); 2010.
13. Tourism by Max Roser. https://ourworldindata.org/tourism.
14. Wilson ME. Travel and the emergence of infectious diseases. Emerg Infect Dis. 1995;1(2): 39–46. https://doi.org/10.3201/eid0102.950201.
15. Ventola CL. The antibiotic resistance crisis: part 1: causes and threats. P T. 2015;40(4):277–83.
16. Michael CA, Dominey-Howes D, Labbate M. The antimicrobial resistance crisis: causes, consequences, and management. Front Public Health. 2014;2:145.
17. Kotwani A, Holloway K. Trends in antibiotic use among outpatients in New Delhi, India. BMC Infect Dis. 2011;11(1):99.
18. Luyt CE, Bréchot N, Trouillet JL, Chastre J. Antibiotic stewardship in the intensive care unit. Crit Care. 2014;18(5):480.
19. Bartlett JG, Gilbert DN, Spellberg B. Seven ways to preserve the miracle of antibiotics. Clin Infect Dis. 2013;56(10):1445–50.
20. Golkar Z, Bagazra O, Pace DG. Bacteriophage therapy: a potential solution for the antibiotic resistance crisis. J Infect Dev Ctries. 2014;8(2):129–36.
21. Michael CA, Dominey-Howes D, Labbate M. The antibiotic resistance crisis: causes, consequences, and management. Front Public Health. 2014;2:145.
22. Al-garadi MA, et al. Using online social networks to track a pandemic: a systematic review. J Biomed Inform. 2016;62:1–11.
23. Ratkiewicz J, et al. Detecting and tracking political abuse in social media. In: ICWSM, 2011.
24. Lee K, Agrawal A, Choudhary A. Real-time disease surveillance using twitter data: demonstration on flu and cancer. In: Proceedings of the 19th ACM SIGKDD international conference on knowledge discovery and data mining, ACM, 2013.
25. Odlum M, Yoon S. What can we learn about the Ebola outbreak from tweets? Am J Infect Control. 2015;43(6):563–71.
26. World Health Organization. Fact Sheet No. 237: food safety and foodborne illness. www.who.int/inf-fs/en/fact237.html. (Version current at September 8, 2003).
27. Duff SB, Scott E, Malfios MM, et al. Cost effectiveness of a targeted disinfection program in household kitchens to prevent foodborne illness in the United States, Canada and the United Kingdom. J Food Protect. 2003;66:2103–15.
28. Scott E. A review of foodborne disease and other hygiene issues in the home. J Appl Bacteriol. 1996;80:5–9.
29. Mead PA, Finelli L, Lambert-Fair MA, et al. Risk factors for sporadic infection with Escherichia coli O157:H7. Arch Intern Med. 1997;157:204–8.
30. Jay L, Comar D, Govenlock LD. A video study of Australian domestic food-handling practices. J Food Protect. 1999;62:1285–96.
31. Health Canada. Outbreaks, hospitalizations and deaths: exposure setting (National Notifiable Diseases Individual Case). http://www.hc-sc.gc.ca/pphb-dgspsp/publicat/ccdr-rmtc/03vol29 /29s1/29s1_7e.html (Version current at September 8, 2003).
32. Delgado CL, Courbois CB, Rosegrant MD. Global food demand and the contribution of livestock as we enter the new millenium. Washington, DC: International Food Policy Research Institute; 1998.
33. USDA Foreign Agricultural Service Export/Import Statistics. www.fas.usda.gov/scriptsw/ bico/bico.asp?Entry=lout&doc=1266. (Version current at September 8, 2003).
34. Whittake M. How infectious diseases have shaped our culture, habits and language. July 12, 2017.   https://theconversation.com/how-infectious-diseases-have-shaped-our-culture-habits-and-language-75061.

Chapter 2
Evolution and Globalization of Antimicrobial Resistance

Laila Woc-Colburn and Daniel Godinez

Objectives
After reading this chapter, the reader should be able to:

1. Define and explain what "antimicrobial resistance" (AMR) and "globalization" in the context of AMR mean
2. Explain the reasons or factors that have led to antimicrobial resistance and its globalization
3. Understand strategies designed to reduce antimicrobial resistance and its global spread

Introduction

Infectious diseases have been the scourge of humanity for millennia. Currently, they are the second most common cause of death worldwide [1].

The Black Death (Bubonic Plague, Yersinia Pestis) in the Middle Ages, which is estimated to have killed up to 200 million people worldwide [2]; the Pox (Smallpox, Variola virus) with a mortality rate of 30% (leaving many survivors with scars and blindness) and which was officially declared eradicated in 1980 [3]; malaria ("the blackwater fever," *Plasmodium*) which has infected and killed millions in the tropics, particularly in Africa (in 2017, there were 219 million estimated cases with 435,000

L. Woc-Colburn
Section Infectious Diseases, Department of Medicine, National School of Tropical Medicine, Baylor College of Medicine, Houston, TX, USA

D. Godinez (✉)
Department of Internal Medicine, Belize Healthcare Partners Limited, Belize City, Belize

© Springer Nature Switzerland AG 2020
J. Hidalgo, L. Woc-Colburn (eds.), *Highly Infectious Diseases in Critical Care*,
https://doi.org/10.1007/978-3-030-33803-9_2

deaths) [4]; dengue fever (the "breakbone disease," *Flavivirus*) which is still common in 110 countries and affects anywhere between 50 and 500 million persons every year [5]; tuberculosis (consumption or phthisis, *M. tuberculosis*) which is estimated to infect one-quarter of the world's population and to have killed 1.6 million in 2017 [6]; and the HIV/AIDS pandemic which started in the 1980s (in 2016, approximately 37 million people were living with HIV, with over one million deaths) [7] are just some of the most dramatic and conspicuous examples of such diseases.

It is, therefore, no surprise that in the course of history scientists, biologists, sociologists, epidemiologists, nurses, doctors, and many other rational and educated individuals have tried to find a cure for many of these conditions, to alleviate suffering, and to extend the lifespan and improve the quality of life of their fellow humans.

From the early efforts by Edward Jenner in 1798 to vaccinate against smallpox [8] and of Robert Koch in 1882 to isolate and treat the causative germ of tuberculosis [9] to the development of antiretroviral medications (ARVs) for the treatment of HIV infection in the 1980s and 1990s [10], much has been done to try to overcome and eliminate these nemeses of humankind, with limited success.

One of the most fascinating (and frightening) chapters in this fight has been the development of antibiotics to combat and cure bacterial infections.

Since the identification of these unicellular microorganisms by van Leeuwenhoek (the "Father of Microbiology") in the 1670s [11] and the demonstration by Louis Pasteur of the relationship between germs and disease (the Germ Theory) in 1864 [12], there was no effective way to treat bacterial infections until Alexander Fleming's discovery of penicillin (Penicillium notatum) in 1928 and its commercial, widespread use in the early 1940s [13], even though it has been known for long that bacteria and fungi produce antibiotics which are capable of killing or inhibit competing microbial species.

Penicillin heralded the dawn of the antibiotic age. Before its introduction, there was no effective treatment for infections such as syphilis, pneumonia, gonorrhea, staphylococcal infections, or rheumatic fever. Hospitals were full of people with "blood poisoning" (now known as sepsis), and doctors could do little for them but wait and hope [14].

Between the 1930s and 1960s, most of the antibiotics we use today were discovered and developed, including sulfas, tetracyclines, macrolides (erythromycin), aminoglycosides (streptomycin), and antituberculous drugs [15].

Later on, semisynthetic antimicrobials (such as fluoroquinolones and beta-lactams) were added to this arsenal to fight infections. Its widespread availability and affordability and its initial effectiveness led some health authorities to believe that "bacterial infections would be virtually eliminated" and the United Nations and World Health Organization to state as a goal the eradication of certain infectious diseases (such as tuberculosis) by a certain date in the future [16, 17].

Unfortunately, sometime after the initial success of antibiotics, reports started arising that over time they were not as effective as before to treat the same infections, that every time the dose of the medication had to be increased to obtain the same effect, and that bacteria were developing resistance to some of them as proven by culture and sensitivity tests. The trend of resistance has spread out rapidly in the last decades, thanks to the rise of rapid, frequent, and relatively cheap international travel that allows diseases to leap from continent to continent [18].

As a microbiologist/immunologist said: "Not only we are unable to eradicate bacterial infections, we are losing the battle as we speak….we are entering an era of 'superbugs' – bacteria resistant to all known antibiotics. In a few decades we will probably find ourselves back in a point where people will die following simple infections" [19]. In a sobering analysis, another microbiologist pointed out that the only two diseases that have been truly eradicated (smallpox and rinderpest) were viral in origin [20].

Definition of Terms

The term *antimicrobial* includes drugs or chemicals that either kill or slow down the growth of microbes. From that definition, we have antibacterial, antiviral, antifungal, and antiparasitic drugs, although, in everyday use, antimicrobials tend to be equated to antibiotics (although, technically, that is not completely correct) [20].

Antimicrobial resistance (AMR) is the ability of a microbe to remain unharmed by the effects of a medication that once could successfully treat that microbe [21]. It refers to the fact that an adequate dose of the antimicrobial is incapable to eliminate or affect significantly the population of said germ. The term *antibiotic resistance* (ABR) is a subset of AMR, and it applies only to bacteria becoming resistant to antibiotics. Even though this article will focus mainly on ABR, it must be kept in mind that bacteria are not the only germs that have developed resistance (viruses, fungi, and protozoa have also done so) [20].

Globalization is the connection of different parts of the world resulting in the expansion of international cultural, economic, and political activities. It is the integration of goods and people among different countries, and it means complying with global standards in economy, politics, culture, education, environment, or other matters. It describes the way countries and people of the world interact and integrate [22].

Factors that Affect the Appearance and Development of Antimicrobial Resistance and Its Globalization

Antimicrobial resistance (AMR) and global warming have at least one similarity: both are man-made phenomena. The evolution of antimicrobial resistance is a multifaceted issue that is influenced by numerous factors.

This growing healthcare problem has significantly impacted the public welfare and has substantially burdened the economic system on a global scale [23].

One of the main reasons for the appearance and development of AMR is the indiscriminate use of antimicrobials. Overuse, misuse, and nonuse of antimicrobials are identified as key factors in the emergence of antimicrobial resistance [1]. In developing countries, antimicrobials are frequently available over the counter in pharmacies. The quality and potency of antibiotics are often suspected, with unregulated import, registration, and distribution [24].

Antibiotics kill or inhibit the growth of susceptible bacteria. When populations of bacteria are repeatedly exposed to an antibiotic, eventually one or more of them survive because of its ability to evade or neutralize the effect of the drug. Those bacteria can then multiply and replace the ones that were killed off, with new specimens that are now impervious to the antibiotic. Exposure to the antibiotic therefore provides what is called "selective pressure" [21, 23].

Bacteria can acquire resistance through mutation of their genetic material or by acquiring pieces of DNA that code for resistance properties. Bacteria that have become resistant can transfer that property to other bacteria through the following:

Transformation When a bacterium dies, it lyses, releasing their intracellular contents, including fragments of DNA, to the environment. These fragments can be taken up and incorporated into the chromosome of a living bacterium to provide the recipient with new characteristics (including AMR).

Conjugation Many bacteria have *plasmids*, which are small circular pieces of DNA separate from the primary bacterial chromosome. These plasmids can carry genes that provide resistance to antibiotics, and bacteria that contain plasmids are able to conjugate with other bacteria and pass a replicate to recipient bacteria.

Transduction Genetic information can also be carried from one bacterium to another by a virus. This virus is called a *bacteriophage* [21].

Once a bacterium has become resistant to a particular antibiotic, it passes the resistant characteristic to subsequent daughter cells that result from binary fission.

Another reason for the development of AMR is the following: In the 1950s, studies were published showing that animals given low doses of antibiotics gained weight more rapidly, and the practice of including antibiotics in grain to promote the growth of cattle, poultry, and swine became widespread, further compounding the problem of bacterial resistance. Up to now, the practice of giving antibiotics routinely to animals, including fish, is still common [26].

Additional factors that contribute to the development of antibiotic resistance include the following:

• Patients not finishing the entire antibiotic course
• Poor infection control in healthcare settings
• Poor hygiene and sanitation
• Absence of new antibiotics being discovered [27]

Viral resistance can be better understood using HIV as an example. HIV is a retrovirus consisting of a single strand of RNA inside a protein coat. When the virus enters a CD4 lymphocyte, it sheds its protein coat and uses a viral enzyme called reverse transcriptase to create a segment of DNA using the viral RNA as a template. This double-stranded DNA version of HIV then gets incorporated into the DNA of the infected host cell, and this process is called "reverse transcription." This has important consequences for the development of drug resistance because of several key characteristics of HIV:

1. HIV replicates at a prodigious rate producing billions of new virus particles each day.
2. Reverse transcription is notoriously error prone, leading to frequent mutations.
3. Current antiviral treatment regimens control the infection, but they do not completely eliminate the virus.

Given the persistence of HIV with high rates of replication and high error rates during reverse transcription, mutations in HIV are inevitable, and some of these mutations lead to the eventual development of drug resistance [21, 22].

Fungi and parasites have also developed resistance to antimicrobials. In April 2019, a CNN report highlighted *Candida auris*, a yeast that has become multiresistant to antifungal medications and has spread to over 30 countries. The same report estimated that by the year 2050, drug-resistant infections could claim 10 million lives per year worldwide [27].

The globalization of antimicrobial resistance is a reality. International travel has increased enormously over the recent years resulting in the multiplication of opportunities for resistant microorganisms to be carried rapidly from one geographic location to another. Population mobility is a main factor in globalization of public health threats and risks, specifically distribution of antimicrobial drug-resistant organisms. Furthermore, the globalization of trade and the increased contribution that developing countries are making to the global market in, for example, meat provide additional chances for the spread of resistant strains (and/or resistance genes) [26].

Each year, over 3 billion persons move across large geographic distances, about half cross international boundaries. The International Air Transport Association (IATA) reported that their member carried 3.1 billion passengers in 2018, with over 100,000 flights every day worldwide [28]. The United Nations World Tourism Organization (UNWTO) estimated 1.32 billion international tourist arrivals in 2018 [29].

International movements for permanent resettlement by immigrants, refugees, asylum seekers, or refugee claimants and temporary movement by migrant workers and others augment the total international movements each year. The International Labor Organization estimates that in 2014 there were 214 million international migrant workers worldwide [30].

Once imported by travelers, resistant strains vary in their propensity for spread according to the route of transmission of the species [21, 24, 25].

Antimicrobial resistance is a global problem that requires local, national, and global responses; surveillance is key to understanding the magnitude and trends of resistance and to evaluating the impact of interventions [31].

Unfortunately, our ability to detect the emergence and global spread of resistant microorganisms is hampered by the weakness or total lack of adequate surveillance of antimicrobial resistance [32].

Considerable effort and resources are being committed by the World Health Organization and other partners including the pharmaceutical industry, to improve surveillance capacity through training, laboratory strengthening, and provision of external quality assurance schemes, but there is still much to do [33].

Strategies to Mitigate or Resolve Antibiotic Resistance and Its Globalization

The basic requirement for controlling antimicrobial resistance in developed and developing countries is multifaceted strategies, which include increase awareness of the antibiotic resistance problem, surveillance of antimicrobial resistance and usage, prudent antimicrobial use in community and hospitals, infection control measures, ongoing education, research, and intersectorial coordination [24].

The most important key to successful implementation of interventions in these countries is a strong governmental commitment and support. Focusing on containment of antimicrobial resistance, countries with limited resources can improve the quality of healthcare in the future [26].

The development and spread of bacterial resistance to antibiotics is inevitable, but it could be greatly curtailed through relatively simple measures. These include the following:

- Preventing infection (general infection control)
- Hand washing among healthcare workers, food handlers, and the general public (the WHO has stated that "hand hygiene is the most effective measure for infection prevention and control, with demonstrated impact on quality of care and patient safety across all levels of the healthcare delivery system" [34])
- Modern sanitation: effective systems for dealing with sewage and providing clean water
- Proper food preparation practices
- Rapid identification and isolation of new cases of infection, e.g., new cases of TB (this is particularly important with drug-resistant cases)
- Continued development of new antibiotics
- Decreased agricultural use of antibiotics to enhance growth
- Physician education to reduce inappropriate prescriptions and inappropriate use of broad-spectrum antibiotics
- Educating physicians and patients about the importance of taking the appropriate dose of an antibiotic for the full period of treatment that is indicated
- Consumer education regarding the importance of bacterial resistance and the uselessness of taking antibiotics for viral infections such as the common cold [21, 25, 26, 35, 36]

A novel idea that has gathered interest over the last decade is the use of bacteriophages (phages) to fight bacterial infections. These small viruses would selectively target and kill specific bacteria (without attaching to the host cells) to cause them to lyse. Even though human trials of phage therapy are lacking so far, there are features that make this modality of treatment attractive: (1) it has the natural ability to target and lyse bacterial walls; (2) it has specificity to the host; (3) it has not been reported to cause side effects or secondary infections, and (4) it is potentially cheaper than antibiotics [37].

Also, there has been a recent surge of interest in the use of probiotics [38] and even bacterial transplants to combat certain types of infections (such as resistant *C. difficile* in pseudomembranous colitis) [39].

Whether or not phage therapy, probiotics, or germ transplants will become the next big steps in the armamentarium against harmful bacteria remains to be seen. One thing is certain: The battle to prevent, slow down, or minimize antimicrobial resistance and its globalization is ongoing and, given the changing nature of germs and the current patterns of human behavior, one that will be very much alive for years to come.

References

1. Dave NG, Trivedi AV, et al. International conference & exhibition on vaccines and vaccination. Philadelphia, November 2011.
2. Wheeler L. Kip. "The black plague: the least you need to know" from Dr. Wheeler's website, August 2015.
3. Centers for Disease Control and Prevention website. www.cdc.gov/smallpox.
4. World Malaria Report 2018, World Health Organization website. https://www.who.int/malaria. Accessed 20 July 2019.
5. Bhatt S, Gething PW. The global distribution and burden of dengue. Nature. 2011;496(7446):504–7.
6. Global Tuberculosis Report, World Health Organization. February 2018. Website: https://apps. who.int/iris/bitstream/handle/10665/329368/9789241565714-eng.pdf?ua=1. Accessed 18 July 2019.
7. UNAIDS data 2018. www.avert.org. Accessed 22 July 2019.
8. Riedel S. Edward Jenner and the history of smallpox and vaccination. Proc (Baylor Univ Med Cent). 2005;18(1):21–5.
9. McIntosh J. Medical News Today (reviewed by University of Illinois – Chicago, School of medicine, November 2018.
10. Fauci AS, Folker GK. Towards an AIDS-free generation. JAMA. 2012;308(4):343–4.
11. Explorable.com. 2010. Discovery of bacteria. https://explorable.com/discovery-of-bacteria. Accessed 19 July 2019.
12. Pasteur L. On the extension of the germ theory to the etiology of certain common diseases. Compttes Rendus de L'Academia des Sciences. 1880, p. 1003–44. (translated from the French).
13. https://www.acs.org/. Alexander Fleming discovery and development of Penicillin. American Chemical Society 1999. Retrieved July 2019.

14. USDA National Center for Agricultural Utilization Research. Penicillin: opening the era of antibiotics. https://www.ars.usda.gov/midwest-area/peoria-il/national-center-for-agricultural-utilizationresearch/docs/penicillin-opening-the-era-of-antibiotics/.
15. University of Minnesota, Michigan State University. Antibiotic resistance learning. 2014. Site: https://amrls.umn.edu/antimicrobial-resistance-learning-site. Accessed 18 July 2019.
16. UN aims to eradicate Tb by 2030, article published 18 September 2018. https://www.mdedge.com/chestphysician/article/175092/pulmonology/un-aims-eradicate-tb-2030. Accessed 18 July 2019.
17. WHO – The End TB Strategy. https://www.who.int/tb/strategy/End_TB_Strategy.pdf?ua=1. Accessed 18 July 2019.
18. Bordowitz, A. Will we be able to eradicate all bacterial infection in the world? Quora, December 2015.
19. Clark DR. Eradicating infectious disease: can we and should we? Front Immunol. 2011;2:53.
20. LaMorte WW. The evolution of antimicrobial resistance. Boston University School of Public Health. http://sphweb.bumc.bu.edu/otlt/MPH-Modules/PH/DrugResistance/DrugResistance2.html.
21. CDC Report. About antimicrobial resistance. www.cdc.gov. October 2017.
22. Daly H. Globalization versus internationalization – some implications. Ecol Econ. Elsevier. 1999:31–7.
23. Hawkey P. The 2017 Garrod lecture: genes, guts and globalization. J Antimicrob Chemother. 2018;73(10):2589–600. https://doi.org/10.1093/jac/dky277.
24. Williams R. Globalization of antimicrobial resistance: epidemiological challenges. Clin Infect Dis. 2001;33(Issue Supplement):S116–7. https://doi.org/10.1086/321835.
25. Hwang A, Gums J. The emergence and evolution of antimicrobial resistance: impact on a global scale. Bioorg Med Chem. 2016;24(24):6440–5.
26. MacPherson D, et al. Population mobility, globalization and antimicrobial drug resistance. Emerg Infect Dis. 2009;15(11):1727–31.
27. CNN Report. 10 April 2019. Website: https://edition.cnn.com/2019/04/09/health/candida-auris-fungus-drug-resistance/index.html. Accessed 21 July 2019.
28. Air Transport Statistics IATA 2018. https://www.iata.org/pressroom/pr/Pages/2019-07-31-01.aspx.
29. UNWTO. Website: www.unwto.org. Accessed 21 July 2019.
30. Mainstreaming of migration in development policy and integrating migration in the post-2015 UN development agenda. From website: www.ilo.org. Accessed 21 July 2019.
31. Williams RJ, Heymann DL. Containment of antibiotic resistance. Science. 1998;279:1153–4.
32. Williams RJ, Ryan MJ. Surveillance of antimicrobial resistance: an international perspective. Br Med J. 1998;317:651.
33. Tenover FC, Mohammed MJ, Stelling J, O'Brien TO, Williams R. Ability of laboratories to detect emerging antimicrobial resistance: proficiency testing and quality control results from the World Health Organization's external quality assurance system for antimicrobial suscepti-bility testing. J Clin Microbiol. 2000;39:241–50.
34. Peters A, et al. "Clean care for all – It's in your hands" The 5 May 2019 WHO SAVE LIVES: Clean your Hands campaign. Clin Infect Dis. pii: ciz236. https://doi.org/10.1093/cid/ciz236, published 5 May 2019.
35. Centers for Disease Control Website. Public health action plan to combat antimicrobial resis-tance   https://www.cdc.gov/drugresistance/pdf/public-health-action-plan-combat-antimicro-bial-resistance.pdf.
36. Centers for Disease Control Website. Public health action plan to combat antimicrobial resistance.
37. Golkar Z, Bagasra O, Pace D. Bacteriophage therapy: a potential solution for the antibiotic resistance crisis. J Infect Dev Ctries. 2014;8(2):129–36. (Golkar, Bagasra & Pace 2014).
38. Dorval E. Probiotics as treatment for infectious diseases. US Pharm. 2015;40(4):20–5.
39. Rupnik M. Toward a true bacteriotherapy for Clostridium difficile infection. N Engl J Med. 2015;372:1566–8.

Chapter 3
Emergency Triage of Highly Infectious Diseases and Bioterrorism

Sarah Bezek, Michael Jaung, and Joy Mackey

Introduction

Effective triage systems that protect patients and staff require a well-functioning health system with integrated referral and communication pathways between community/prehospital, outpatient, emergency department, and hospital settings.

The 2009 pandemic influenza and 2014 Ebola virus disease (EVD) outbreaks had a global impact, and they revealed gaps in triage and health surveillance systems in low- and high-resource countries alike. Other high-visibility events are attacks with biological and chemical agents such as the 1995 sarin nerve gas attack in Tokyo, the 2001 anthrax attacks in the USA, and the ongoing use of chemical weapons in conflicts in the Middle East. No community is immune to a future outbreak or attack, and preparations require proper planning among healthcare workers, government officials, private businesses, and community leaders.

This chapter will approach the triage of highly infectious diseases and terrorist attacks in two sections. The first will focus on general considerations at each point of the health system with examples of specific triage practices from select disease outbreaks. The second will emphasize biological agents of interest and the use of decontamination units and personal protective equipment.

Triage of Highly Infectious Diseases by Health System Point

Health systems in all communities are complex networks with many actors unique to each context. In addition to healthcare facilities, these networks include the emergency response system, community health workers, local government and public

S. Bezek (✉) · M. Jaung · J. Mackey
Department of Emergency Medicine, Baylor College of Medicine, Houston, TX, USA
e-mail: bezek@bcm.edu; jaung@bcm.edu; jmmackey@bcm.edu

© Springer Nature Switzerland AG 2020   23
J. Hidalgo, L. Woc-Colburn (eds.), *Highly Infectious Diseases in Critical Care*,
https://doi.org/10.1007/978-3-030-33803-9_3

health departments, pharmacies and medical supply manufacturers, traditional healers and alternative medicine practitioners, universities and research laboratories, and schools and childcare centers. These health systems may interact with or be a part of larger systems at local, regional, national, and international levels.

Disease control policies and programs can strengthen infectious disease and bioterrorist attack care and surveillance at each of these levels. This chapter will focus on system points staffed by health workers: prehospital response and transport, outpatient facilities, emergency departments, hospitals and specialized treatment units, facilities in response to disasters and conflict, and the public health surveillance service.

Prehospital Response, Triage, and Transport

In health systems with established prehospital emergency medical service (EMS) systems, EMS health providers and other responders are an essential first point of contact for ill patients seeking care. There is a wide variance in the structure of EMS systems and training of responders from country to country as well as means of transport, dispatch, and communication (Fig. 3.1). The World Health Organization (WHO) Emergency Care Framework identifies the key prehospital components of bystander response, EMS dispatch, on-scene provider response, and patient transport with on-board transport care.

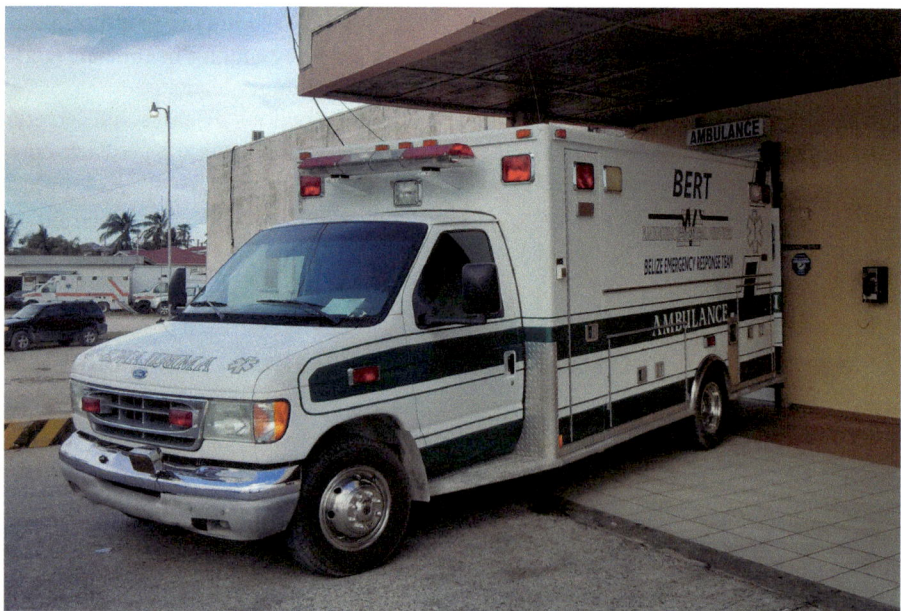

Fig. 3.1 Emergency medical services in Belize City, Belize. (Source: Michael Jaung)

During the 2014 EVD outbreak, governmental agencies like the US Centers for Disease Control and Prevention (CDC) developed specific recommendations to guide local EMS systems in responding to possible cases and prevent spread of the infection [1–3]. The modifications occur at multiple points of care:

- Developing a case definition for person under investigation
- Standardized questions for dispatchers to identify possible infection
- Preparation for and evaluation upon arrival on scene by EMS personnel
- Precautions while transporting patients and contacting appropriate receiving hospital
- Monitoring of potentially exposed EMS personnel
- Maintenance of transportation vehicles and equipment
- Decontamination processes

Similar peer-reviewed frameworks have been proposed for a pandemic of influenza and other respiratory illnesses [4]. During a pandemic or a surge in patients that requires rationing of EMS response, an additional consideration is the implementation of minimal resuscitation criteria for patients in possible cardiac arrest on initial call to the dispatcher or other inclusion and exclusion criteria for care and transport. An algorithm that is decided at the local level, well-communicated to the public, and uniformly followed by EMS system and healthcare facilities is necessary for equitable rationing. Although it is out of the scope of this book chapter, separate and effective mortuary services to transport deceased patients from the prehospital setting can be important to prevent overwhelming EMS dispatch and response systems.

In the event of a biological or chemical terrorist attack, the prehospital EMS systems may respond differently if it is an overt or covert attack. A set of algorithms was developed from military and civilian sources for use to evaluate patients from an attack with known or unknown agents [5]. Initial triage and treatment are based on symptomatology without a definitive diagnosis, and they highlight the importance of isolation and decontamination to prevent further spread or exposure to patients and responders while transporting patients for definitive treatment.

Appropriate implementation of these principles can potentially help prevent further spread of disease or agent exposure, initiate appropriate care of ill patients, protect essential EMS responders, and promote efficient use of healthcare resources.

Outpatient Facility

Ambulatory clinics are often the first place that patients seek medical care. This may be a clinic for primary care, pediatrics, antenatal care, urgent care, or specialist care, or it could be the general outpatient department of a hospital. In many health systems, patients may reach a clinic's nurse-on-call and undergo triage by telephone. This is an opportunity to direct the patient to an appropriate care facility for evaluation and give hygiene and isolation instructions at home for cases that may not need immediate attention. During an outbreak, additional screening questions can be instituted for patient presenting to any outpatient facility.

One example is the screening protocol was described by a multifacility academic health system in the USA during the 2014 EVD outbreak [6]. All patients presenting to the facilities were asked screening questions, and patients that met the CDC definition for "person under investigation" were then triaged to either a tropical medicine clinic, emergency department, or specialized EVD treatment unit depending on symptomatology and time of day of presentation. Of the 25 patients who met the inclusion definition, the majority were triaged to the clinic or emergency department, and no patients were diagnosed with EVD.

Patients may seek care at clinics following a terrorist attack by biological or chemical agents either in the event of a widespread attack with varying degrees of illness or a covert attack with an agent that has an insidious onset of symptoms. Facilities should have reporting and referral pathways in place if healthcare workers detect a pattern in presenting cases.

Emergency Department

Many emergency departments (ED) use standardized and validated triage tools in order to prioritize patients who are most sick on presentation. Examples of commonly used instruments include the Emergency Severity Index, the South African Triage Score, and the Emergency Triage Assessment and Treatment for pediatric patients. These and other similar tools use easily observable physical exam signs, with or without measured vital signs and rapid diagnostic tests such as a fingerstick glucose measurement, to quickly identify patients needing immediate evaluation and treatment. Additionally, specific triage instruments and scores such as the systemic inflammatory response syndrome (SIRS) criteria, quick sepsis-related organ failure assessment (qSOFA), and the national early warning score (NEWS) are tools that have been used in the ED to identify patients who have infection resulting in sepsis or septic shock (Table 3.1) [7, 8].

Initial ED triage includes early identification of patients for isolation and decontamination. At the beginning of the outbreak of severe acute respiratory syndrome (SARS) in 2003, an ED in Singapore activated the decontamination area outside its entrance as a screening and consultation area of at-risk patients identified by triage nurses immediately on arrival and registration [9]. Similarly, a mobile pediatric emergency response team was stationed outdoors during the 2009 influenza pandemic in the USA to evaluate low acuity patients with influenza-like symptoms [10]. The rationale of both of these responses was to prevent disease transmission and absorb increased patient volumes with minimal impact on the care for other ED patients.

The ED has also been used as a place for continued treatment in cases that require prolonged isolation while awaiting confirmation of a diagnosis. During the 2014 EVD outbreak, a referral hospital in the USA developed a mobile containment unit staffed with EMS personnel adjacent to the ED as an extended treatment area for

Table 3.1 Triage instruments for evaluating sepsis and septic shock

Sepsis scoring system	Vital signs	Laboratory values
Systemic inflammatory response syndrome (SIRS)	Temperature	Complete blood count with white blood cell differential
	Heart rate	
	Respiratory rate	
Quick sepsis-related organ failure assessment (qSOFA)	Respiratory rate	None
	Blood pressure	
	Mental status	
National early warning score (NEWS)	Temperature	None
	Heart rate	
	Respiratory rate	
	Blood pressure	
	Mental status	
	Oxygen saturation	

Source: [8]

patients under investigation for EVD [11]. By separating the unit from the ED and integrating the unit with the EMS referral system, the arrival and initial evaluation of patients were more confidential and streamlined. The resource-intense unit also had dedicated laboratory, portable radiology, and staff decontamination equipment.

In the event of a bioterrorist attack, ED needs will depend on the extent of exposure and agent used. Bioterrorist attacks can be covert or announced. The detection of a covert attack can be delayed depending on incubation period, access to healthcare facility, and location of the attack [12]. Triage systems should alert providers in the case of unusual patterns of illness, such as geographical clusters, an unusual number of deaths or critically ill patients, or sudden rise in a specific syndromic presentation. Once a bioterrorist attack is suspected, local and national authorities should be notified, and an emergency preparedness plan should be initiated. This is discussed in greater detail in the section "The Threat of Bioterrorism: Triage in Setting of Suspected Attack".

Additional triage after initial entry into the ED may be implemented to stratify treatments for patients who may present with similar symptoms and to formalize the criteria for hospitalization. These triage systems can assist in prioritizing available resources based on patient needs in an equitable manner and not solely relying on clinical judgment.

In Mexico during the 2009 pandemic influenza, a large referral hospital implemented an adapted scoring system for adults presenting with an influenza-like illness (ILI) to determine hospitalization and oseltamivir use [13]. The ILI score elements included patient symptoms, comorbidities, number of previous healthcare facility visits, and results from labs and imaging, and they found the score complemented clinical judgment. In the UK, the simple triage scoring system (STSS) was applied retrospectively to patients admitted for pandemic influenza [14]. The STSS adds mental status and age to vital signs and had similar predictive value for intensive care unit (ICU) admission and mechanical ventilation compared to the full sepsis-related organ failure assessment (SOFA) score which requires laboratory exam values.

General and Specialized Treatment Units

There is also a role for critical care triage for patients requiring hospitalization in general or specialized wards such as ICUs or isolation units. The American College of Chest Physicians published a consensus statement on tertiary triage for the critically ill and injured in pandemics and disasters in 2014 [15]. They recommended critical care and acute care physicians be designated as triage officers or in triage teams, and they emphasized the role of clinical decision support tools that are agreed upon at the health facility and regional levels. In pandemics and disasters that result in severe resource scarcity, triage teams may need to consider excluding patients from intensive care units who have a predicted mortality of greater than 90% but allow for reassessment and an appeal mechanism.

Identifying patients who will require intensive care should also be accompanied by streamlining and increasing available hospital resources to treat the influx of patients. This has been characterized as surge capacity and is a basic element of disaster and epidemic preparedness and described further in the section on bioterrorism [16].

Another mechanism for increasing resources among hospitals is regional coordination of treatment centers. In response to the 2014 EVD outbreak, the US Department of Health and Human Services created a regional treatment network for EVD and other special pathogens [17]. Hospitals across the country were designated as frontline facilities that provide stabilizing treatment for the first 12–24 hours after presentation, assessment hospitals capable of evaluation and treatment in the initial 96 hours to confirm or rule out illness, treatment centers that can care for patients during the entire duration of illness, and regional treatment centers with enhanced capabilities for multiple patients. This tiered plan allowed for distribution of regional resources and limits healthcare worker exposure to patients with confirmed illness.

Ports of Entry, Mass Gatherings, and Humanitarian Emergencies

Triage for highly infectious diseases and bioterrorism attacks may occur in non-health facilities in specific contexts such as at ports of entry, during mass gatherings, and among populations displaced by humanitarian emergencies.

Health screening at ports of entry is a public health surveillance function aimed at delaying and reducing the spread of disease by international travelers (Fig. 3.2). Modeling for screening of passengers arriving on international flights at 18 US airports during a simulated pandemic influenza estimated that the program would identify about half of infected individuals and reduce the rate of new US cases [18]. During the 2014 EVD outbreak, the CDC implemented health border screening of passengers coming from other EVD-affected countries arriving at select US airports with referral to designated health facilities for possible cases, and the agency also

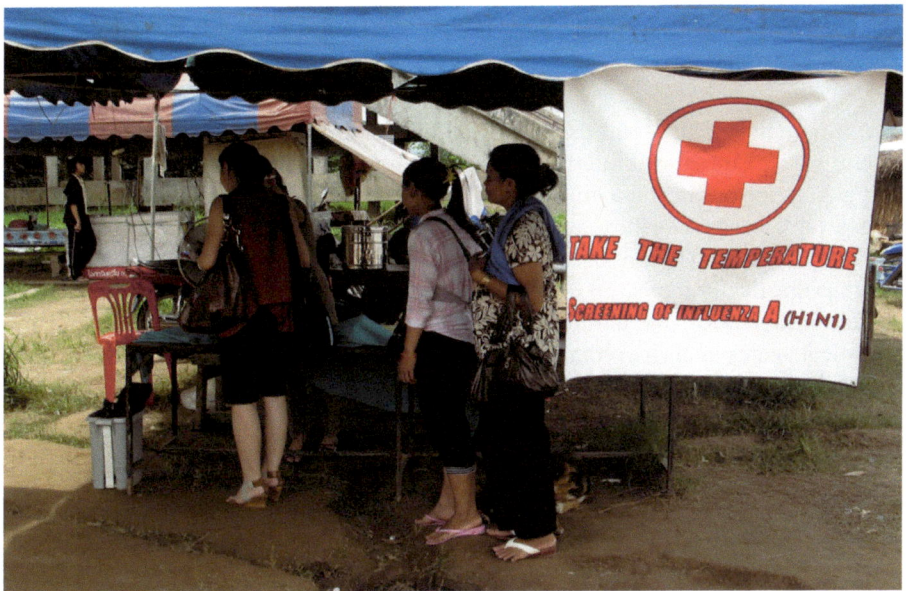

Fig. 3.2 Influenza screening at Thai-Laotian border. (Source: Christopher Lee)

worked with multiple West African countries to strengthen ground and air border health strategies [19, 20].

Another special consideration for triage is surveillance during anticipated mass gatherings and migrations. One example is the annual Hajj pilgrimage to Saudi Arabia. A systematic review of prevalence studies of acute respiratory infections among pilgrims while in Saudi Arabia and on return to their origin countries spanned the 2009 pandemic influenza and 2012 emergence of Middle East Respiratory Syndrome Coronavirus (MERS-CoV) [21]. Although there was a high incidence of acute respiratory infections among pilgrims, there was a low prevalence of pandemic influenza, and no cases of MERS-CoV were reported among Hajj pilgrims during the review period.

Humanitarian emergencies from man-made and natural disasters can lead to large and unexpected population displacement within and between countries. Disease surveillance, prevention, and treatment can be challenging in informal communities and during times of protracted conflict with disruption of governmental health services [22]. Although the burden of disease during the crisis often reflects pre-crisis disease prevalence, populations affected by humanitarian disasters are vulnerable to specific respiratory and diarrheal illnesses such as measles and cholera because of crowded living conditions, malnutrition, and lack of adequate water and sanitation. The Sphere project is a multiorganizational effort to establish minimum standards for health, nutrition, shelter, and water and sanitation interventions to improve quality and accountability [23]. Although there is specific emphasis on implementation of vaccine measures to prevent disease, surveillance and triage are essential to identify and manage health risks in these vulnerable populations.

The Threat of Bioterrorism: Triage in Setting of Suspected Attack

The use of biological agents as weapons of war or terrorism has been in practice for centuries. The threat of bioterrorism has heightened in the past several decades as our population has become highly mobile and the means to implement a bioterrorist attack have become readily accessible due to increased access to technology and biological agents. The use of chemical and biological weapons as means of terrorism has drastically increased in the past three decades, including the Japanese sarin attack in the 1990s, the anthrax attacks in the USA in the 2000s, and the use of chemical agents against civilians in the Syrian civil war this decade all demonstrate the need for emergency preparedness and a clear triage protocol for healthcare settings in the setting of a suspected attack.

Mass Casualty Incidents/Surge Capacity

Densely populated areas, such as urban centers, are traditionally at higher risk of bioterrorism threat due to easier dissemination and greater exposure than more sparsely populated rural areas, leading to a potential mass casualty incident. In the event of a mass casualty incident due to a recognized bioterrorist attack, it is imperative that hospitals have adaptability to divert resources and space to accommodate the influx of patients, e.g., "surge capacity." Surge capacity is generally divided into three components: human resources, physical space, and equipment [16]. The most impactful of the three is human resources, such as calling in off-duty staff to increase the personnel on site in anticipation or response to a mass casualty event. In addition to increasing personnel, streamlining hospital resources, such as expediting inpatient discharges to increase available beds, cancelling elective procedures, and mobilizing equipment to the areas where it is most needed (such as the emergency department and critical care units), is also key to a successful response.

With the exception of the plague (*Yersinia pestis*), anthrax (*Bacillus anthracis*), and smallpox (*Variola major*), the majority of biological agents utilized in bioterrorist attacks are not aerosolized or spread from person-to-person contact and do not require strict isolation protocols aside from typical universal precautions, so open spaces such as parking lots or cafeterias can be converted into temporary triage or patient treatment areas to increase the physical space utilized for patient care. National agencies including the CDC recommend cohorting patients who present with similar syndromes, limiting access or transportation to what is necessary to provide patient care, and exercising standard precautions while cleaning equipment or utilizing personal protective gear [24]. In addition, hospital protocols that allow for deviation from standard of care in order to provide basic critical care for the maximum number of people, including utilizing noncritical care providers, converting noncritical care areas to critical care treatment areas, and having access to basic mechanical ventilation, intravenous fluids, and vasopressors for at least the first 48 hours without outside support, have been advocated by expert working groups in the setting of a mass bioterrorist attack [25].

Surveillance Network and System

Bioterrorist attacks can be covert or announced. An established surveillance network and reporting system is key to enable early detection of potential covert attacks. Surveillance typically takes place at the state (health department) and national (CDC or equivalent agency) level. Once notified of an unusual presentation or pattern or disease, an epidemiological investigation is initiated to determine the underlying cause and potential exposures. Initial notification has historically relied upon the individual practitioner to recognize an aberrant or concerning presentation and notify the respective authorities. However, recognition of covert bioterrorist attacks can be delayed depending on incubation period, access to healthcare facility, and location of the attack. Surveillance systems should account for response time, incubation period, and population density [12]. Initial cases can present with vague, generalized complaints that can be difficult to distinguish from seasonal illnesses such as influenza.

In addition to relying on the individual practitioner to recognize potential covert attacks, triage systems should also be designed to alert the appropriate personnel in the case of unusual patterns of illness, such as geographical clusters, an unusual number of deaths or critically ill patients, or sudden rise in a specific syndromic presentation. This is also known as a "sentinel monitoring system" [12]. Once a bioterrorist attack is suspected, local and national authorities should be notified, and an emergency preparedness plan should be initiated. This would include a case definition that should be disseminated and utilized for screening purposes and infection control measures specific to the suspected agent.

Specific Gaps in Management of Children

Children are disproportionately affected by bioterrorist attacks due to differences in their anatomy, physiology, and development as well as a lack of pediatric-specific research and planning in the event of an attack. Children have higher metabolic and respiratory rates, an immature immune system, decreased physiological reserve, and underdeveloped cognitive capacity (leading to a child being less likely to recognize or flee a dangerous situation). For instance, aerosolized agents that are heavier than air are more toxic to children than adults due to a higher concentration at the child's stature and greater intake due to a child's faster respiratory rate compared to an adult [26]. Children have more permeable skin and a proportionally greater body surface ratio and eat more food and drink more milk on a per-kilogram basis than adults, making them more vulnerable to biological agents spread via contact or ingestion.

In addition to having a greater risk via exposure, most current public health surveillance and treatment systems in the event of a bioterrorist attack have major gaps in the management of children. Schools and childcare facilities have been largely ignored in planning for a bioterrorist event, and most lack an emergency preparedness protocol or personnel trained in the initial triage or stabilization of children following an attack. Likewise, common medications utilized by first responders in the event of an attack, such as the rapid administration of antidotes by autoinjectors, are not available in pediatric appropriate dosing [26]. Other antidotes or antibiotics may have unknown pharmacokinetics in children, having only been tested in adults, or may not be available in liquid formulations for children who have difficulty swallowing pills [27]. National organizations, such as the American Association of Pediatrics (AAP), have made great strides in advocating for pediatric inclusion in future bioterrorism research and strategic planning and creating pediatric-specific resources.

Possible Agents

The CDC classifies biological agents into three categories: A, B, and C. Category A agents are most concerning as they can be easily disseminated and are highly fatal. These will be the agents addressed in this section, with the exception of ricin, which is a Category B agent. The most alarming of these potential biological agents are those that can be disseminated via aerosol and persist in the environment. These include the plague (*Yersinia pestis*), anthrax (*Bacillus anthracis*), and ricin. Other agents are disseminated via direct contact or ingestion. For the purposes of triage, a brief syndromic description, route of dissemination, and recommended contact precautions are summarized (Table 3.2). Please refer to Chap. 7 for more detailed descriptions of syndromes and treatments.

Decontamination Unit

A decontamination unit is designed to remove any gross contamination from the clothing and body of patients or exposed first responders to an aerosolized, liquid, or solid agent prior to further contact with other patients or healthcare personnel. Ideally, a unit should be located near the receiving area of the healthcare facility and have access to running water, detergent, and clean linens [30]. Patients presenting with a suspected exposure should be quickly triaged for emergent interventions (e.g., impending respiratory or cardiac failure, seizure) and then directed to the decontamination unit to remove all items of clothing. Patients should also remove contact lenses. Some exposures also require cutting off hair that would otherwise

Table 3.2 Possible bioterrorism agents, syndrome, and recommended contact precautions

Agent	Route	Person-to-person transmission	Syndrome	Contact precautions
Plague (*Yersinia pestis*)	Airborne	Yes	Fever, cough, chest pain, hemoptysis	Droplet + standard
Anthrax (Bacillus anthracis)	Airborne	No	Prodrome of flu-like symptoms followed by respiratory failure, meningitis	Standard
	Cutaneous		Localized pruritic lesion to papular/vesicular to eschar	Standard
	Ingestion (GI)		Fever and abdominal pain, profuse nausea, vomiting	Standard
Smallpox (*Variola major*)	Airborne	Yes	Prodrome of fever, myalgias followed by synchronous onset centrifugal vesicular rash (face/extremities>trunk)	Airborne + standard
Tularemia (*Francisella tularensis*)	Inhalation	No	Fever, cough, dyspnea progressing to respiratory failure and septic shock	Standard
	Cutaneous		Ulcer + lymphadenopathy	
Botulism (*Clostridium botulinum*)	Inhalation	No	Symmetric descending weakness (proximal to distal), cranial nerve abnormalities, blurred vision, respiratory failure	Standard
	Ingestion (GI)		Above + nausea, vomiting, diarrhea, and abdominal pain	
Ricin (Ricin*us* communis)	Inhalation	No	Fever, cough, pulmonary edema, and respiratory failure	Standard
	Cutaneous		Skin erythema	
	Ingestion (GI)		Profuse nausea, vomiting, diarrhea followed by multiorgan failure or seizures	

Sources: [24, 28, 29]

serve as a reservoir for the agent (typically, chemical or radiation exposures). After disrobing, patients should wash from head to toe in soap and clean water before dressing in clean linens and entering the rest of the healthcare facility.

Personal Protection

The usual standard precautions should be utilized for personal protection in all cases while triaging potential highly infectious diseases. This includes handwashing and personal protective equipment (PPE). PPE will vary depending on the exposure. When contact with blood or bodily fluids is expected, gloves and a gown should be worn. When splashing of blood or bodily fluids is expected, PPE should be expanded to include a mask and eye protection such as goggles. For aerosolized sources, a respirator such as an N95 or hood should also be worn [31]. For the initial triage of most highly infectious suspected respiratory or CNS illnesses, full precautions should be taken. With the exception of the plague, anthrax, and smallpox, most biological agents used in a terrorist attack are not transmittable person to person and do not require specialized PPE aside from the usual standard precautions [24]. Hemorrhagic fevers require more extensive PPE and is covered in Chap. 8.

Summary

Effective triage practices at all levels of the health system is essential in the management of highly infectious diseases and response to bioterrorism attacks. Strong emergency triage systems require well-trained health workers; adequate infrastructure and equipment for isolation, decontamination, and treatment; and clear communication and referral pathways. Early identification and management of suspected cases can improve patient outcomes and protect healthcare workers.

References

1. Centers for Disease Control and Prevention. Emergency medical services for management of patients who present with possible Ebola virus disease [Internet]. 2015. Available from: http://www.cdc.gov/quarantine/.
2. McCoy C, Lotfipour S, Chakravarthy B, Schultz C, Barton E. Emergency medical services public health implications and interim guidance for the Ebola virus in the United States. West J Emerg Med. 2014;15(7):723–7.
3. Lowe JJ, Jelden KC, Schenarts PJ, Rupp LE, Hawes KJ, Tysor BM, et al. Considerations for safe EMS transport of patients infected with Ebola virus. Prehosp Emerg Care. 2015;19(2):179–83.
4. Bielajs I, Burkle FM, Archer FL, Smith E. Development of prehospital, population-based triage-management protocols for pandemics. Prehosp Disaster Med [Internet]. 2007;23(5):420–30. Available from: http://pdm.medicine.wisc.
5. Subbarao I, Johnson C, Bond WF, Schwid HA, Wasser TE, Deye GA, et al. Symptom-based, algorithmic approach for handling the initial encounter with victims of a potential terrorist attack. Prehosp Disaster Med. 2005;20(5):301–8.
6. Fairley JK, Kozarsky PE, Kraft CS, Guarner J, Steinberg JP, Anderson E, et al. Ebola or not? Evaluating the ill traveler from Ebola-affected countries in West Africa. Open Forum Infect Dis. 2016;3:ofw005.
7. Brink A, Alsma J, Verdonschot RJCG, Rood PPM, Zietse R, Lingsma HF, et al. Predicting mortality in patients with suspected sepsis at the Emergency Department; a retrospective cohort study comparing qSOFA, SIRS and National Early Warning Score. PLoS One. 2019;14(1):1–14.
8. Usman OA, Usman AA, Ward MA. Comparison of SIRS, qSOFA, and NEWS for the early identification of sepsis in the Emergency Department. Am J Emerg Med [Internet]. 2018;37:1490. Available from: https://doi.org/10.1016/j.ajem.2018.10.058.
9. Tham KY. An emergency department response to severe acute respiratory syndrome: a prototype response to bioterrorism. Ann Emerg Med. 2004;43(1):6–14.

10. Cruz AT, Patel B, DiStefano MC, Codispoti CR, Shook JE, Demmler-Harrison GJ, et al. Outside the box and into thick air: implementation of an exterior mobile pediatric emergency response team for North American H1N1 (swine) influenza virus in Houston, Texas. Ann Emerg Med. 2010;55(1):23–31.
11. Sugalski G, Murano T, Fox A, Rosania A. Development and use of mobile containment units for the evaluation and treatment of potential Ebola virus disease patients in a United States Hospital. Acad Emerg Med. 2015;22(5):616–22.
12. Grundmann O. The current state of bioterrorist attack surveillance and preparedness in the US. Risk Manag Healthc Policy. 2014;4:177–87.
13. Rodriguez-Noriega E, Gonzalez-Diaz E, Morfin-Otero R, Gomez-Abundis GF, Briseño-Ramirez J, Perez-Gomez HR, et al. Hospital triage system for adult patients using an influenza-like illness scoring system during the 2009 pandemic-Mexico. PLoS One. 2010;5(5):e10658.
14. Adeniji KA, Cusack R. The simple triage scoring system (STSS) successfully predicts mortality and critical care resource utilization in H1N1 pandemic flu: a retrospective analysis. Crit Care. 2011;15:R39.
15. Christian MD, Sprung CL, King MA, Dichter JR, Kissoon N, Devereaux AV, et al. Triage care of the critically ill and Injured during pandemics and disasters: CHEST consensus statement. Chest. 2014;146(4):e61–74.
16. Sheikhbardsiri H, Raeisi AR, Nekoei-Moghadam M, Rezaei F. Surge capacity of hospitals in emergencies and disasters with a preparedness approach: a systematic review. Disaster Med Public Health Prep. 2017;11:612.
17. US Department of Health and Human Services. Regional treatment network for Ebola and other special pathogens [Internet]. 2017. Available from: http://www.cdc.gov/vhf/ebola/outbreaks/2014-west-africa/case-counts.html.
18. Malone JD, Brigantic R, Muller GA, Gadgil A, Delp W, McMahon BH, et al. U.S. airport entry screening in response to pandemic influenza: modeling and analysis. Travel Med Infect Dis [Internet]. 2009;7(4):181–91. Available from: https://doi.org/10.1016/j.tmaid.2009.02.006.
19. Centers for Disease Control and Prevention. Enhanced Ebola screening to start at five U.S. airports for all people entering U.S. from Ebola-affected countries [Internet]. 2014. Available from: https://www.dhs.gov/news/2014/10/08/enhanced-ebola-screening-start-five-us-airports-all-people-entering-us-ebola.
20. Ward S, Bamsa O, Garba H, Oppert M, MacGurn A, Kone I, et al. Responding to communicable diseases in internationally mobile populations at points of entry and along porous borders, Nigeria, Benin, and Togo. Emerg Infect Dis. 2017;23:S114.
21. Al-Tawfiq JA, Benkouiten S, Memish ZA. A systematic review of emerging respiratory viruses at the Hajj and possible coinfection with Streptococcus pneumoniae. Travel Med Infect Dis. 2018;23(February):6–13.
22. Leaning J, Guha-Sapir D. Natural disasters, armed conflict, and public health. N Engl J Med. 2013;369:1836–42.
23. Sphere Association. The sphere handbook: humanitarian charter and minimum standards in humanitarian response [Internet]. 4th ed. Geneva: The Sphere Handbook; 2018. Available from: https://www.spherestandards.org/handbook-2018/.
24. APIC Bioterrorism Task Force and CDC Hospital Infections Program Bioterrorism Working Group. Bioterrorism readiness plan: a template for healthcare facilities [Internet]. 1999. Available from: https://emergency.cdc.gov/bioterrorism/pdf/13apr99APIC-CDCBioterrorism.pdf.
25. Rubinson L, Nuzzo JB, Talmor DS, O'Toole T, Kramer BR, Inglesby TV. Augmentation of hospital critical care capacity after bioterrorist attacks or epidemics: recommendations of the Working Group on Emergency Mass Critical Care. Crit Care Med. 2005;33(10):e2393.
26. AAP Committee on Environmental Health and Committee on Infectious Diseases. Chemical-biological terrorism and its impact on children. Pediatrics. 2006;118(3):1267–78.
27. AAP Disaster Preparedness Advisory Council. Medical countermeasures for children in public health emergencies, disasters, or terrorism. Pediatrics. 2016;137(2):e20154273.

28. Siegel JD, Rhinehart E, Jackson M, Chiarello L. Guideline for isolation precautions: preventing transmission of infectious agents in healthcare settings [Internet]. 2007. Available from: https://www.cdc.gov/infectioncontrol/pdf/guidelines/isolation-guidelines-H.pdf.
29. Adalja AA, Toner E, Inglesby TV. Clinical management of potential bioterrorism-related conditions. N Engl J Med. 2015;372(10):954–62.
30. Houston M, Hendrickson RG. Decontamination. Crit Care Clin. 2005;21:653–72.
31. Suri AP, Gopaul R. Emergency Department and Receiving Areas. In: Guide to Infection Control in the Healthcare Setting [Internet]. Brookline, MA: International Society for Infectious Diseases; 2018. Available from: https://isid.org/guide/infectionprevention/emergency/.

Chapter 4
Diagnostics: The Role of the Laboratory

Azka Afzal, Holland Kaplan, Tina Motazedi, Talha Qureshi, and Laila Woc-Colburn

Introduction

The laboratory can be the physician's most valuable tool in clinical management. The results provided by the laboratory can help provide diagnostics, guide management, and demonstrate prognostic value to the clinician. With the advent of automation and the integration of genomics and proteomics in microbiology, physicians have the opportunity to diagnose quickly and focus treatment earlier in the stage of disease than ever before. However, interpretation of results still depends on the correct test being ordered by the physician and quality of the specimen received by the laboratory. To assure high-quality results, sample handling requires appropriate selection, collection, and transportation. Enhancing the quality of a specimen requires communication between the physician, nurse, and laboratory staff. The physician should first answer whether he or she believes the patient has an infection and, if so, what type of organism is suspected. The physician can then tailor his or her work to that group of organisms and can coordinate the collection and processing of specimens with the staff. The diagnosis of infectious disease is best achieved by applying in-depth knowledge of both medical and laboratory science. In addition, understanding the principles of epidemiology and pharmacokinetics of antibiotics is essential for guiding management.

A. Afzal (✉)
Department of Internal Medicine, University of Chicago, Chicago, Illinois, USA

H. Kaplan · T. Qureshi
Department of Internal Medicine, Baylor College of Medicine, Houston, TX, USA

Department of Infectious Diseases, Baylor College of Medicine, Houston, TX, USA

T. Motazedi
Massachusetts General Hospital, Boston, Massachusetts, USA

L. Woc-Colburn
Section Infectious Diseases, Department of Medicine, National School of Tropical Medicine, Baylor College of Medicine, Houston, TX, USA

© Springer Nature Switzerland AG 2020   37
J. Hidalgo, L. Woc-Colburn (eds.), *Highly Infectious Diseases in Critical Care*,
https://doi.org/10.1007/978-3-030-33803-9_4

By integrating a strategic view of host-parasite interactions, the physician can tackle disease early and prevent clinical deterioration. Clearly, the best outcomes for patients are the result of strong partnerships amongst the medical team composed of the physicians, nurses, and laboratory personnel.

This chapter will begin by describing the various laboratory instruments used to identify microorganisms. For physicians to order specific tests, they must understand the mechanisms and tools available to them in the laboratory to address their diagnostic dilemmas. Furthermore, the understanding of specific specimen sites and specimen handling will be essential in providing high-quality and accurate results. This chapter will be unique in that it will discuss tests based on specific organisms. Bacterial, viral, fungal, and parasitic infections will be separated, and each individual group of organisms will be addressed for laboratory workup.

Laboratory Instruments

Cultures

Bacterial

Hospitals should optimize best practice in the collection, handing, and management of blood cultures. This is an often overlooked but essential component in providing optimal care of patients in all settings and populations, reducing financial burdens, and increasing the diagnostic accuracy of bacterial infections. Blood cultures are a critical diagnostic tool in identifying bacteremia and severe sepsis which can help identify targeted treatment regimen for specific bacteria [1]. Proper collection and handling is essential to identify a true pathogen. Errors in collection or handling can result in inadvertent introduction of bacteria into the specimen which can be a detriment to patient care. In addition, central line-associated bloodstream infections (CLABSI) are a reportable event for most hospitals across the world [2]. Therefore, the impact of proper blood culture collection is significant for quality of care recognition at most hospitals.

There are many reasons to optimize blood culture collection and handling. First, the medical team would like to avoid false-negative blood cultures. Enhancing the identification of the true pathogen allows the physician to tailor antibiotics and reduce length of hospital stays. In addition, reducing contaminated, or false positive, blood cultures can have a large financial and safety impact on patient care. One study has shown that contaminated cultures over a period of 1 year resulted in an average of 2000 extra hospital days and cost approximately $1.9 million [3]. In addition, the literature has shown that up to 50% of patients with contaminated cultures will get treated with antimicrobials. This leads to exposure to inappropriate therapy resulting in increased complications such as allergic reactions, increased *Clostridium difficile* infections, and emergence of antibiotic-resistant organisms [4]. Also, for many hospitals across the world, especially in the United States, CLABSI is detrimental to hospital quality metrics. Thus, false-positive blood cultures can result in decreased hospital funding and increased inspection of quality metrics at the institution.

Blood cultures should be drawn in any patient with fever (≥ 38 °C), leukocytosis, absolute granulocytopenia, or a combination of these factors. Specific indications include sepsis, meningitis, catheter-related bacteremia, endocarditis, septic arthritis, osteomyelitis, and fever of unknown origin. Blood cultures are not always indicated in patients with pneumonia or soft tissue infections but can be performed on a case-by-case basis.

When collecting blood cultures, it is ideal to collect them before empiric antibiotics are initiated. The collector should use proper hand hygiene and use gloves to prevent contamination. Most organisms identified as contaminants arise from the skin. It is crucial that antisepsis of the skin is performed. Alcohol-, chlorhexidine-, and iodine-based products can be used to clean the puncture site [5]. Meta-analysis of six randomized control trials showed that alcohol-based products were associated with the lowest rates of contamination [6]. It is recommended that a 2×2 area of the skin should be cleaned in a circular fashion prior to puncture. The blood cultures should come from prepackaged kits and should also be disinfected at the rubber tops prior to inoculation. Blood cultures should always be drawn from peripheral venipuncture unless clearly necessary. Higher rates of contamination have been reported when cultures are drawn from intravascular catheters [7]. Avoid drawing blood cultures near a site of infusion or areas where recent surgery or radiation therapy has occurred [8]. However, there are indications when catheter-drawn blood cultures are indicated and have shown greater sensitivity and negative predictive value. The Infectious Disease Society of America (IDSA) recommends that when catheter-associated bloodstream infection is suspected, paired blood samples from the catheter and peripheral vein should be drawn. The best yield from blood cultures occurs when at least two sets of cultures are drawn, increasing rates of recovery from 73% at one site to >99% at 3 sites [9]. Most infection requires two sets of blood cultures, while suspected endocarditis requires at least three sets of blood cultures. It is also important to note that each set of culture should be drawn from different sites. Blood cultures should be delivered to the laboratory within 2 hours at room temperature and should never be refrigerated or frozen. It is also important to note that aerobic bottles should be inoculated before anaerobic cultures to optimize yield as anaerobic organisms are reported to account for less than 4% of infections. It is also important to label the blood culture bottles with the time, name of collector, and site of collection. If these proper techniques are upheld in the collection and processing of blood cultures, the hospital can benefit from improved quality, safety, and financial measures in the care of its patients.

Viral

The use of viral cultures has gained significance in the era of newly developed targeted antiviral therapeutics. Multiple techniques are used for the identification of the isolated viral pathogen, which will aid in choosing the right antiviral therapy, early discontinuation of antibiotics, and further diagnostic data for public health purposes [10].

Methods available for viral detection include cell culture, antigen detection, nucleic acid detection, and serological tests. Cell culture allows for identification of multiple viruses with the ability for further characterization. Laboratories are equipped with several cell lines to allow for growth and isolation of different viruses (i.e., human fibroblast cell line can be used for isolation of rhinovirus). The growth and identification of the virus can be achieved by looking at the cytopathic effect (CPE), which is the distinct morphological changes in the cell. The time from incubation to identification depends on the type of virus [10].

Fungal

Fungi are not typically fastidious in their nutritional requirements and will readily grow on media used for bacterial isolation. However, growth on traditional bacterial media can be slow. For this reason, laboratories adjust media specifications based on the suspected organism. Selective media can be included if there is concern for the presence of other microorganisms in the sample [11].

It is traditionally recommended that fungal cultures be incubated at 3 degrees Celsius for a minimum of 4 weeks. If primary suspicion was for *Candida* from a genital site or mucosal surface, growth may occur as soon as 7 days. If there is suspicion for *Histoplasma capsulatum* or *Blastomyces dermatitidis*, 6–8 weeks of incubation may be needed. In areas where dimorphic fungi are endemic, it may be worthwhile to implement default incubation periods of 5 weeks [12].

A unique concern for growing fungal cultures is the chance of a low fungal load, leading to false negatives. This challenge can be overcome by sending as much specimen as possible for culture. Whenever possible, the fungal specimen should be collected before antifungal is given.

Given this potential for a low fungal load, it is important to recognize that a single colony of a potentially pathogenic mold does not necessarily represent a contaminant. The organism identified should be correlated with the clinical presentation to determine if it is the likely cause of the pathogenic process. Some organisms are more frequently identified as pathogenic or as contaminant. For example, *Histoplasma capsulatum* or *Trichophyton rubrum* are often a representative of true infection. However, when opportunistic organisms such as *Aspergillus fumigatus* or *Candida albicans* are identified, they may not be clinically relevant unless there is evidence suggesting they are part of the disease process [13]. Correlating culture findings with histopathology can be helpful in these cases.

Fungal cultures can be used to identify features specific to types of fungi. For yeasts, cultures can allow for identification of a capsule, budding characteristics, size, morphology, and colony color, all of which aids in more specific identification of the yeast. For molds, cultures can reveal culture characteristics, sporulation characteristics, the presence or absence of septa, and hyphal or conidial color [14].

While nucleic acid techniques will likely be the primary diagnostic modality for fungi in the future, there is still utility in using culture techniques for most fungi.

PCR

Polymerase chain reaction (PCR) is a well-developed molecular technique with a wide range of clinical applications for specific and broad-spectrum pathogen detection, evaluation of novel infections, antimicrobial resistance profiling, and early detection of biothreat agents. PCR is an enzyme-driven process for amplifying short sequences of DNA in vitro. It relies on prior knowledge of at least partial sequences of the target DNA/RNA allowing for design of oligonucleotide primers that hybridize specific pathogen DNA/RNA sequences. A DNA polymerase enzyme can then be used to rapidly amplify target DNA into millions of copies. Quantitative real-time PCR allows for this to occur in a single reaction vessel providing advantages in speed, simplicity, reproducibility, and quantitative capacity in which detection can occur. The sensitivity, specificity, and speed of amplification have made PCR a top choice for infectious disease experts for identifying organisms that cannot grow in vitro or when prolonged incubation periods are needed. Multiplex PCR has enabled the simultaneous detection of multiple target sequences of organisms allowing for better sensitivity and specificity. Reverse transcription PCR (RT-PCR) has also been created and allows for RNA-only organisms to be detected [15].

In addition to speed and improved sensitivity, the concept of the broad-ranged PCR can be used to identify classes of pathogens. For example, sequences of the 16s rRNA, exclusively seen in bacterial species, can be designed to quickly identify bacterial organisms in cerebrospinal fluid (CSF) or whole blood, otherwise sterile areas of the body [16]. In a time when antimicrobial resistance is on the rise, PCR can provide information of antimicrobial resistance profiling. For example, the mecA gene has been used to identify methicillin resistance and has become the most reliable tool for identifying methicillin-resistant *Staphylococcus aureus* (MRSA) [17]. PCR-based techniques are also being used to identify resistance testing in *Mycobacterium tuberculosis* and HIV. By early identification of resistance, the practitioner can tailor antibiotic regimens for specific pathogens. Furthermore, with the increasing threat of bioterrorism, rapid detection with PCR has become more of a necessity. Refinements are being made to PCR-based assays for category A bioterrorism agents including *Variola major, Bacillus anthracis, Yersinia pestis*, and *Francisella tularensis* [18].

One limitation of PCR is the cost of PCR reagents, equipment, personnel training, and labor to run each reaction. Each reaction run can cost up to US $125. There are also technical challenges as most thermocyclers cannot do multiple runs of PCR simultaneously which has prevented around-the-clock testing in the clinical setting. False positives are also a large concern of PCR given its high sensitivity. Background contamination of exogenous sources of DNA, even in minute amounts, can lead to false positives. Contamination is most common in universal assays such as in assays that use eubacterial 16s ribosomal RNA gene. PCR can also lead to false-negative results primarily because of the small sample volume permissible in the PCR device. DNA extraction and purification can be performed prior to amplification as a means to concentrate total DNA [15].

PCR has revolutionized the rapid detection of pathogens allowing for early detection and rapid tailored treatment for many organisms. As specific PCR assays are being developed, this technique can change the way medical practitioners approach infection in the critical care unit.

Western Blot

Western blot is an essential technique in molecular and cell biology as it allows for protein detection and quantification of protein expression. There are three major steps in this technique, which include (1) separation of proteins based on molecular weight using gel electrophoresis, (2) transferring results onto a solid support which creates bands for each protein, and (3) using antibodies to detect proteins of interest [19].

ELISA

ELISA is a highly sensitive tool for rapid detection of an antigen or antibody using an enzyme-linked antibody. A variety of ELISA assays have been developed and marketed for the purpose of detecting desired targets. ELISA is the most commonly used immunological technique and has many applications in diagnosis of infectious agents [20].

One area in which ELISA has particularly been utilized is in the detection of sexually transmitted infections. ELISA platforms have been developed that are sensitive and specific in identifying HIV, chlamydia, hepatitis, and syphilis.

ELISA can also be a useful tool in the early diagnosis of tropical diseases, such as dengue fever, borreliosis, yellow fever, and Chagas disease. Given the nonspecific clinical course of these diseases, development of techniques for early and timely diagnosis is important.

Additionally, ELISA has been used to identify pathogens that can cause prenatal infections. ELISA platforms have been developed that can detect *Toxoplasma*, *Treponema pallidum*, and viruses such as rubella, cytomegalovirus, herpes simplex, hepatitis B, Epstein-Barr, varicella zoster, and HIV [21].

Blood Smear

Examination of the peripheral blood smear is an underutilized laboratory investigation in clinical practice. The visual search for intracellular organisms on a peripheral blood smear is a simple and readily available diagnostic approach that has the potential for establishing an immediate diagnosis. Certain bacterial, fungal, and protozoan infections all have the potential to be diagnosed quickly with the use of a peripheral blood [3]. There are many examples in which the presence of atypical cells can aid in diagnosis. The presence of atypical lymphocytosis and large granular lymphocytes has been seen in infectious mononucleosis. Lymphocytosis with atypical cells showing convoluted nuclei has been associated with pertussis. In a young neonate with laboratory finding of thrombocytopenia and blood smear showing polymorphic atypical lymphocytes, cytomegalovirus infection was detected [22].

There are studies showing the utility of blood smears in fever of unknown origin (FUO). In a retrospective study of over 2800 patients at a Chinese hospital presenting with FUO, a significant difference in the presence of abnormal cells such as atypical lymphocytes, nuclear left shift, toxic granulation, or malaria was found between the FUO and the healthy control group [23]. Causative organisms of diseases such as malaria, babesiosis, and bartonellosis can be directly visualized within red blood cells. Many bacteria (such as *Ehrlichia*) and fungi can be found within white blood cells. Still there are organisms such as spirochetes, microfilariae, and trypanosomes that can lie between cells.

Finally, there has been reported utility for peripheral blood smears in identifying organisms during sepsis. A patient with splenectomy had presented with meningitis and was found to have diplococci on the peripheral blood smear allowing for prompt diagnosis of *Streptococcus pneumoniae* prior to the lumbar puncture. In another case report, an immunocompromised patient had presented with respiratory and neurological symptoms *Histoplasma capsulatum* within neutrophils in the blood smear [24]. Thus, the peripheral blood smear can be a powerful adjunct to guide diagnostic tests, provide rapid preliminary diagnosis, and strengthen the empirical antibiotic armamentarium.

Metagenomics

Metagenomics refers to the practice of sequencing all nucleic acid material in a clinical specimen for the purpose of identifying a pathogenic organism. Also referred to as next-generation sequencing, metagenomics has broad potential applications.

Metagenomics can be applied to a broad variety of clinical samples, such as blood, cerebrospinal fluid, respiratory secretions, stool, and tissue. In the setting of rapidly improving sequencing technology, it has the potential to quickly identify potential pathogens. Genetic sequences obtained for pathogenic organisms can also be used to develop antimicrobial resistance profiles. The costs and processing time for metagenomics have improved, making its application increasingly more practical.

However, broader implementation of metagenomics has been limited by several challenges. When all organisms in a sample are sequenced, standardized limits must be set for detection of different specimens. The presence of several organisms in a sample can pose the challenge of distinguishing contaminants and nonpathogenic colonizers from pathogenic organisms. A broad database of existing sequence data needs to be created and maintained to enable accurate identification of organisms [25].

As technology continues to evolve, metagenomics will likely have an increasing role in the identification of pathogens.

BioFire FilmArray

The BioFire FilmArray is a multiplex PCR that has revolutionized the speed at which results can be delivered [26]. This system integrates sample preparation, amplification, detection, and analysis into one device with minimal hands-on time. Results can be delivered to the medical team in about 60 minutes. The device has been approved for detection of viral organisms that infect the upper respiratory tract and gastrointestinal tracts. It can also detect bacterial species in positive blood cultures and gastrointestinal tract. It can help detect antimicrobial resistance genes. It also allows for the simultaneous detection of bacterial, fungal, and viral organisms involved in meningitis or encephalitis. In a multicenter prospective trial involving the BioFire FilmArray GI panel for the simultaneous detection for the 22 most common bacterial and viral causes of gastroenteritis, it was found that the assay had 100% sensitivity for more than half the organisms. For 7/22 organisms, it had a sensitivity of 94.5%. The specificity for all panel targets was 97.1% [27]. Given the speed at which this tool can provide such sensitivity and specificity, it can help clinicians in the critical care unit target specific organisms quickly for better outcomes.

GeneXpert

In 2010, GeneXpert was endorsed by the World Health Organization (WHO) as a novel test for rapid diagnosis of tuberculosis (TB), especially in difficult cases such as multidrug-resistant TB and HIV-associated TB [28]. GeneXpert is a nucleic acid amplification test (NAAT) which can be readily performed on a clinical sputum sample in under 2 hours. Collected sputum is transferred to an instrument where the specific genomic DNA are released through ultrasonic lysis. The sample is then amplified through polymerase chain reaction (PCR) [29, 30]. This method allows for simultaneous detection of MTB and antibiotic susceptibility to rifampin [31].

Lateral Flow

Lateral flow immunoassays (LFA) are performed by passing a liquid sample containing the target of interest through a polymeric strip. While the liquid passes through the strip, small molecules interact with the sample and provide a visual signal indicating a positive or negative result.

LFAs are rapid, accurate, cost-effective tools for use at the point of care in primary screening. There are many features of LFAs that make them particularly desirable for use in low-resource settings. Specific equipment is not needed, and LFAs do not require special storage. The visual result seen on LFA is easily identified by anyone using the assay. For example, a sensitive and specific LFA has been developed for preliminary screening of cryptococcal meningitis through detection of the cryptococcal antigen polysaccharide [32].

While the simplicity of LFAs is appealing, it also presents limitations. An LFA can only provide qualitative bimodal results, for example, indicating "positive" or "negative." A confirmatory test is thus required to make a final diagnosis, giving LFAs a role mainly in primary screening.

LFAs are becoming more sophisticated and may have broader uses in the future. Current research is underway to develop different types of labels, integrate simultaneous detection of multiple targets, and create new strategies for signal amplification [33].

Specimen Sites

Blood

Blood is the most widely used specimen due to its simplicity of collection and stability over time of analyte concentration. Proper preanalytical treatment and handling of blood is essential for quality and accuracy of results. The most important aspect of collection is the correct identification of the patient. Proper safety and identification should be implemented in all quality measures at every hospital. The appropriate containers used for blood collection are essential for allowing transportation and permitting analysis of the blood and derivatives (plasma and serum) [34]. Preservatives and additives are added to containers to prevent clotting and other catabolic activities. Additives to containers include citrate, heparin, EDTA, and glycolysis inhibitors. It is important that sample volume is sufficient for each collection. Samples requiring larger amounts of blood should be drawn first. Volume is not only important for the lab to run tests effectively, but the volume-to-additive ratio is important to prevent blood clotting. For example, the ratio between sodium citrate and blood in the tube should be 1:9. Clotting is important to prevent and can be caused by prolonged venipuncture or failing to mix the tube after collection [35]. By using proper technique, trained personnel, and appropriate vehicles to collect and store blood, the laboratory can run a myriad of tests used to aid the clinician in the critical care unit.

Urine

Urine is usually available in abundant quantity and easy to collect and store, making it an excellent diagnostic specimen for infectious diseases. Beyond culture results, the detection of specific elements within the urine (color, inflammatory markers, antigen, STDs) allows for a broad range of infectious disease diagnoses. Urine color such as hematuria can indicate a urinary tract infection or suggest viral zoonotic infections in addition to other noninfectious causes. Antigen detection in urine through enzyme immunoassay (EIA) allows for diagnosis of disseminated infectious diseases such as histoplasmosis. Urine can also be useful in diagnosis of community-acquired pneumonia or legionellosis by detecting *Streptococcus pneumoniae or Legionella pneumophila* polysaccharides in the specimen, respectively. Urine is now being used as a noninvasive test to check for sexually transmitted diseases such as chlamydia trachomatis and *Neisseria gonorrhoeae* [36].

Sputum (Holland)

Recommendations for collection of sputum prioritize noninvasive over invasive approaches. In patients who are not ventilated, specimens can be obtained by sputum induction or by spontaneous expectoration. The first morning expectorated sputum is most desirable for bacterial culture. In mechanically ventilated patients, endotracheal aspirates or bronchoscopically obtained samples can be used. Bronchial washes are not considered sufficient for routine bacterial culture. For immunocompromised patients, an invasively obtained specimen is recommended [37].

Laboratories should have a procedure for screening sputum samples for acceptability given the high rate of contamination. If a sample is heavily contaminated with oropharyngeal fauna, it should not proceed to routine bacterial culture. Inadequate screening can lead to misleading results.

An appropriate number of sputum samples should be collected based on the clinical suspicion of the etiologic organism. For example, in a cystic fibrosis patient experiencing an exacerbation, additional samples for mycobacterial and fungal cultures may also be desired. For fastidious pathogens such as *Bordetella pertussis*, the clinician collecting the sample should confer with the laboratory prior to collection for specific instructions [38].

Stool (Azka)

Observational studies show that stool cultures are only positive up to 5.6% of the time in the general population. However, a randomized controlled trial in the United Kingdom that assessed stool culture performance in cases of severe diarrheal illness (defined as four fluid stools per day for more than 3 days) detected bacterial pathogens in 87% of patients [39]. Since most acute gastroenteritis is viral and self-limited, stool cultures should typically only be used in severe cases that are more likely to be caused by bacterial pathogens. Patients who are hypovolemic or requiring hospitalization are considered to have severe diarrheal illness. However, if a patient develops diarrhea 3 days after being hospitalized for another cause, stool cultures are lower yield and testing for *Clostridium difficile* is recommended instead.

The enteric pathogens that routine stool cultures can identify are *Salmonella, Campylobacter,* and *Shigella,* which are the most common bacterial causes of acute diarrhea in the United States. However, if a different bacterium is suspected based on a patient's clinical history and exposures, clinicians should notify the laboratory about the suspected pathogen since specific plating techniques are required to identify *Yersinia, Vibrio, Listeria,* and *Aeromonas* [40].

Of note, stool specimens should be placed in sterile containers without preservative and be transported to the laboratory within 2 hours. Obtaining a rectal swab sample and collecting fresh stool have been shown to be equivalent in terms of bacterial yield. If a rectal swab is done, it should be obtained within 5 minutes after a bowel movement, and the sterile swab should be inserted 1–2 cm past the anal verge and lightly rotated 360 degrees [41].

Wound (Tina)

Identifying pathogenic bacteria based on wound cultures (tissues, aspirates, swabs) can often be challenging. Some of this challenge is secondary to improper collection or contamination of samples. In addition, given the long processing time (2 days), the bacterial burden can change in the interim, affecting treatment plan. Surface environmental or host microbiota can also complicate results, making it difficult to see which bacteria are pathogenic [42].

With the rise of obesity and diabetes, chronic wounds have become a major problem in healthcare. These wounds often occur in immunocompromised patients and most commonly include non-healing surgical wounds, venous ulcers, diabetic ulcers, and pressure sores. These wounds present a diagnostic challenge as they have bacterial biofilms that are polymicrobial in nature. Both molecular and culture studies are available for identification of bacteria in wounds, though molecular technologies have proven to be more sensitive [43].

CSF (Holland)

Three or four tubes of CSF should be collected by lumbar puncture for diagnostic studies. At least 0.5–1.0 mL of CSF is required for bacterial testing. However, larger volumes of 5–10 mL increase the specificity in culture for detection of bacteria and are required for detection of fungi and mycobacteria. The first specimen collected is the most likely to be contaminated and should not be used for molecular studies, smears, or cultures. The last specimen should have fewer RBCs than earlier specimens unless the patient has frank hemorrhage. CSF should not be refrigerated [37].

The most commonly ordered assays of CSF include cell count, total protein, glucose, Gram stain, and culture. If fastidious organisms, such as Nocardia, fungi, or mycobacteria, are suspected in the CSF, the laboratory should be informed [44].

Handling of Bioterrorism Organisms (Holland)

The safety of lab personnel in the handling of bioterrorism organisms is of paramount importance. Preparation of suspected bioterrorism organisms should be done in a laminar flow hood at biological safety level (BSL) 2 or greater. The samples may ultimately require delivery to a BSL-3 facility for inactivation prior to electron microscopic assessment. Laboratory personnel handling bioterrorism specimens must have been recently vaccinated or not have contraindications to post-exposure vaccination. Guidance on handling of specific organisms can be found on the CDC website or the American Society of Microbiology website [45–49].

Types of Organisms

Viral

Respiratory Illnesses (Azka)

Several laboratory methods have been established for the detection of respiratory viruses. For the influenza virus specifically, these methods can be divided into rapid influenza diagnostic tests (RIDTs) and molecular assays (particularly RT-PCR). The RIDTs are immunoassays that use antibodies against influenza A and B nucleoproteins to detect viral antigens. These assays can result within 15 minutes and are more widely available but are not as accurate as the RT-PCR and not recommended in the inpatient setting. If a patient tests negative for influenza using the RIDTs but clinical suspicion is high, the CDC recommends continuing to treat the patient and confirming the negative test with a RT-PCR or viral culture [50]. In general, nasopharyngeal specimens are recommended over nasal or throat swabs individually to increase detection.

Multiple manufacturers have created molecular assays using RT-PCR to detect the influenza virus. The molecular assays vary in their sensitivities and specificities but as a general rule are highly specific but not as sensitive (although more sensitive than the RIDTs), meaning that false negatives can occur based on collection methods but false positives are quite rare. If a hospitalized patient has suspected influenza but tests negative using an upper respiratory tract specimen, the CDC suggests testing a lower respiratory tract specimen using a molecular assay since the virus is detectable for a longer period of time in the lower respiratory tract [51].

For the detection of other respiratory viral pathogens, the BioFire FilmArray Multiplex PCR is a comprehensive method that can be used to detect 20 different viruses, including respiratory viruses, within an hour. Aside from multiplex PCR such as BioFire, multiplex nucleic acid amplification testing (NAAT) is also used to diagnose respiratory viral illnesses [52].

Hemorrhagic Fevers (Tina)

Viral hemorrhagic fevers (VHF) are caused by a group of single-stranded RNA viruses with lipid envelopes that come from four families: *Arenaviridae, Bunyaviridae, Filoviridae, and Flaviviridae*. Given their lipid envelopes, these viruses cannot survive in low pH environments; however, they are stable in environments with neutral pH (such as blood). These viruses are highly infectious in nature and pose endemic disease threats with potential for high morbidity and mortality [53, 54].

Humans can contract the virus through direct contact with infected body fluids, inhalation, or arthropod vectors. Patients often have constitutional symptoms such as high fevers, myalgias, and arthralgias; however, the main damage occurs at the vascular beds. These patients can develop shock and multiorgan damage [54].

As mentioned above, diagnosis takes place at highly specialized laboratories given biosafety concerns. Category 3 organisms are not contagious; however, they do cause significant harm to those who come in contact with them. Treatments are available for this category. In contrary, category 4 are those that cause significant disease and are easily transmittable without available treatment. Research and diagnosis have been limited secondary to VHF classification as biosafety levels 2–4 with potential to cause lethal disease upon inhalation [53, 55].

Virus is present in blood from the first day of fever occurrence. There are several diagnostic methods available for detection of VHF including viral culture, electron microscopy, and nucleic acid detection. Viral culture usually requires microbiological containment and takes 3–10 days for most VHF virus detection. Acute phase immunoglobulins (IgM) can be detected by enzyme-linked immunosorbent assays (ELISA) [53, 55]. Given the high cross-reactivity between related viruses, ELISA assays are not very specific [53, 56].

Electron microscopy can be utilized for direct visualization of the virus after isolation from cell culture [57]. In addition, immunohistochemistry staining of specimen allows for identification of VHF viruses by looking at specific morphologic features and helps identify these viruses in different human tissues [58]. Viral culture and electron microscopy are no longer the gold standard for diagnosis given the lengthy process and needs for specialized resources [53].

The most sensitive diagnostic modality for VHF is reverse transcription polymerase chain reaction (RT-PCR) on the blood, urine, or saliva after RNA extraction. This method is especially useful when isolation of the infectious virus has proven to be difficult using cultures, with assays now available for majority of VHF viruses. In addition, multiplex assays have developed to assist with identification of multiple

VHF viruses [59]. This method requires advanced resources and trained personnel, making it unavailable in resource-limited areas. Efforts are directed toward obtaining sensitive and specific testing that is also rapid to allow for timely quarantine of those affected to prevent the spread of VHF disease [53].

Viral Encephalitides (Holland)

Identification of the infectious agent is the primary challenge in management of suspected viral encephalitis. As many as 60% of cases of presumed viral encephalitis remain unexplained because conventional diagnostic strategies fail to identify a causative organism [60].

Viral cultures are often ordered for these CSF specimens; however, the culprit virus is rarely recovered. Given the low yield of viral cultures of CSF, PCR has largely replaced cultures in diagnosis of viral encephalitis. When viral encephalitis is suspected, CSF PCR for HSV-1, HSV-2, and enteroviruses should be sent. PCR testing for VZV and CMV can also be pursued if clinically suspected [61].

Serologic testing when suspecting viral encephalitis is particularly important when the patient's condition fails to improve. Serological assessment for arboviruses may be pursued in the appropriate clinical context. Of note, many viral pathogens require paired sera for diagnosis, making it important to save serum obtained during the acute phase of illness to be used at a later time if necessary.

The gold standard for the diagnosis of suspected viral encephalitis is brain biopsy. Given its invasive nature, this intervention is pursued only after failure of other options.

Hepatitis (Azka)

Antibodies to the different viral hepatitides are used in the diagnosis of viral hepatitis infection. In the testing for hepatitis B virus (HBV) infection, hepatitis B surface antigen is also tested to see if the patient is currently infected. The surface antibody alone being positive (with a negative surface antigen) represents vaccination or immunity from previous resolved infection [62]. The presence of total core antibody represents an infection, whether in the past or present, instead of vaccination. The IgM fraction of core antibody can show if a person is currently or recently infected. The presence of hepatitis B e antigen indicates active replication in hepatocytes, and antibody to e antigen represents an immune response including response to treatment [63]. Aside from these six serological tests for HBV detection, the other viral hepatitides commonly tested for (A, C, and D) have 1–2 serological tests each available for diagnosis. All serology is done using enzyme immunoassays.

There are also several nucleic acid-based tests (such as PCR) that can detect the presence of HBV DNA or HCV RNA. For accurate results, serum should be removed from clotted blood within 4 hours of collection and then stored at −20 to −70 degrees Celsius. An additional method to avoid the breakdown of nucleic acid in the specimen is to use an EDTA tube which allows for storage at 4 degrees Celsius for up to 5 days [64].

HIV (Tina)

HIV screening has been recommended for all persons between ages 13 and 64 years [65]. Diagnostic tests have been developed not only to screen for disease but also for rapid detection during acute infection, a time with the highest likelihood of transmission [66]. Traditionally, HIV testing has included a two-step process, an immunoassay test followed by confirmatory testing with western blot or immunofluorescence [67].

First-generation enzyme immunoassays (EIA) take the viral lysate as antigen to detect immunoglobulin G (IgG) against HIV type 1 [68]. These tests detected infection within 6–8 weeks and are no longer commonly used due to their lack of sensitivity and specificity [69, 70]. Second-generation immunoassays have increased specificity with the use of recombinant peptides or proteins to produce antigens and detect the IgG antibodies. With this method, antibody detection occurs about a week earlier compared to first-generation assays [69, 70]. Third-generation immunoassays detect both IgM and IgG to confirm HIV-1 and HIV-2 infection within 20–25 days [67]. Fourth-generation immunoassays can detect p24 in addition to HIV-1 and HIV-2 antibodies, allowing for diagnosis within 2 weeks postexposure [67]. Furthermore, it will detect infection in majority of those with positive nucleic acid amplification test who have nonreactive/indeterminate results with other assays [71–73].

Once immunoassays are reactive, HIV confirmatory testing is performed with higher specificity. These tests include the western blot or indirect immunofluorescence assay (IFA). Western blot is more commonly used and looks at IgG antibodies that are attached to fixed HIV proteins [67, 74]. However, this test lags behind immunoassay testing by up to 3 weeks, which can lead to false-negative results. IFA also only detects anti-HIV IgG and is less commonly used [67, 74].

Several rapid HIV tests have been approved by the FDA for point-of-care testing outside the clinical setting with detection times of less than 30 minutes. These tests come in two formats including lateral flow and immune concentration [67]. Some perform similar to third-generation immunoassays [74]. False-negative results remain a concern with rapid testing, which is mostly seen during the window period. The fourth-generation antigen/antibody rapid HIV test (Alere Determine HIV1/2 Ag/Ab combo) is currently not FDA approved in the United States [67] and has low rates of HIV p24 detection [75].

HIV RNA detection through quantitative NAAT is able to detect the viral load. However, it is not FDA approved for diagnosis of HIV infection. These tests often require many resources and are expensive [67].

Other Common Viral Infections

CMV (Holland)

Histologic assessment of biopsy samples can be diagnostic of CMV in tissue-invasive disease. Diagnosis is made based on the presence of inclusion bodies and is confirmed by immunohistochemical staining [76].

CMV can be isolated using traditional culture methods from most specimen types in 1–6 weeks. Shell culture has replaced conventional culture in most laboratories due to rapid turnaround time. In shell culture, samples are centrifuged prior to exposure to a cell monolayer. Antibodies bind the antigen, demonstrating intracellular CMV replication. This process takes 2–3 days, enabling more rapid diagnosis than conventional viral culture methods.

In CMV antigenemia assays, CMV proteins such as pp65 are detected in peripheral leukocytes using fluorescently labeled antibodies. Results are reported as number of cells staining positive among the total number of cells counted. Turnaround time for assessment of CMV antigenemia is about 24 hours.

Quantitative PCR may be preferred over antigenemia assays due to improved assay standardization, specimen stability, and ability to test leukopenic patients. The threshold for a positive CMV viral load varies between laboratories [77, 78].

Serology must be interpreted cautiously in diagnosing CMV as the causative agent of infection. CMV IgM antibodies can be detected in serum from 2 weeks after symptom onset to 4–6 months thereafter. Thus, it is important to have a prior baseline CMV IgM level to assess whether a positive CMV IgM is indicative of prior infection. CMV IgG is detectable 2–3 weeks after infection and persists lifelong [79].

EBV (Azka)

Epstein-Barr virus, or EBV, has a seroprevalence rate of 95% in the Western adult population. The detection of heterophilic IgM antibodies by the well-known heterophile antibody test (also known as the Monospot test) is neither sensitive nor specific for the diagnosis of EBV infection. Thus, EBV-specific serologic assays are preferred for diagnosis in immunocompetent individuals instead. The gold standard is the immunofluorescent antibody (IFA) test, which tests for IgM and IgG viral capsid antigens (VCAs) and the EBV nuclear antigens (EBNA). When a person has been infected with EBV once, the EBNA antibody titers will persistently be elevated lifelong. The presence of VCA antibodies but absence of EBNA IgG indicates an acute infection. If the VCA IgM antibody is negative but the VCA IgG and EBNA IgG are positive, then that is indicative of a past infection [80].

Serology is unreliable in immunocompromised patients, particularly those with a blunted humoral response. In these patients, PCR is used instead to detect viral DNA copies. EBV DNA is also used for detection in most EBV-associated malignancies [81].

Herpes (Tina)

Laboratory diagnosis of herpes simplex virus (HSV) is important to guide treatment. In the presence of vesicles, it is recommended to unroof the vesicles and obtain a swab of the lesion in a sterile fashion. Sample should then immediately be placed in appropriate media and readily transferred to laboratory for viral culture [82]. PCR offers a more rapid and sensitive method for diagnosis of HSV [83, 84]. Serological tests can be used in the absence of vesicular lesions. This is done through detection of IgG antibodies against glycoprotein G of HSV1 or HSV2 [85]. The combination of direct virus testing and serological tests can help determine whether HSV infection is new versus reactivation of disease [86]. Immunofluorescence staining can be used to detect the herpes antigen in prepared slides that include cells from HSV lesions [87].

Bacterial

Identifying Resistant Organisms (Azka)

One of the greatest concerns regarding antibiotic use is emerging bacterial resistance in both hospital-associated and community-acquired strains. In the case of *Staphylococcus aureus*, for instance, methicillin resistance is common and caused by the bacterial presence of the *mec*A gene, which encodes the enzyme PBP2a. The gene can be tested for by PCR. PCR is sensitive but not specific for methicillin resistance because some bacterial strains with the *mec*A gene are still susceptible to methicillin. Thus, phenotypic confirmation of PCR results is required. This is primarily done using a latex agglutination test for PBP2a as this is the most accurate mechanism to ascertain resistance [88].

Additionally, inducible clindamycin resistance has become a concern when interpreting antibacterial susceptibility results. Clindamycin resistance can occur with the presence of *erm* genes and is not always detected on standard susceptibility testing. To test for this gene, the laboratory places an erythromycin susceptibility testing disk next to the clindamycin disk on the agar plate. In *S. aureus* strains that carry the *erm* gene, this results in blunting of the zone of inhibition surrounding the clindamycin disk due to an amplified bacterial expression of resistance. Since the blunting around the clindamycin disk occurs in the region closest to the erythromycin disk, this bears resemblance to the letter D and has thus come to be called the "D-zone test" [89].

The detection of methicillin resistance in *S. aureus* is just one example of many resistance patterns that have emerged. Others include extended-spectrum beta-lactamase-producing and carbapenem-resistant bacteria. Since resistance varies by location, a specific hospital's antibiogram should be consulted when making decisions about antibiotics.

Toxin Identification (Azka)

Toxin identification in the laboratory is most often used in the diagnosis of the Gram-positive obligate anaerobe *Clostridium difficile*. The inflammation and necrosis caused by *C. diff* are due to toxin A, toxin B, and, in some strains, the binary *C. diff* transferase (CDT) toxin. *C. diff* spores are found in normal intestinal tracts and are also found ubiquitously in the environment. Thus, it is important to identify the pathogenic strains, which are the ones that produce toxins [90].

The 2018 Infectious Disease Society of America (IDSA) guidelines recommend using a multistep algorithm for diagnosis of *C. diff* infection. Enzyme immunoassays (EIAs) use antibodies to detect the presence of toxins A and B, but the multiple commercial assays that are available for use vary in their sensitivities and specificities. Thus, it is preferred that glutamate dehydrogenase (GDH) immunoassays be used instead since GDH is invariably present in all *C. diff* strains. GDH immunoassays lack specificity for toxigenic strains so should be combined with a toxin test (two-step algorithm) or toxin test and toxin gene detection (three-step algorithm). These algorithms should be used if a hospital does not have a prespecified policy for stool specimens submitted for *C. diff* testing [91].

If a hospital specifies that a stool sample cannot be submitted if a laxative was given within the previous 48 hours and the stool sample should be liquid or soft, then a one-step nucleic acid amplification testing (NAAT) approach can be used, forgoing toxin detection [91].

Difficult-to-Culture Bacteria (Azka)

There are numerous bacteria that do not grow on routine culture media. An example is the HACEK organisms (*Haemophilus*, *Aggregatibacter*, *Cardiobacterium*, *Eikenella*, and *Kingella* species), which are fastidious, Gram-negative bacteria implicated in infective endocarditis. These bacteria were found to be the cause of previously termed "culture-negative endocarditis." However, that title is misleading because they do grow on culture but may need specific media or prolonged incubation [92].

Haemophilus parainfluenzae (unlike *H. influenzae*, which is the better-known genus but does not cause endocarditis) has been shown in studies to be the most common HACEK organism causing endocarditis. It requires NAD (V factor) for culture growth, unlike *H. influenzae* which requires both NAD and hemin (X factor) for culture growth.

Aggregatibacter grows in aggregate lumps in broth culture. *Cardiobacterium* is a facultative anaerobe and is the HACEK organism that does grow on routine blood culture. However, it needs prolonged incubation to do so. It is oxidase positive and produces indole, both being features that can be used to identify the bacteria [93]. *Eikenella corrodens* is named after its characteristic corrosion into solid agar media. This bacterium is also known for its presence in human bite wound infections. The corrosion is thought to occur due to molecules that aid in adhesion to host tissue. *Kingella* (like *Neisseria*) is a member of the Neisseriaceae family, so growth requires Thayer-Martin agar, which is a selective agar that contains antibiotics that suppress the growth of other bacteria. Of note, matrix-assisted laser desorption/ionization time-of-flight mass spectrometry (MALDI TOF-MS) is a promising, emerging method that can more rapidly identify fastidious organisms such as these [94].

TB (Azka)

Smear and culture are used for the diagnosis of acute tuberculosis (TB) infection. The sensitivity and specificity of AFB smear microscopy are low, so it is recommended that three samples are provided for evaluation. Despite the use of AFB smears inpatient to "rule out" TB, the sensitivity is only 45–80%. The samples need to include an early morning sputum collection, and all three need to be collected at least 8 hours apart. Collecting 5–10 mL of sputum increases the yield of smear microscopy. AFB culture is the gold standard for diagnosis but takes 2–6 weeks to obtain a result. Since both false-positive and false-negative results can occur with smear microscopy, its results need to be confirmed with mycobacterial culture regardless [95, 96].

Nucleic acid amplification testing (NAAT) done on sputum samples can result in 24–28 hours. The NAAT has a higher positive predictive value (>95%) for TB in settings where nontuberculous mycobacteria are present. Thus, NAAT is recommended when an AFB smear is positive. It should also be done when there is an intermediate or high pretest probability for TB despite negative AFB smears, as it can identify 50–80% of true TB cases when AFB smear is negative. The NAAT can also identify rifampin resistance to guide early therapy. However, AFB cultures are still needed to identify sensitivities to all antitubercular medications [95].

Interferon-y release assay (IGRA) can also be used to test for TB. The QuantiFERON-TB Gold and T-SPOT TB tests are IGRAs that assess the release of interferon-y in response to the TB antigens ESAT-6 and CFP-10, respectively. These assays cannot differentiate between active and latent TB and thus have limited value in the inpatient setting.

Atypical Bacterial Infections

Tickborne Infections (Azka)

Rickettsia

Rickettsiae are obligate intracellular Gram-negative bacteria, and this classification includes infections from *Rickettsia*, *Ehrlichia*, and *Anaplasma*. Infection is typically transmitted to humans by ticks, but unrecognized tick bites are common especially since the bite is often painless. There are certain laboratory findings, such as thrombocytopenia, transaminitis, hyponatremia, and elevated creatine kinase and LDH, that are associated with infection. However, diagnosis is confirmed by serologic assays, most commonly IgG indirect immunofluorescence antibody (IFA) assays. These assays are not sensitive during the first week of infection as IgG antibodies are not yet formed. The sensitivity increases 2–3 weeks after the onset of illness. Most laboratories do not have tests for IgM available since the specificity of these tests is low.

With IFA assays, antigens of rickettsial pathogens are fixed on slides and bind to serum antibodies, if present, which are then identified by fluorescein labeling. Since the test is often falsely negative initially, the CDC recommends that an additional repeat test be done 2–4 weeks after the initial. A fourfold increase in antibody titer confirms the diagnosis. A diagnosis cannot be made with a single test [97].

Additionally, since the test can remain positive for years after infection, the testing should only be done in patients with acute illness that has manifestations similar to that of rickettsial disease.

Rash is seen in Rocky Mountain spotted fever (RMSF), which is caused by *Rickettsia rickettsii*, but is less commonly seen in anaplasmosis or ehrlichiosis. Biopsy of cutaneous lesions in RMSF, such as eschar or rash, and subsequent immunostaining and immunofluorescence approach 100% specificity for the diagnosis [98].

Lyme

If a patient has the rash of erythema migrans, then it is considered pathognomonic for the diagnosis of Lyme disease and no further testing is recommended. This is because erythema migrans is an early finding of Lyme disease, and most patients are not seropositive at the time of rash development. In fact, after the rash develops, it takes 1–2 weeks for IgM antibodies to *Borrelia burgdorferi* to appear and 2–6 weeks for the IgG antibodies to develop [99].

However, patients are seropositive by the time they develop either early disseminated or late disease. In such cases, the diagnosis of Lyme disease is made by a two-tier process that can be done on the same sample of blood. The testing typically starts with an enzyme immunoassay (EIA) which, if positive, is followed by an immunoblot (typically a western blot) for confirmation. The western blot tests for both IgM and IgG.

If the initial EIA is negative, no further testing is done. If the EIA is equivocal or positive, the positivity of the western blot confirms the infection since the latter is a more specific test. Of note, since the EIA is more sensitive, it can falsely turn positive by detecting another spirochete, such as *Treponema pallidum*, the causative agent of syphilis.

Serologic results should be interpreted in the setting of the clinical context. If a patient has had symptoms for more than 6 weeks without treatment, a positive IgM but negative IgG EIA and western blot should be viewed as a false positive.

If both parts of the test are positive and a patient is thus diagnosed with Lyme disease, a follow-up test to confirm a decrease in antibody titer should not be done

[100]. This is because patients can have persistent antibodies despite being treated and the acute infection resolving.

Other testing algorithms have been proposed, especially since the western blot is a time-intensive procedure. However, the CDC does not endorse the use of any other tests because their efficacy and clinical use have not yet been established.

Acinetobacter (Holland)

Acinetobacter is easily isolated in standard cultures. However, use of cultures results in delayed identification because this organism is nonreactive to common biochemical tests, including indole, glucose fermentation, and nitrate reduction. Cultures are also limiting because of slow turnaround time and limited sensitivity.

An important role of the lab is detection of carbapenem-resistant *Acinetobacter baumannii* (CRAB). Current approaches to identifying CRAB include culture-based methods such as the modified Hodge test, which is time consuming, and PCR, which is limited by its ability to only detect known carbapenem-resistant genes [101].

New approaches for the identification of CRAB are needed given the spread of this organism. New methods are being developed for extraction of carbapenemase-associated proteins prior to matrix-assisted laser desorption/ionization time-of-flight mass spectrometry (MALDI TOF-MS) [102].

Nocardia (Azka)

The diagnosis of nocardiosis is made by culture of the specific tissue that is infected with the aerobic, acid-fast bacteria. This sample is oftentimes sputum or a skin specimen. *Nocardia* takes longer to grow as compared to other, more prevalent bacteria but will typically grow within 5 days. However, for actinomycete (both *Nocardia* and *Actinomyces*) isolation, culture should be incubated for 2–3 weeks [103]. The smear can be highly suggestive of *Nocardia* since it will commonly show the characteristic Gram-positive coccobacillary (bead-like) branching filaments.

Fusobacterium (Azka)

Fusobacterium is an obligate anaerobic Gram-negative bacillus. *F. necrophorum* is the species that is specifically implicated in pharyngitis leading to Lemierre syndrome. Although rare, *Fusobacterium* infection can be severe with life-threatening metastasis to different organs, most commonly the lungs. Throat swabs do not identify the bacteria since these swabs are typically not cultured in anaerobic media [104].

Diagnosis is often made by blood culture or culture of tissue from a metastatic lesion. *Fusobacterium* has a pleomorphic appearance with irregular staining of rods, cocci, and filamentous forms when isolated in blood culture. Stain is typically only taken up in the center of the organism and its border which is characteristic for this bacterium. If basic blood agar is supplemented with vitamin K and hemin, the organism is likely to grow more robustly.

Fusobacterium colonies growing on culture have a distinctive appearance. The colonies are yellow, smooth, and round. Hemolysis is variable based on strain and culture so cannot contribute to the diagnosis. The bacteria do readily contain indole, so a spot indole reagent can be used to detect its presence. It is beneficial if laboratories are notified if *Fusobacterium* is suspected, so that they can use these methods for improved detection [105].

Fungal

Candida (Holland)

In suspected local *Candida* infections, Gram stain or potassium hydroxide preparation of scrapings reveals budding yeasts with or without pseudohyphae. Direct examination of punch biopsies shows microabscesses.

For invasive infections and candidemia, blood cultures are the gold standard for diagnosis. Unfortunately, blood cultures in patients with suspected candidemia are negative about half of the time. Additionally, cultures require 1–3 days for growth and often several more days for identification. New techniques have been developed for more rapid identification; peptide nucleic acid fluorescence in situ hybridization can be used to detect *C. albicans* and *C. glabrata* within hours of culture growth [106]. If blood cultures are incidentally positive for *Candida* when assessing for other organisms, the clinician should obtain a biopsy in patients with focal findings such as a skin lesion. *Candida* is rarely a contaminant in the blood but may be a local colonizer in the urine [107].

The limitations of culture methods in detection of *Candida* have necessitated development of other diagnostic methods. Matrix-assisted laser desorption ionization-time-of-flight mass spectrometry (MALDI-TOF MS) enables detection and identification of *Candida* proteins grown in culture. Results are available in about 30 minutes [108].

The antigen assay for beta-D-glucan, found in the cell wall of many fungi, may be used in conjunction with other techniques to bolster detection of *Candida*.

PCR and antibody detection are not typically used in diagnosis of suspected *Candida* infections. While PCR would be desirable for fast, accurate identification of specific *Candida* species, there is no commercially available PCR test available. An antibody assay for *Candida* would not be useful since healthy people have *Candida* as a normal component of their microbiome and thus produce antibodies [109].

The T2Candida panel is a newer strategy for the diagnosis of candidemia. In this assay, the yeast cells are broken apart. *Candida* DNA is then amplified and detected using magnetic resonance technology [107].

Histoplasmosis (Azka)

Histoplasma capsulatum is a thermally dimorphic endemic fungus, meaning that it exists as a yeast at body temperature but as a mold in its native environment. Gold standard for detection is a demonstration of the yeast on histopathology slides or of the mold in fungal cultures. This can take up to 8 weeks, so the most common test used for detection of *Histoplasma* in the clinical setting is antigen detection by enzyme immunoassay [110].

Antigen testing provides a noninvasive and rapid method for diagnosis and can be done on serum, urine, cerebrospinal fluid, and fluid from bronchoalveolar lavage. In cases of acute or disseminated histoplasmosis, urine antigen testing is over 85% sensitive and specific. However, sensitivity and specificity of antigen testing decrease in chronic infections, so culture is often required to make the diagnosis.

Culture is typically incubated at 25–30 degrees Celsius. If incubated at higher temperatures, it transforms to yeast, but this transformation should not be used to make the diagnosis. Calcofluor white is a stain that adheres to chitin in fungal cell walls so can be used for identification. Culture is less sensitive than antigen testing in the acute setting [111].

Coccidioidomycosis (Azka)

There are several methods that have been standardized and can be used for the detection of *Coccidioides* species, the most common method being serology. Enzyme immunoassay can detect both IgM and IgG antibodies against the fungus and is very sensitive for the diagnosis. Other serologic methods include immunodiffusion, complement fixation, and lateral flow assay. Lateral flow assay is the most rapid test and can accurately detect IgM and IgG antibodies within 30 minutes [112].

PCR is useful for detection from lower respiratory tract specimens obtained by bronchoscopy. Testing on sputum, however, has low sensitivity for the diagnosis, in part due to the cough often being nonproductive. Culture can also be performed but should be handled in biosafety level 3 laboratories only [112]. *Coccidioides* can grow on most fungal culture media and even routine bacterial cultures in less than a week [113].

Cryptococcus (Holland)

Stains such as mucicarmine and methenamine silver can be used to identify *Cryptococcus* in histopathological specimens. The polysaccharide capsule can be visualized when stained with India ink. Evaluation is usually performed on specimens that have been grown in culture. However, the cryptococcal antigen test is more rapid than histopathologic identification and should be readily available for use in both serum and CSF [114].

Commercial identification systems such as Vitek, AuxaColor, and API systems are currently being used in clinical microbiology laboratories. MALDI-TOF has also been shown to successfully identify *Cryptococcus* and should be considered in favor of commercial identification systems where available [115].

Blastomycosis (Azka)

Blastomyces, just like the other endemic fungi, is thermally dimorphic. In vivo, it is in its yeast form, so direct examination of a bodily specimen – such as sputum, cerebrospinal fluid, pleural fluid, or skin scrapings – under a microscopic will show broad-based budding. This direct examination can be done on wet prep with special staining with Calcofluor white or potassium hydroxide. Calcofluor white is more commonly used because it causes the yeast wall to fluoresce under fluorescence microscopy. Such direct examination when positive can provide rapid diagnosis. *Blastomyces* species can be differentiated from other yeast by its size, which is 8–15 microns. *Blastomyces* – unlike *Candida* or *Aspergillus* – are never contaminants when isolated from body fluid or tissue [116].

Although direct examination is always done due to its capability for rapid diagnosis, the actual diagnostic yield is only 36% for a single specimen. The gold standard for diagnosis is by culture growth or histopathology [117]. *Blastomyces dermatitidis* will typically grow as a mold in culture at 25 degrees Celsius within 1–4 weeks but can be detected sooner in culture using a DNA probe (AccuProbe). Sputum culture – and particularly culture obtained from bronchoscopy – has a high sensitivity up to 80% and 92%, respectively, and 100% specificity [116].

Mucormycosis (Azka)

Mucorales molds, most commonly *Mucor* and *Rhizopus* species, are typically the cause of mucormycosis. The diagnosis requires histopathologic or culture confirmation from an affected tissue [118]. Infections are typically rhinocerebral, pulmonary, cutaneous, or disseminated, so biopsy of a lesion can yield the diagnosis. For pulmonary mucormycosis, a sputum or bronchoalveolar culture can confirm the diagnosis. The filamentous mold looks similar to other fungi, so an experienced pathologist is needed to make the diagnosis from histopathology or culture [119]. Since early surgical debridement is the standard of care, the surgical specimens can often be submitted for histopathology and culture. PCR typically uses fungal ribosomal genes to detect Mucorales. PCR is not yet standardized in laboratories but can be used to support the diagnosis made by the other approaches [118].

Aspergillosis (Holland)

Aspergillus can be identified in biopsy specimens as having narrow, septated hyphae branching at acute angles. Methenamine silver or periodic acid-Schiff staining can be used.

Aspergillus grows rapidly in culture and may be seen within 1–3 days. However, identification requires sporulation for evaluation of spore-bearing structures.

Cell wall components may be used in conjunction with other identification methods for *Aspergillus*. Galactomannan is a component of the *Aspergillus* cell wall that can be detected through ELISA. Sensitivity ranges from 40% to 70% but can improve with serial testing. Specificity is high. Thus, this test should be ordered only in situations in which there is high clinical suspicion of aspergillosis. 1,3-Beta-D-glucan is a polysaccharide present in the cell wall of *Candida, Aspergillus,* and *Pneumocystis*. Of note, it is not found in *Mucor* or *Cryptococcus* [120, 121].

Parasites

Malaria (Azka)

The four species of the parasite *Plasmodium* that infect humans are *P. falciparum, P. malariae, P. vivax,* and *P. ovale*. The parasite can be identified on microscopy with the use of thick and thin slides. The thick slide consists of more blood on the slide and is used to detect the presence of the parasite. The thin slide can then identify the actual species of *Plasmodium* since it looks at a smaller sample of blood and can appreciate the subtle differences in cellular structure between the four species. Either smear can be used to quantify the burden of parasitemia as a percentage of the blood sample that contains the parasite. Giemsa staining is used for both the thick and thin smears.

Microscopy is the gold standard for the detection of malaria but is not always able to differentiate between the morphologic characteristics between species such as *P. vivax* and *P. ovale* which often appear similar. In such cases, a PCR assay can use parasitic DNA extracted from a blood sample to identify the species [122].

In addition to microscopy, an indirect fluorescent antibody (IFA) can also be used to detect the presence of the parasite. This method is not preferred for diagnosing acute malarial infection since the antibody testing takes longer to perform. However, it can be used if microscopy results are ambiguous in order to clarify the diagnosis [122].

Protozoa (Tina)

Intestinal

The most common pathogenic protozoans include *Giardia, Cryptosporidium, Dientamoeba fragilis, Entamoeba* species, *Blastocystis* species, and *Cyclospora cayetanensis* [123, 124]. Stool ova and parasite testing, though time consuming and labor intensive, has been the most common way to test for these species [123]. Stool antigen detection tests have been approved by the FDA for recognition of *Giardia*,

Cryptosporidium, and *Entamoeba histolytica* [123]. Stool collection and preservation (with need of preservatives) become important for proper detection of protozoa in the laboratory. Microscopic detection of protozoa is aided by their distinctive morphology [123].

Blood Specimen

Microscopic examination of blood smears for detection of malaria has remained the gold standard of diagnosis. This method is fast and cost-effective and allows for speciation in addition to the quantification of the amount of parasites [125]. Species-specific PCR is also available for detection of malaria and Babesia [126–130].

For other parasitic infections such as toxoplasmosis, where identification through host tissue is not possible, the detection of antibodies can help identify the timing of infection [130, 131].

Helminths (Holland)

Histopathologic examination is the most important diagnostic tool for parasitic infections. However, its usefulness is limited by the required technical expertise. A small number of organisms may be present in samples, and distinguishing between similar-appearing organisms can be challenging.

Nucleic acid amplification tests are particularly useful when microscopic identification of a helminth fails. However, these methods should not be utilized to monitor response to treatment, as antigens and DNA can persist weeks after treatment [14, 132, 133].

Serological assays are considered an adjunctive method for diagnosis of helminths. These panels have limited sensitivity and specificity, largely due to cross-reaction of antibodies from one helminth with antibodies of another.

References

1. Garcia RA, Spitzer ED, Beaudry J, et al. Multidisciplinary team review of best practices for collection and handling of blood cultures to determine effective interventions for increasing the yield of true-positive bacteremias, reducing contamination, and eliminating false-positive central line-associated bloodstream infections. Am J Infect Control. 2015;43:1222–37.
2. Fenner L, Widmer AF, Straub C, Frei R. Is the incidence of anaerobic bacteremia decreasing? Analysis of 114,000 blood cultures over a ten-year period. J Clin Microbiol. 2008;46: 2432–4.
3. Lee CC, Lin WJ, Shih HI, et al. Clinical significance of potential contaminants in blood cultures among patients in a medical center. J Microbiol Immunol Infect. 2007;40:438–44.
4. McDonald LC, Gerding DN, Johnson S, et al. Clinical Practice Guidelines for Clostridium difficile Infection in Adults and Children: 2017 Update by the Infectious Diseases Society of America (IDSA) and Society for Healthcare Epidemiology of America (SHEA). Clin Infect Dis. 2018;66:987–94.

5. Calderia D, David C, Sampaio C. Skin antiseptics in venous puncture-site disinfection for prevention of blood culture contamination: systematic review with meta-analysis. J Hosp Infect. 2011;77:223–32.
6. Malani A, Trimble K, Parekh V, et al. Review of clinical trials of skin antiseptic agents used to reduce blood culture contamination. Infect Control Hosp Epidemiol. 2007;28:892–5.
7. Willems E, Smismans A, Cartuyvels R, et al. The preanalytical optimization of blood cultures: a review and the clinical importance of benchmarking in 5 Belgian hospitals. Diagn Microbiol Infect Dis. 2012;73:1–8.
8. Alahmadi YM, Aldeyab MA, McElnay JC, et al. Clinical and economic impact of contaminated blood cultures within the hospital setting. J Hosp Infect. 2011;77:233–6.
9. Clinical and Laboratory Standards Institute. Principles and procedures for blood cultures: approved guideline. CLSI document M47-A. Wayne, PA: Clinical and Laboratory Standards Institute; 2007.
10. Storch GA. Diagnostic virology. Clin Infect Dis. 2000;31(3):739–51. https://doi.org/10.1086/314015.
11. Kauffman CA, Pappas PG, Sobel JD, Dismukes WE. Essentials of clinical mycology. New York: Springer; 2011.
12. Leber AL. Clinical microbiology procedures handbook. Washington, DC: American Society for Microbiology, ASM Press; 2016.
13. Sangoi AR, Rogers WM, Longacre TA, Montoya JG, Baron EJ, Banaei N. Challenges and pitfalls of morphologic identification of fungal infections in histologic and cytologic specimens: a ten-year retrospective review at a single institution. Am J Clin Pathol. 2009;131:364–75.
14. Miller JM, Binnicker MJ, Campbell S, et al. A Guide to Utilization of the Microbiology Laboratory for Diagnosis of Infectious Diseases: 2018 Update by the Infectious Diseases Society of America and the American Society for Microbiology. Clin Infec Dis. 2018;67(6):e1–e94.
15. Yang S, Rothman RE. PCR-based diagnostics for infectious diseases: uses, limitations, and future applications in acute-care settings. Lancet Infect Dis. 2004;4:337–48.
16. Greigen K, Loeffelholz M. A Purohit PCR primers and probes for the 16S rRNA gene of most species of pathogenic bacteria, including bacteria found in cerebrospinal fluid. J Clin Microbiol. 1994;32:335–51.
17. Tenover FC, Jones RN, Swenson JM, et al. Methods for improved detection of oxacillin resistance in coagulase-negative staphylococci: results of a multicenter study. J Clin Microbiol. 1999;37:4051–8.
18. Bell CA, Uhl JR, Hadfield TL, et al. Detection of Bacillus anthracis DNA by LightCycler PCR. J Clin Microbiol. 2002;40:2897–902.
19. Mahmood T, Yang PC. Western blot: technique, theory, and trouble shooting. North Am J Med Sci. 2012;4:429–34.
20. Arora DK, Das S, Sukumar M. Analyzing microbes: manual of molecular biology techniques. Heidelberg: Springer; 2013.
21. Hosseini S, Vázquez-Villegas P, Rito-Palomares M, Martinez-Chapa SO. Enzyme-linked immunosorbent assay (ELISA): from A to Z. Singapore: Springer; 2018.
22. Lehmann LS, Spivak JL. Rapid and definitive diagnosis of infectious diseases using peripheral blood smears. J Intensive Care Med. 1992;7:36–47.
23. Lv J, Zong H, Ma G, et al. Predictive significance of peripheral blood smears in patients with fever of unknown origin: a retrospective study of 2871 cases. Clin Lab. 2015;61:1643–52.
24. Fred HL, Hassan Y. Eyeing pathogens in the peripheral blood film. Hosp Pract. 1999;34:124–6.
25. Forbes JD, Knox NC, Peterson C, Reimer AR. Highlighting clinical metagenomics for enhanced diagnostic decision-making: a step towards wider implementation. Comput Struct Biotechnol J. 2018;16:108–20.
26. "BIOFIRE® FILMARRAY®." BioMérieux, www.biomerieux-usa.com/clinical/biofire-film-array.
27. Buss SN, Leber A, Chapin K, et al. Multicenter evaluation of the BioFire FilmArray gastrointestinal panel for etiologic diagnosis of infectious gastroenteritis. J Clin Microbiol. 2015;53:915–25.

28. World Health Organization. WHO endorses new rapid tuberculosis test; 2010. Dec 8., Available: http://www.who.int/mediacentre/news/releases/2010/tb_test_20101208/en/index. html. Accessed 15 June 2011.
29. Boehme CC, et al. Rapid molecular detection of tuberculosis and rifampin resistance. NEJM. 2010;363:1005–15.
30. Blakemore R, et al. Evaluation of the analytical performance of the Xpert MTB/RIF Assay. J Clin Microbiol. 2010;48(7):2495–501.
31. Helb D, Jones M, Story F, et al. Rapid detection of Mycobacterium tuberculosis and rifampin resistance by use of on demand, near-patient technology. J Clin Microbiol. 2010;48:229–37.
32. Ma Q, Yao J, Yuan S, Liu H, Wei N, Zhang J, Shan W. Development of a lateral flow recombinase polymerase amplification assay for rapid and visual detection of Cryptococcus neoformans/C. gattii in cerebral spinal fluid. BMC Infect Dis. 2019;19(1):108.
33. Koczula KM, Gallotta A. Lateral flow assays. Essays Biochem. 2016;60(1):111–20.
34. Giavarina D, Lippi G. Blood venous sample collection: recommendations overview and a checklist to improve quality. Clin Biochem. 2017;50:568–73.
35. Clinical Laboratory Standards Institute. Procedures for the Collection of Diagnostic Blood Specimens by Venipuncture Approved Standard. 6th ed. Wayne, PA: CLSI document H3-A6. Clinical Laboratory Standards Institute; 2007.
36. Tuuminen T. Urine as a specimen to diagnose infections in twenty-first century: focus on analytical accuracy. Front Immunol. 2012;3:45. https://doi.org/10.3389/fimmu.2012.00045.
37. Miller JM, Binnicker MJ, Campbell S, et al. A Guide to Utilization of the Microbiology Laboratory for Diagnosis of Infectious Diseases: 2018 Update by the Infectious Diseases Society of America and the American Society for Microbiology. Clin Infect Dis. 2018;67(6):e1–e94.
38. Kalil AC, Metersky ML, Klompas M, et al. Management of adults with hospital-acquired and ventilator-associated pneumonia: 2016 clinical practice guidelines by the Infectious Diseases Society of America and the American Thoracic Society. Clin Infect Dis. 2016;63:e61–111.
39. Dryden MS, Gabb RJ, Wright SK. Empirical treatment of severe acute community-acquired gastroenteritis with ciprofloxacin. Clin Infect Dis. 1996;22(6):1019–25.
40. Shane AL, Mody RK, Crump JA, et al. Infectious Diseases Society of America Clinical Practice Guidelines for the Diagnosis and Management of Infectious Diarrhea. Clin Infect Dis. 2017;65(12):e45–80.
41. Bassis CM, Moore NM, Lolans K, et al. Comparison of stool versus rectal swab samples and storage conditions on bacterial community profiles. BMC Microbiol. 2017;17(1):78.
42. Kallstrom G. Are quantitative bacterial wound cultures useful? J Clin Microbiol. 2014;52(8):2753–6. https://doi.org/10.1128/jcm.00522-14.
43. Rhoads DD, et al. Comparison of culture and molecular identification of bacteria In chronic wounds. Int J Mol Sci. 2012;13(3):2535–50. MDPI AG. https://doi.org/10.3390/ijms13032535.
44. Christie LJ, Loeffler AM, Honarmand S, et al. Diagnostic challenges of central nervous system tuberculosis. Emerg Infect Dis. 2008;14:1473–5.
45. American Society of Microbiology. https://www.asm.org/ASM/media/Policy-and-Advocacy/LRN/Sentinel%20Files/AnthraxLRN-Sept2017.pdf. Accessed 5 Feb 2019.
46. American Society of Microbiology. https://www.asm.org/ASM/media/Policy-and-Advocacy/LRN/Sentinel%20Files/Botulism-July2013.pdf. Accessed 5 Feb 2019.
47. American Society of Microbiology. https://www.asm.org/ASM/media/Policy-and-Advocacy/LRN/Sentinel%20Files/Smallpox_July2013.pdf. Accessed 5 Feb 2019.
48. Centers for Disease Control. https://www.cdc.gov/vhf/ebola/laboratory-personnel/safe-specimen-management.html. Accessed 5 Feb 2019.
49. Hazelton PR, Gelderblom HR. Electron microscopy for rapid diagnosis of emerging infectious agents. Emerg Infect Dis. 2003;9(3):294–303.
50. Information on Collection of Respiratory Specimens for Influenza Virus Testing | CDC. Centers for Disease Control and Prevention. https://www.cdc.gov/flu/professionals/diagnosis/info-collection.htm. Accessed 20 May 2019.

51. Ginocchio CC, McAdam AJ. Current best practices for respiratory virus testing. J Clin Microbiol. 2011;49(9 Supplement):S44–8.
52. Azar MM, Landry ML. Detection of Influenza A and B Viruses and Respiratory Syncytial Virus by Use of Clinical Laboratory Improvement Amendments of 1988 (CLIA)-Waived Point-of-Care Assays: a Paradigm Shift to Molecular Tests. J Clin Microbiol. 2018;56(7).
53. Racsa LD, et al. Viral hemorrhagic fever diagnostics. Clin Infect Dis. 2016;62(2):214–9. https://doi.org/10.1093/cid/civ792.
54. Marty AM, et al. Viral hemorrhagic fevers. Clin Lab Med. 2006;26(2):345–86. Elsevier BV. https://doi.org/10.1016/j.cll.2006.05.001.
55. World Health Organization. Laboratory biosafety manual. Geneva, CH: World Health Organization; 2004. Available at: http://www.who.int/csr/resources/publications/biosafety/Biosafety7.pdf?ua=1. Accessed 9 Jun 2015.
56. Fajfr M, Ruzek D. Laboratory diagnosis of viral hemorrhagic fevers. In: Viral hemorrhagic fevers. Boca Raton, FL: CRC Press; 2013. https://doi.org/10.1201/b15172-14.
57. Geisbert TW, Jahrling PB. Differentiation of filoviruses by electron microscopy. Virus Res. 1995;39(2–3):129–50. Elsevier BV. https://doi.org/10.1016/0168-1702(95)00080-1.
58. Zaki SR, et al. A novel immunohistochemical assay for the detection of ebola virus in skin: implications for diagnosis, spread, and surveillance of ebola hemorrhagic fever. J Infect Dis. 1999;179(s1):S36–47. Oxford University Press (OUP). https://doi.org/10.1086/514319.
59. Drosten C, et al. Rapid detection and quantification of RNA of Ebola and Marburg viruses, Lassa Virus, Crimean-Congo hemorrhagic fever virus, Rift Valley fever virus, dengue virus, and yellow fever virus by real-time reverse transcription-PCR. J Clin Microbiol. 2002;40(7):2323–30. American Society For Microbiology. https://doi.org/10.1128/jcm.40.7.2323-2330.2002.
60. Kennedy P, Quan P, Lipkin W. Viral encephalitis of unknown cause: current perspective and recent advances. Viruses. 2017;9(6):138.
61. Kupila L, Vuorinen T, Vainionpaa R, Hukkanen V, Marttila RJ, Kotilainen P. Etiology of aseptic meningitis and encephalitis in an adult population. Neurology. 2006;66(1):75–80.
62. Krajden M, McNabb G, Petric M. The laboratory diagnosis of hepatitis B virus. Can J Infect Dis Med Microbiol. 2005;16(2):65–72.
63. Yang H, Lu S, Liaw Y, et al. Hepatitis B e antigen and the risk of hepatocellular carcinoma. N Engl J Med. 2002;347(3):168–74.
64. Test Center. Viral hepatitis: laboratory support of diagnosis and management. https://www.questdiagnostics.com/testcenter/testguide.action?dc=CF_ViralHepatitis. Accessed 28 May 2019.
65. Centers for Disease Control and Prevention. Revised recommendations for HIV testing of adults, adolescents, and pregnant women in health-care settings. MMWR Recomm Rep. 2006;55. RR-14:1–17.
66. Brenner BG, Roger M, Routy JP, et al. High rates of forward transmission events after acute/early HIV-1 infection. J Infect Dis. 2007;195:951–9.
67. Cornett JK, Kim TJ. Laboratory Diagnosis of HIV in adults: a review of current methods. Clin Infect Dis. 2013;57(5).
68. Murphy G, Atiken C. HIV testing-the perspective from across the pond. J Clin Virol. 2011;52 suppl 1:S71–6.
69. Owen SM. Testing for acute HIV infection: implications for treatment as prevention. Curr Opin HIV AIDS. 2012;7:125–30.
70. Owen SM, Yang C, Spira T, et al. Alternative algorithms for human immunodeficiency virus infection diagnosis using tests that are licensed in the United States. J Clin Microbiol. 2008;46:1588–95.
71. Pandori MW, Hackett J Jr, et al. Assessment of the ability of a fourth generation immunoassay for HIV antibody and p24 antigen to detect both acute and recent HIV infection in a high-risk setting. J Clin Microbiol. 2009;47:2639–42.
72. Chavez P, Wesolowski L, Patel P, et al. Evaluation of the performance of the Abbott ARCHITECT HIV Ag/Ab Combo Assay. J Clin Virol. 2011;52 Suppl 1:S51–5.

73. Bentsen C, Mclaughlin L, et al. Performance evaluation of the Bio-Rad Laboratories GS HIV Combo Ag/Ab EIA, a 4th generation HIV assay for the simultaneous detection of HIV p24 antigen and antibodies to HIV-1 (groups M and O) and HIV-2 in human serum or plasma. J Clin Virol. 2011;52 Suppl 1:S57–61.
74. Delaney KP, Branson BM, Uniyal A, et al. Evaluation of the performance characteristics of 6 rapid HIV antibody tests. Clin Infec Dis. 2011;52:257–63.
75. Fox J, O'Shea S. Low rates of p24 antigen detection using a fourth generation point of care HIV test. Sex Transm Infect. 2011;87:178–9.
76. Chou S. Newer methods for diagnosis of cytomegalovirus infection. Clin Infect Dis. 1990;12 Suppl 7:S727–36.
77. Kotton CN, Kumar D, Caliendo AM, et al. Transplantation Society International CMV Consensus Group. International consensus guidelines on the management of cytomegalovirus in solid organ transplantation. Transplantation. 2010;89:779–95.
78. Razonable RR, Paya CV, Smith TF. Role of the laboratory in diagnosis and management of cytomegalovirus infection in hematopoietic stem cell and solid-organ transplant recipients. J Clin Microbiol. 2002;40(3):746–52.
79. Wreghitt TG, Teare EL, Sule O, Devi R, Rice P. Cytomegalovirus infection in immunocompetent patients. Clin Infect Dis. 2003;37(12):1603–6.
80. Hess R. Routine Estein-Barr virus diagnostics from the laboratory perspective: still challenging after 35 years. J Clin Microbiol. 2004;42(8):3381–7.
81. De Paschale M, Pierangelo C. Serological diagnosis of Epstein-Barr virus infection: problems and solutions. World. J Virol. 2012;1(1):31–43.
82. Singh A, et al. The laboratory diagnosis of herpes simplex virus infections. Can J Infect Dis Med Microbiol. 2005;16(2):92–8. https://doi.org/10.1155/2005/318294.
83. Filen F, et al. Duplex real-time polymerase chain reaction assay for detection and quantification of herpes simplex virus type 1 and herpes simplex virus type 2 in genital and cutaneous lesions. Sex Transm Dis. 2004;31:331–6.
84. Ramaswamy M, McDonald C, et al. Diagnosis of genital herpes by real time PCR in routine clinical practice. Sex Transm Infect. 2004;80:406–10.
85. Bhattarakosol P, et al. Intratypic variation of herpes simplex virus type 2 isolates detected by monoclonal antibodies against viral glycoproteins. Arch Virol. 1990;115:89.
86. Sauerbrei A. Herpes Genitalis: diagnosis, treatment and prevention. Geburtshilfe und Frauenheilkunde. 2016;76(12):1310–7. https://doi.org/10.1055/s0042-116494.
87. Lafferty WE, Krofft S, et al. Diagnosis of herpes simplex virus by direct immunofluorescence and viral isolation from samples of external genital lesions in a high prevalence population. J Clin Microbiol. 1987;25:323–6.
88. Vitko NP, Richardson AR. Laboratory maintenance of methicillin-resistant Staphylococcus aureus (MRSA). Curr Protoc Microbiol. 2013;Chapter 9:Unit 9C.2.
89. Lewis JS, Jorgensen JH. Inducible clindamycin resistance in staphylococci: should clinicians and microbiologists be concerned? Clin Infect Dis. 2005;40(2):280–5.
90. Smits WK, Lyras D, Lacy DB, Wilcox MH, Kuijper EJ. Clostridium difficile infection. Nat Rev Dis Primers. 2016;2(1):16020.
91. McDonald LC, Gerding DN, Johnson S, et al. Clinical Practice Guidelines for Clostridium difficile Infection in Adults and Children: 2017 Update by the Infectious Diseases Society of America (IDSA) and Society for Healthcare Epidemiology of America (SHEA). Clin Infect Dis. 2018;66(7):e1–e48.
92. Smith K. Who Are the HACEK Organisms? American Society for Microbiology. https://www.asm.org/Articles/2019/February/Who-are-the-HACEK-organisms. Published February 11, 2019. Accessed 28 May 2019.
93. Walkty A. Cardiobacterium hominis endocarditis: a case report and review of the literature. Can J Infect Dis Med Microbiol. 2005;16(5):293–7.
94. Chambers ST, Murdoch D, Morris A, et al. HACEK infective endocarditis: characteristics and outcomes from a large, multi-national cohort. PLoS ONE. 2013;8(5):e63181.

95. Centers for Disease Control and Prevention. Updated guidelines for the use of nucleic acid amplification testing in the diagnosis of tuberculosis. https://www.cdc.gov/mmwr/preview/mmwrhtml/mm5801a3.htm?s_cid=mm5801a3_e. Accessed 24 May 2019.
96. Lewinsohn DM, Leonard MK, LoBue PA, et al. Official American Thoracic Society/Infectious Diseases Society of America/Centers for Disease Control and Prevention Clinical Practice Guidelines: Diagnosis of Tuberculosis in Adults and Children. CLINID. 2017;64(2):e1–e33.
97. Biggs HM, Behravesh CB, Bradley KK, et al. Diagnosis and Management of Tickborne Rickettsial Diseases: Rocky Mountain Spotted Fever and Other Spotted Fever Group Rickettsioses, Ehrlichioses, and Anaplasmosis — United States. MMWR Recomm Rep. 2016;65(2):1–44.
98. Walker DH. Rickettsiae. In: Baron S, editor. Medical microbiology. 4th ed. Galveston, TX: University of Texas Medical Branch at Galveston; 1996. Chapter 38. Available from: https://www.ncbi.nlm.nih.gov/books/NBK7624/.
99. Branda J, Aguero-Rosenfeld M, Ferraro M, Johnson B, Wormser G, Steere A. 2-tiered antibody testing for early and late lyme disease using only an immunoglobulin G blot with the addition of a VlsE band as the second-tier test. Clin Infect Dis. 2010;50(1):20–6.
100. Centers for Disease Control and Prevention. Two-step laboratory testing process. https://www.cdc.gov/lyme/diagnosistesting/labtest/twostep/index.html. Accessed 24 May 2019.
101. Viau R, Frank KM, Jacobs MR, Wilson B, Kaye K, Donskey CJ, et al. Intestinal carriage of carbapenemase-producing organisms: current status of surveillance methods. Clin Microbiol Rev. 2015;29(1):1–27.
102. Chang K, Chung C, Yeh C, Hsu K, Chin Y, Huang S, et al. Direct detection of carbapenemase-associated proteins of Acinetobacter baumannii using nanodiamonds coupled with matrix-assisted laser desorption/ionization time-of-flight mass spectrometry. J Microbiol Methods. 2018;147:36–42.
103. Saubolie M, Sussland D. Nocardiosis. J Clin Microbiol. 2003;41(10):4497–501.
104. Riordan T. Human infection with Fusobacterium necrophorum (Necrobacillosis), with a Focus on Lemierre's syndrome. Clin Microbiol Rev. 2007;20(4):622–59.
105. Bank S, Nielsen HM, Mathiasen BH, Leth DC, Kristensen LH, Prag J. Fusobacterium necrophorum- detection and identification on a selective agar. APMIS. 2010;118(12):994–9.
106. Gherna M, Merz WG. Identification of Candida albicans and Candida glabrata within 1.5 hours directly from positive blood culture bottles with a shortened peptide nucleic acid fluorescence in situ hybridization protocol. J Clin Microbiol. 2008;47(1):247–8.
107. Clancy CJ, Nguyen MH. Diagnosing invasive candidiasis. J Clin Microbiol. 2018;56(5).
108. Spanu T, Posteraro B, Fiori B, Dinzeo T, Campoli S, Ruggeri A, et al. Direct MALDI-TOF mass spectrometry assay of blood culture broths for rapid identification of Candida species causing bloodstream infections: an observational study in two large microbiology laboratories. J Clin Microbiol. 2011;50(1):176–9.
109. McMullan R, Metwally L, Coyle PV, Hedderwick S, Mccloskey B, Oneill H, et al. A prospective clinical trial of a real-time polymerase chain reaction assay for the diagnosis of candidemia in nonneutropenic, critically Ill adults. Clin Infect Dis. 2008;46(6):890–6.
110. Centers for Disease Control and Prevention. Information for Healthcare Professionals about Histoplasmosis. https://www.cdc.gov/fungal/diseases/histoplasmosis/health-professionals.html. Accessed 24 May 2019.
111. Azar MM, Hage CA. Laboratory diagnostics for histoplasmosis. J Clin Microbiol. 2017;55(6):1612–20. https://doi.org/10.1128/JCM.02430-16.
112. Centers for Disease Control and Prevention. Information for Healthcare Professionals about Valley Fever (Coccidioidomycosis). https://www.cdc.gov/fungal/diseases/coccidioidomycosis/health-professionals.html#ten. Accessed 24 May 2019.
113. Saubolle MA. Epidemiologic, clinical, and diagnostic aspects of coccidioidomycosis. J Clin Microbiol. 2007;45(1):26–30.
114. Posteraro B, Efremov L, Leoncini E, Amore R, Posteraro P, Ricciardi W, Sanguinetti M. Are the conventional commercial yeast identification methods still helpful in the era of new

clinical microbiology diagnostics? A meta-analysis of their accuracy. J Clin Microbiol. 2015;53(8):2439–50.

115. Firacative C, Trilles L, Meyer W. MALDI-TOF MS enables the rapid identification of the major molecular types within the Cryptococcus neoformans/C. gattii species complex. PLoS ONE. 2012;7(5):e37566.

116. Martynowicz MA, Prakash UB. Pulmonary blastomycosis: an appraisal of diagnostic techniques. Chest. 2002;121(3):768.

117. Frost HM, Novicki TJ. Blastomyces antigen detection for diagnosis and management of blastomycosis. J Clin Microbiol. 2015;53(11):3600–36002.

118. Centers for Disease Control and Prevention. Information for Healthcare Professionals about Mucormycosis. https://www.cdc.gov/fungal/diseases/mucormycosis/health-professionals. html. Accessed 24 May 2019.

119. Riley TT, Muzny CA, Swiatlo E, Legendre DP. Breaking the Mold. Ann Pharmacother. 2016;50(9):747–57.

120. Miceli MH, Kauffman CA. Aspergillus galactomannan for diagnosing invasive aspergillosis. JAMA. 2017;318(12):1175.

121. Ostrosky-Zeichner L, Alexander BD, Kett DH, Vazquez J, Pappas PG, Saeki F, et al. Multicenter clinical evaluation of the (1-3)-D-glucan assay as an aid to diagnosis of fungal infections in humans. Clin Infect Dis. 2005;41(5):654–9.

122. Centers for Disease Control and Prevention. Malaria – diagnostic tools. Atlanta, GA: CDC; 2017.

123. McHardy IH, et al. Detection of intestinal protozoa in the clinical laboratory. J Clin Microbiol. 2013;52(3):712–20. American Society For Microbiology. https://doi.org/10.1128/ jcm.02877-13.

124. Fletcher SM, Stark D, Harkness J, Ellis J. Enteric protozoa in the developed world: a public health perspective. Clin Microbiol Rev. 2012;25:420–49. https://doi.org/10.1128/ CMR.05038-11.

125. Moody A. Rapid diagnostic tests for malaria parasites. Clin Microbiol Rev. 2002;15:66–78.

126. Bonnet S, Jouglin M, Malandrin L, Becker C, Agoulon A, L'Hostis M, Chauvin A. Transstadial and transovarial persistence of Babesia divergens DNA in Ixodes ricinus ticks fed on infected blood in a new skin-feeding technique. Parasitology. 2007;134:197–207.

127. Snounou G, Viriyakosol S, Zhu XP, Jarra W, Pinheiro L, do Rosario VE, et al. High sensitivity detection of human malaria parasites by the use of nested polymerase chain reaction. Mol Biochem Parastiol. 1993;61:315–20.

128. Rougemont M, Van Saanen M, Sahli R, Hinrikson HP, Bille J, Jaton K. Detection of Four Plasmodium Species in Blood from Humans by 18S rRNA Gene Subunit-Based and Species-Specific Real-Time PCR Assays. J Clin Microbiol. 2004;42(12):5636.

129. Hojgaard A, Lukacik G, Piesman J. Detection of Borrelia burgdorferi, Anaplasma phagocytophilum and Babesia microti, with two different multiplex PCR assays. Ticks Tick Borne Dis. 2014;5:349–51.

130. CDC - Dpdx - Serum/Plasma Specimens. Cdc.Gov; 2019. https://www.cdc.gov/dpdx/diagnosticprocedures/serum/antibodydetection.html.

131. Wilson M, Schantz P, Nutman T, Tsang VCW. Clinical immunoparasitology. In: Rose NR, Hamilton RG, Detrick B, editors. Manual of clinical laboratory immunology. 6th ed. Washington: American Society for Microbiology; 2002.

132. Centers for Disease Control and Prevention. DPDx—laboratory identification of parasitic diseases of public health concern. Atlanta, GA: CDC; 2017.

133. Garcia LS. Diagnostic medical parasitology. 5th ed. Santa Monica, CA: ASM Press; 2007.

Chapter 5
Influenza, Measles, SARS, MERS, and Smallpox

Daniel S. Chertow and Jason Kindrachuk

The Viruses

Influenza Biology

Influenza viruses are spherical or filamentous, enveloped, negative-sense, single-stranded RNA viruses of family *Orthomyxoviridae* of approximately 100 nm to 300 nm in diameter that include types A, B, C, and D [1, 2]. Influenza A and B viruses cause mild to severe illness during seasonal epidemics, and influenza A viruses cause intermittent pandemics. Influenza C viruses cause mild infections but not epidemics, and influenza D virus may cause subclinical infection [3, 4]. Influenza A viruses are classified into subtypes based on the combination of the surface glycoproteins hemagglutinin and neuraminidase, with 18 H and 11 N known subtypes [5–7]. Specific influenza strains are named according to the World Health Organization (WHO) convention designating influenza virus type, host of origin (if not human), geographic origin, strain number, year of isolation, and subtype (for influenza A viruses) (e.g., Influenza A/California/7/2009[H1N1]) [8].

Influenza A viruses have eight genome segments that code for structural and nonstructural proteins (Fig. 5.1a) [9]. Surface glycoproteins include hemagglutinin (HA), required for viral binding and entry, and neuraminidase (NA), required

D. S. Chertow (✉)
Critical Care Medicine Department, National Institutes of Health Clinical Center and Laboratory of Immunoregulation, National Institute of Allergy and Infectious Diseases, Bethesda, MD, USA
e-mail: chertowd@cc.nih.gov

J. Kindrachuk
Laboratory of Emerging and Re-Emerging Viruses, Department of Medical Microbiology, University of Manitoba, Winnipeg, MB, Canada
e-mail: Jason.Kindrachuk@umanitoba.ca

© Springer Nature Switzerland AG 2020
J. Hidalgo, L. Woc-Colburn (eds.), *Highly Infectious Diseases in Critical Care*,
https://doi.org/10.1007/978-3-030-33803-9_5

a

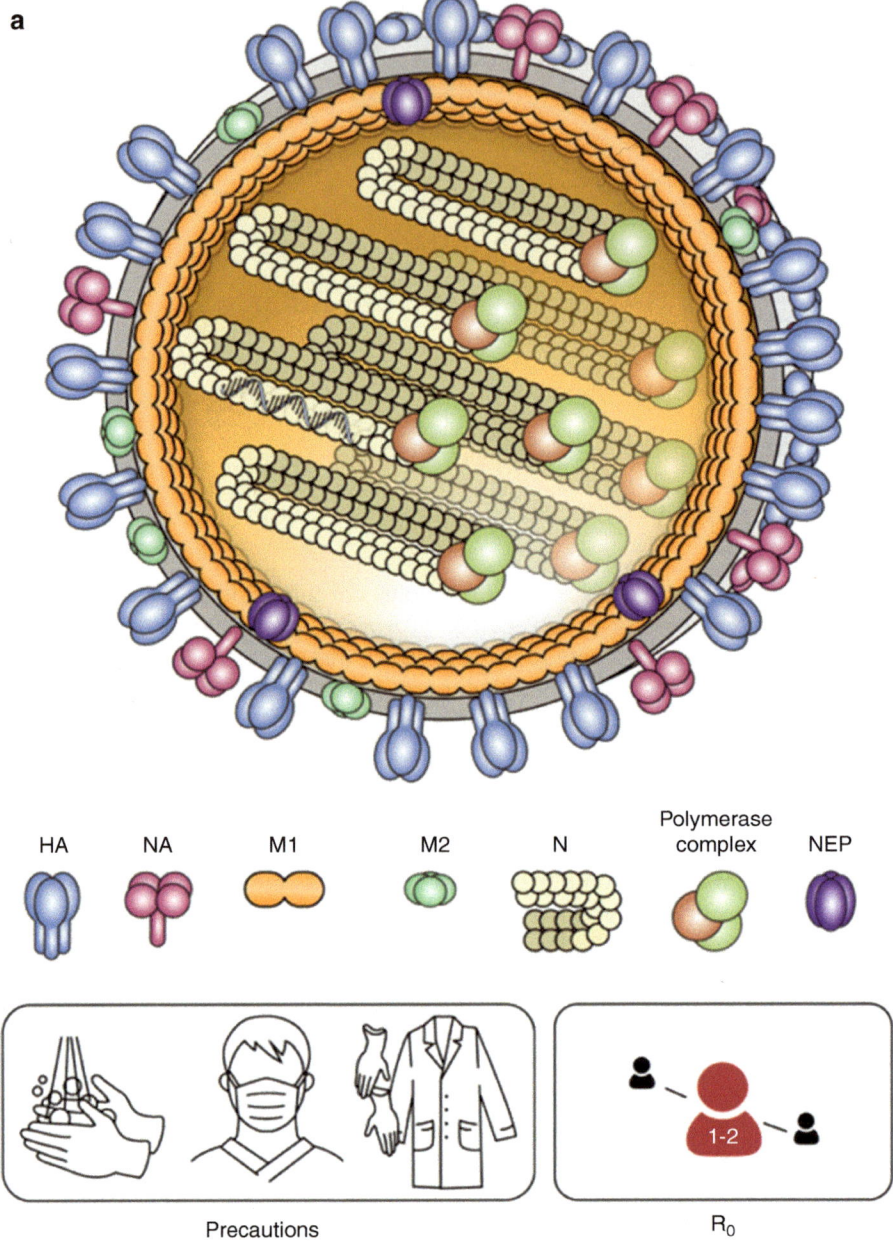

HA	NA	M1	M2	N	Polymerase complex	NEP

Precautions

R_0

Fig. 5.1 Schematic of viral structures and key epidemiological features. (**a**) *Influenza* virus is spherical or filamentous in shape. Hemagglutinin (HA) and neuraminidase (NA) proteins are integrated into the host-derived lipid envelope and project from the viral surface. Matrix (M1) protein underlies the envelope, and M2 forms an ion channel within the envelope. Eight single-stranded RNA genome segments are coated with nucleoprotein (NP) and bound by the polymerase complex. Nuclear export protein (NEP) mediates export of viral RNA. Influenza has estimated reproductive number (R_0) between 1 and 2. Standard, droplet, and contract precautions are recommended to prevent nosocomial transmission. (**b**) *Measles* virus is pleomorphic in shape. Hemagglutinin (H) and fusion (F) proteins are integrated into the host-derived lipid envelope, and matrix (M) protein underlies the envelope. The single-stranded RNA genome is coated with nucleoprotein (N) and bound by the polymerase complex. Measles has an estimate R_0 between 9 and 18. Standard, airborne, and contact precautions are recommended to prevent nosocomial transmission. (**c**) *Coronaviruses* are spherical in shape. Spike (S), membrane (M), and envelope (E) proteins are integrated into the host-derived lipid envelope. The single-stranded RNA genome is coated with nucleoprotein (N). SARS and MERS have an estimated R_0 of <1–2. Standard, airborne, and contact precautions are recommended to prevent nosocomial transmission. (**d**) *Poxviruses* are oval to brick shaped. The biconcave viral core contains double-stranded DNA and several proteins organized as a nucleosome and surrounded by a core membrane. Two proteinaceous lateral bodies flank the core, and a single lipid membrane surrounds the cell-associated form of the mature virion (MV). A second host-derived lipid envelope covers the extracellular virion (EV). Smallpox has an estimated R_0 between 4 and 6. Standard, airborne, and contact precautions are recommended to prevent nosocomial transmission of smallpox

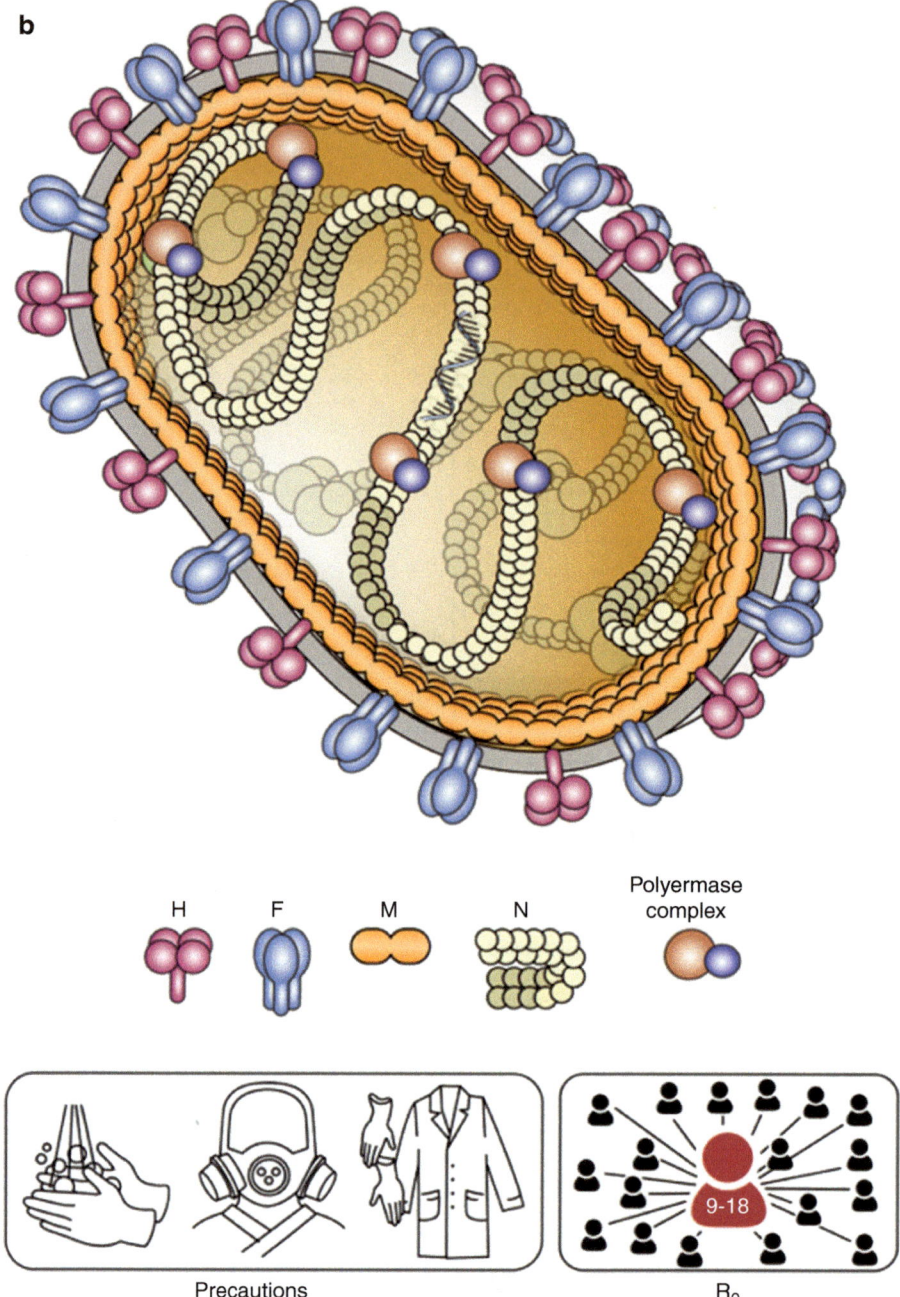

b

H   F   M   N   Polyermase
                                            complex

Precautions   R₀

Fig. 5.1 (continued)

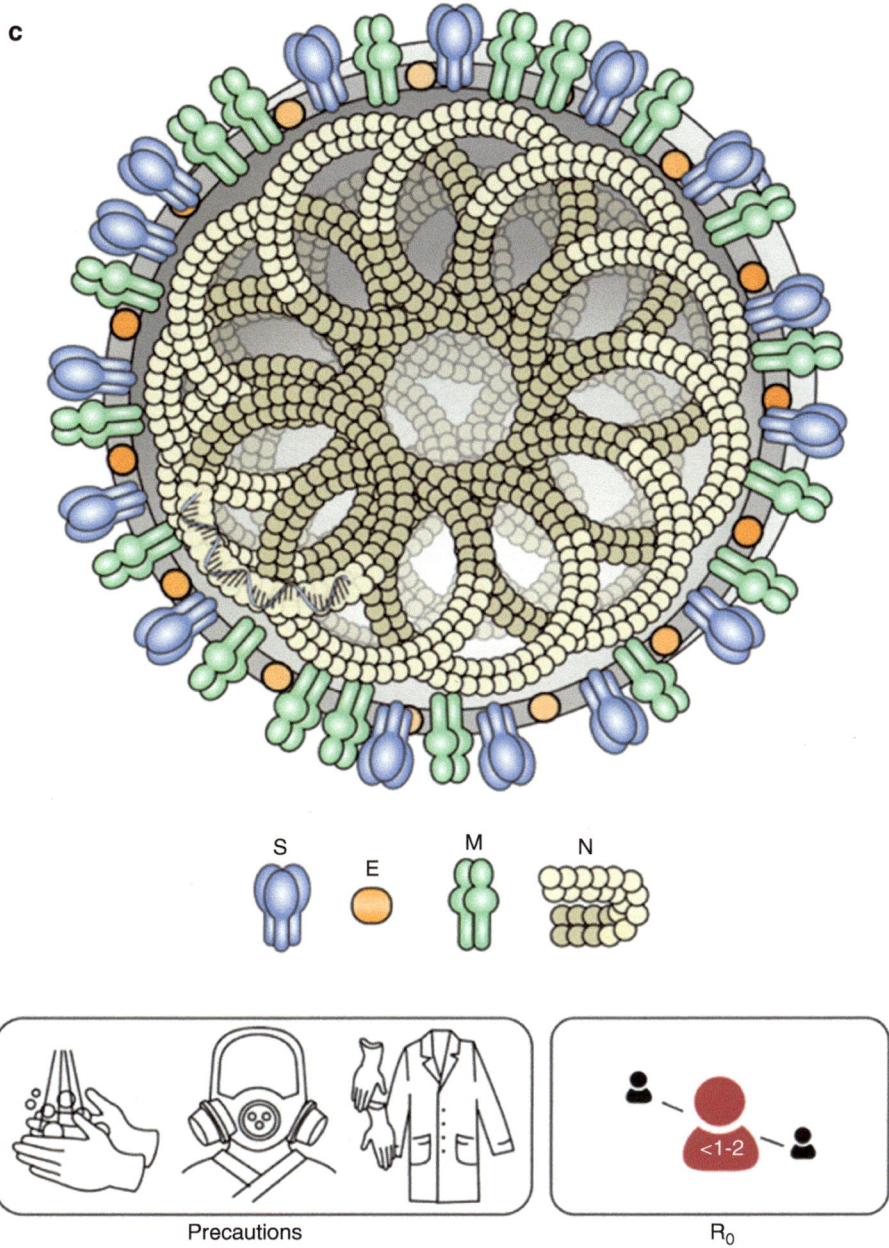

Fig. 5.1 (continued)

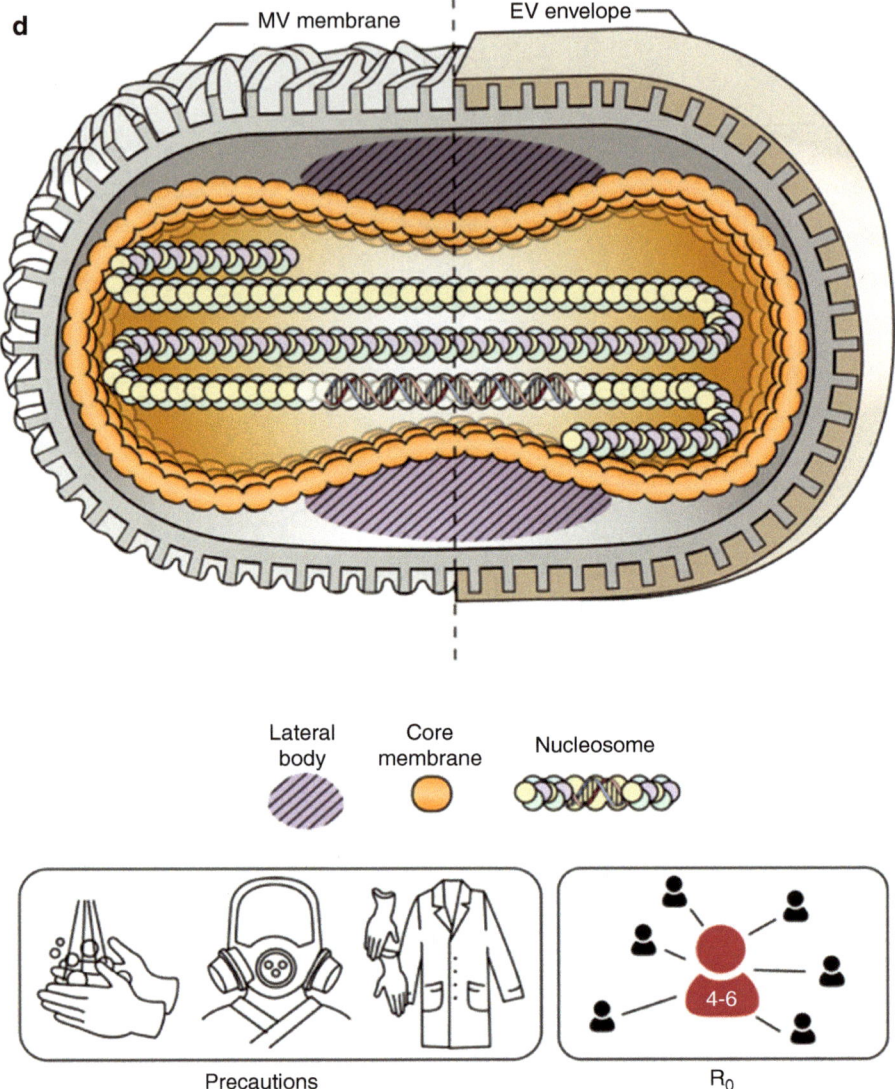

Fig. 5.1 (continued)

for viral budding. Matrix (M1) protein underlies the host-derived lipid envelope providing structure, and M2 protein is an ion channel integrated into the envelope. Eight single-stranded RNA viral genome segments are coated with nucleoprotein (N) and bound by the polymerase complex, composed of basic polymerase 1 (PB1), PB2, and acidic polymerase (PA). Nuclear export protein (NEP) mediates trafficking of viral RNA segments and nonstructural protein (NS1) inhibits host antiviral responses. The virus can also express accessory proteins PB1-F2 and PA-x.

Measles (Rubeola Virus) Biology

Measles virus is a pleomorphic, enveloped, negative-sense, single-stranded RNA virus of family *Paramyxoviridae* of approximately 100 nm to 300 nm in diameter [2]. Measles virus causes mild to severe illness during seasonal outbreaks in endemic areas and intermittent outbreaks in nonendemic area [10]. Measles virus codes for six structural and two nonstructural proteins (Fig. 5.1b) [11]. Hemagglutinin (H) and fusion (F) glycoproteins project from the viral surface and facilitate viral binding to cellular receptors and fusion with the host cell membrane, respectively. Matrix (M) protein underlies the envelope providing structure. The inner nucleocapsid is composed of RNA coated by nucleoprotein (N), bound by the polymerase complex which includes the large (L) polymerase protein, and phosphoprotein (P), a polymerase cofactor. The remaining nonstructural proteins include C and V.

Coronavirus Biology

Coronaviruses are spherical, enveloped, positive-sense, single-stranded RNA viruses of family *Coronaviridae* of approximately 120 nm in diameter [12]. Coronaviruses are the causative agents of an estimated 30% of upper and lower respiratory tract infections in humans resulting in rhinitis, pharyngitis, sinusitis, bronchiolitis, and pneumonia [13]. While coronaviruses are often associated with mild disease (e.g., HCoV-229E, HCoV-OC43, HCoV-NL63, HCoV-HKU1), severe acute respiratory syndrome coronavirus (SARS-CoV), a lineage B betacoronavirus, and Middle East respiratory syndrome coronavirus (MERS-CoV), a lineage C betacoronavirus, are associated with severe and potentially fatal respiratory infection [14, 15].

SARS- and MERS-CoV transcribe 12 and 9 subgenomic RNAs, respectively, which encode for the spike (S), envelope (E), membrane (M), and nucleocapsid (N) structural proteins (Fig. 5.1c) [14]. S, E, and M are all integrated into the host-derived lipid envelope, and S facilitates host cell attachment to angiotensin-converting enzyme (ACE)-2 receptors for SARS-CoV and dipeptidyl peptidase (DPP)-4 receptors for MERS-CoV [16, 17]. The N protein encapsidates the viral genome to form the helical nucleocapsid. The viral replicase-transcriptase complex is made up of 16 nonstructural proteins (nsp1–16) including a unique proofreading exoribonuclease that reduces the accumulation of genome mutations [12].

Smallpox (Variola Virus) Biology

Poxviruses are oval-to-brick-shaped double-stranded DNA viruses of family *Poxviridae* that range in size from 200 to 400 nm [2]. Viruses within genus *Orthopoxvirus* that cause human disease include cowpox virus (CPXV), monkeypox virus (MPXV), vaccinia virus (VACV), and variola virus (VARV), the etiologic agent of smallpox [18].

Poxviruses contain a biconcave viral core where the DNA genome, DNA-dependent RNA polymerase, and enzymes necessary for particle uncoating reside (Fig. 5.1d) [19]. This nucleosome is surrounded by a core membrane that is flanked by two proteinaceous lateral bodies. A single lipid membrane surrounds the cell-associated form of the mature virion (MV·). A second host-derived lipid envelope covers the extracellular virion (EV) [2, 19]. Poxvirus genomes are comprised of a large, linear double-stranded viral DNA genome that encodes ~200 genes. Highly conserved structural genes are predominantly found in the middle of the genome, whereas variable virulence factor genes that function in immune evasion, virulence, and viral pathogenesis are found at the termini of the genome [20].

Ecology and Epidemiology

Avian, Swine, Seasonal, and Pandemic Influenza A Viruses

Wild aquatic birds are natural reservoirs for nearly all influenza A virus subtypes, which spread to domestic avian species and mammals, including humans [5]. H17N10 and H18N11 subtypes are exceptions in that they have only been isolated from bats [6, 7]. Certain H5 and H7 subtypes are highly pathogenic to domestic poultry when transmitted from wild birds, known as highly pathogenic avian influenza (HPAI) viruses [21]. HPAI viruses cause spillover infections in humans that may be severe or fatal. Examples include outbreaks of H5N1 and H7N9 HPAI viruses in Asia with high case fatality among humans, although limited human-to-human transmission [22, 23] has been reported. HPAI virus adaptations might lead to sustained human-to-human transmission, and so poultry outbreaks are managed by flock depopulation [24]. Influenza A subtypes isolated in swine include H1 to H5, H9, and N1 and N2. Subtypes that spillover into humans cause mild to severe illness and are known as swine "variant" viruses [25].

Currently circulating seasonal influenza A subtypes H1N1 and H3N2 and influenza B viruses, Yamagata or Victoria lineage, cause annual epidemics during fall through spring in temperate regions and infections throughout the year in the tropics [26]. Antigenic drift of H and N surface glycoproteins drives annual epidemics. From 2017 to 2018, seasonal influenza caused approximately 49 million illnesses, 1 million hospitalizations, and 79,000 deaths in the United States alone [27]. When two or more influenza A viruses infect a common host, such as a bird or pig, individual gene segments may recombine to form a novel virus, known as antigenic shift. Influenza pandemics occur when novel viruses emerge into an immunologically naïve population and become adapted for sustained human-to-human spread. The 1918 "Spanish" influenza pandemic was the most severe on record, resulting in an estimated 50 million deaths [28]. Less severe pandemics occurred in 1957, 1968, and 2009. In an effort to improve preparedness and response to seasonal, pandemic, and zoonotic influenza, the World Health Organization (WHO) conducts global surveillance of influenza A and B isolates (Fig. 5.2a) [29].

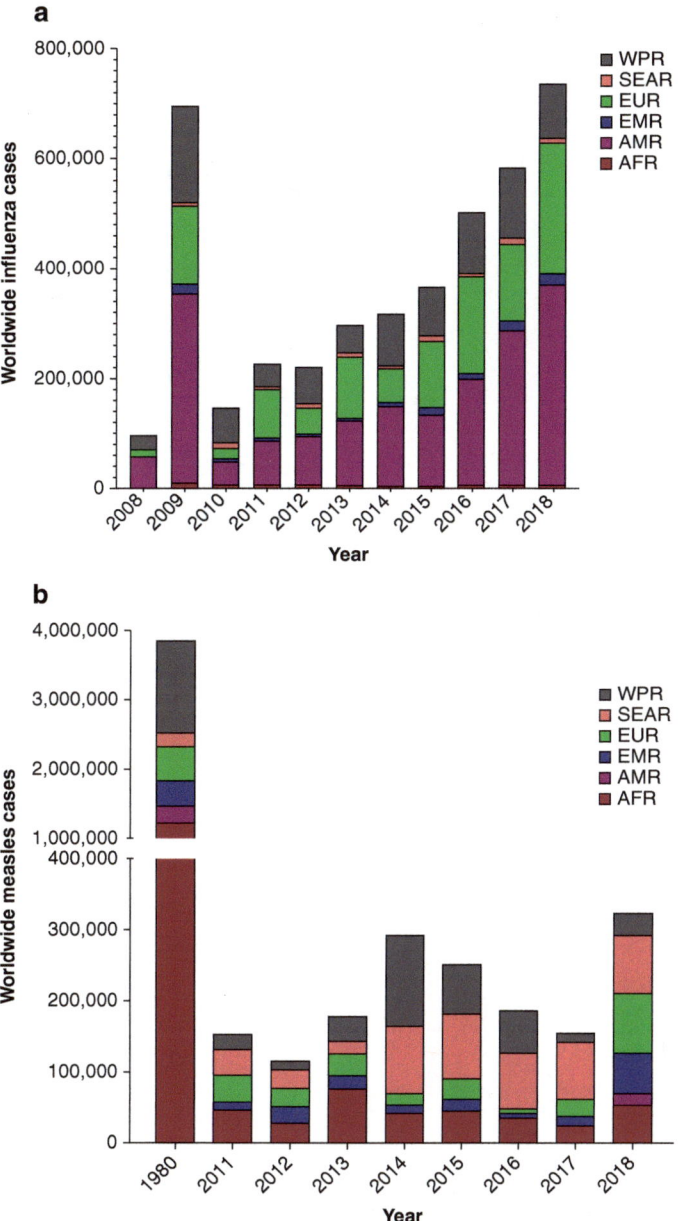

Fig. 5.2 Viral disease burden reported by WHO region. (**a**) WHO global influenza surveillance of laboratory confirmed influenza A and B infections, 2008–2018. (**b**) Global measles cases reported to WHO, 2011–2018. Reported cases from 1980 are used as a reference. (**c**) Global cases of SARS- and MERS-CoV infections. (**d**) Global cases of smallpox from 1920 to 1970. Data represents the cumulative cases for that year. WHO regions are as follows: WPR Western Pacific Region, SEAR South-East Asia Region, EUR European Region, EMR Eastern Mediterranean Region, AMR Region of the Americas, AFR African Region. (Data courtesy of WHO)

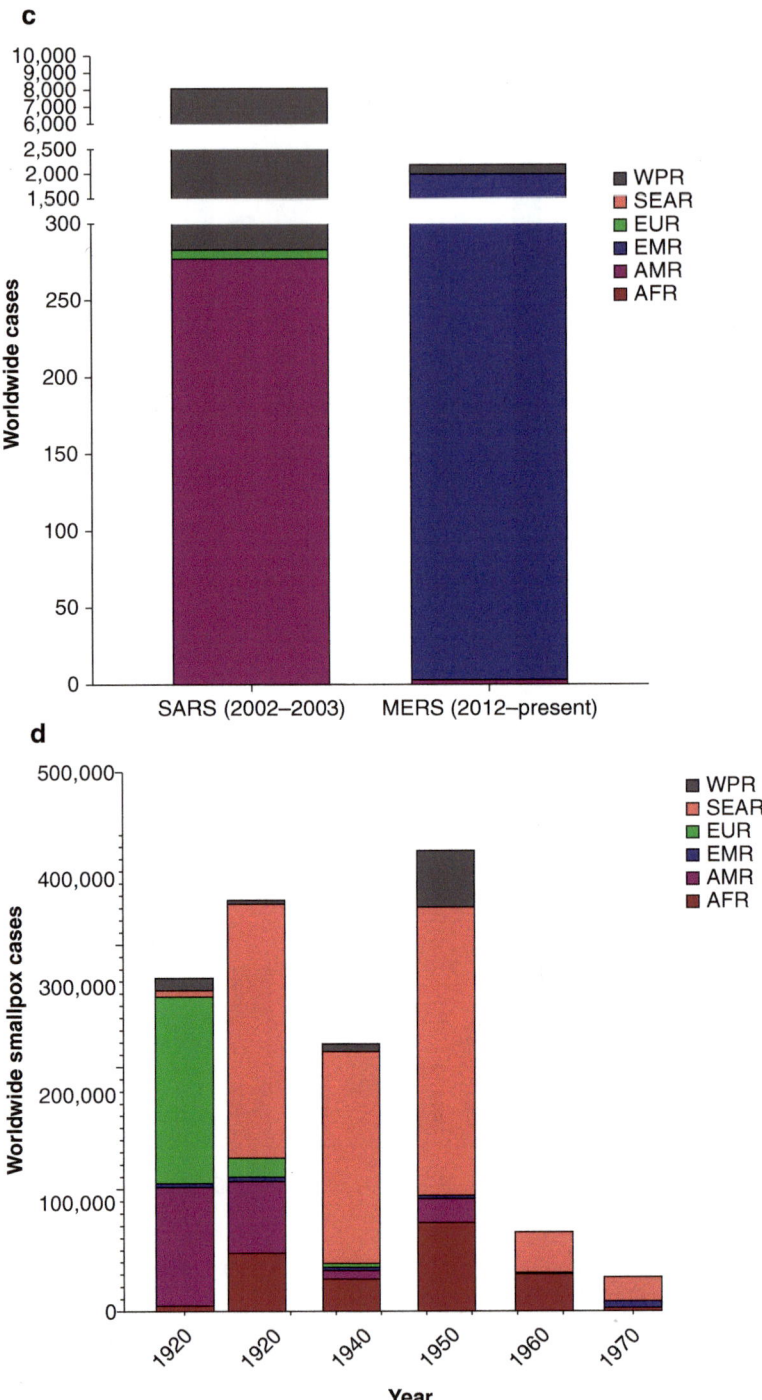

Fig. 5.2 (continued)

Endemic and Epidemic Measles

Measles is pathogenic for humans and nonhuman primates, although sustained transmission occurs only among humans raising potential for global elimination [30]. Historically, measles infected an estimated 90% of children by age 5 years, resulting in approximately 2 million global deaths each year [10]. With the introduction of the measles vaccine in 1963 and advances in global vaccination programs, measles cases and mortality have drastically declined (Fig. 5.2b). By 2017, 85% of children worldwide had received at least one dose of the measles vaccine by age 1 year, and during 2000–2017, global measles mortality decreased by 80%, preventing an estimated 21 million deaths [31]. Of the 24 known measles genotypes, only five were detected in circulation during 2016–2017. Despite these gains, measles remains endemic in many regions of the world including Africa, Western Pacific, South East Asia, and Europe, and measles has resurged in previously low-incidence areas (e.g., regions within Europe and the Americas) with epidemics attributable to importation of cases and suboptimal immunization coverage [32–34]. An estimated 93% population immunity is required to prevent measles transmission within communities, a prerequisite for global elimination [35].

SARS and MERS Epidemics

Chinese horseshoe bats are the putative reservoir for SARS-CoV, and dromedary camels are thought to be the reservoir for MERS-CoV [36–43]. Animal-to-human transmission likely occurs following direct contact with intermediate hosts [38, 44]. During the 2003–2004 SARS epidemic, 8096 cases and 774 deaths were reported from 26 countries with no cases reported since (Fig. 5.2c) [45]. Human-to-human transmission of SARS-CoV occurred primarily in healthcare settings with healthcare workers comprising 22% and >40% of reported cases in China and Canada, respectively [45]. MERS was first reported in Saudi Arabia in 2012 with >2000 cases and >800 deaths reported from 27 countries through 2018 [46]. While most cases have been reported from the Arabian Peninsula, an imported case to South Korea in 2015 resulted in a large outbreak in multiple healthcare facilities [47]. MERS transmission occurs primarily in healthcare facilities and to a lesser degree within households [48, 49].

Smallpox Eradication

While the only known reservoir for VARV is humans, it has been postulated that the virus emerged from an ancestral rodent-borne poxvirus more than 10,000 years ago [18, 50]. Numerous smallpox epidemics have occurred throughout recorded history including more than 300 million fatalities during the twentieth century alone [51–53]. Smallpox was eventually eradicated following the implementation of the Smallpox Eradication Program by the WHO from 1966 to 1980 (Fig. 5.2d) which was facilitated by the absence of a zoonotic reservoir for VARV [51].

Pathogenesis

Influenza Transmission and Mechanisms of Disease

Influenza viruses are transmitted by large respiratory droplets by coughing, sneezing, or talking or through contact with infected surfaces [54]. Influenza viruses bind to sugar moieties on the surface of airway epithelial cells where early viral replication, propagation, and shedding occur during an average 1–2 days of incubation period [55–57]. Peak viral replication typically occurs within 4 days of symptom onset and resolves within 7–10 days, lasting longer in children and immunocompromised hosts [58–60]. On average one person infects —one to two additional people; however, this reproductive number (R_0) varies by viral strain and social and environmental factors [61]. Viral infection impairs the airway mucosal barrier and disrupts the alveolar-capillary membrane contributing to leakage of fluid and inflammatory cells into the alveolar space which impairs gas exchange resulting in hypoxemia [62, 63]. Bacterial coinfection often complicates severe cases contributing to respiratory failure and death, with *Staphylococcus aureus* and *Streptococcus species* as predominant copathogens [64]. Seasonal influenza virus infection is largely limited to the respiratory tract; however, H5 and H7 HPAI viruses have a polybasic cleave site within the hemagglutinin allowing for replication outside of the respiratory tract [65, 66]. Infection with one strain of influenza does not confer complete immunity to other strains or subtypes [67].

Measles Transmission and Mechanisms of Disease

Measles is among the most highly contagious respiratory infections, spread by exposure to large respiratory droplets through coughing, sneezing, or talking; by indirect contact with infected surfaces; or by small infectious droplets that can remain suspended in air for up to 2 hours [10, 68]. Respiratory tract dendritic cells, lymphocytes, and alveolar macrophages are early targets of infection where during an average 8- to 12-day incubation period measles replicates and spreads to local lymphatics and respiratory epithelium and then disseminates in blood via infected lymphocytes to epithelial and endothelial cells in most organs [69–71]. The infectious period begins with fever onset and extends for several days after rash appears

[72]. The estimated R_0 of measles is 9–18 dependent upon host susceptibility and social and environmental factors [73]. Measles infects and disrupts tissues throughout the body; however, severe disease is primarily due to lower respiratory tract and neurological complications [72]. Natural measles infection confers lifelong immunity, and passive transfer of maternal antibodies protects newborns during the early postnatal period [74]. Individuals who recover from measles infection are at increased risk of secondary infection [75, 76].

SARS- and MERS-CoV Transmission and Mechanisms of Disease

SARS-CoV is transmitted by large respiratory droplets and by contact with infected surfaces. Epidemiologic data also support small droplet airborne transmission of SARS-CoV although the estimated R_0 of 0.86–1.83 argues against this being a predominate route of spread [77, 78]. SARS-CoV binds to angiotensin-converting enzyme (ACE)-2 receptors on respiratory epithelial cells, pneumocytes, and alveolar macrophages resulting in diffuse alveolar damage and respiratory failure [79, 80]. SARS is a systemic infection with viremia detected in most cases affecting multiple cell types and organs [81, 82]. Acute kidney injury is multifactorial with evidence of acute tubule necrosis, vasculitis, and glomerular fibrosis, and central nervous system manifestations are at least in part attributable to direct infection of neurons resulting in edema and degeneration [83].

MERS-CoV is transmitted by large respiratory droplets and by contact with infected surfaces with an estimated R0 of <1 to >1 outside of versus within healthcare settings, respectively [84]. MERS-CoV binds dipeptidyl peptidase 4 (DPP4) on respiratory epithelial cells and pneumocytes where it undergoes productive replication during a 2–14 days incubation period [16]. Viral shedding from the lower respiratory tract may persist for weeks [85, 86]. Viremia, while not documented in all cases, is associated with severe disease and productive infection of DCs, and macrophages is thought to facilitate immune dysregulation [87, 88]. DPP4 is broadly expressed on cells outside of the lung; however, few autopsy data are available to define viral distribution [16, 89].

Variola Virus Transmission and Mechanisms of Disease

VARV is transmitted primarily by large respiratory droplets and to a lesser degree through contact with contaminated objects such as scabs, bedding, or clothing or by airborne small respiratory droplets [90, 91]. VARV is thought to replicate in airway epithelium and spread to regional lymph nodes [92, 93]. VARV replicates within lymph nodes and disseminates via the bloodstream seeding distant sights including skin, spleen, bone marrow, liver, kidney, and other organs [94]. Fever manifests following an average 12 days incubation, and rash follows fever by 3–4 days, concurrent with high-level viral shedding from oropharyngeal secretions [95, 96]. The estimated R_0 of smallpox is between 3.5 and 6 [97]. High-level viremia is detected more often with hemorrhagic compared with ordinary type smallpox, although exact mechanisms of organ failure observed in fatal case are not well defined [98–101].

Clinical Findings

Influenza Illness and Complications

Influenza infection manifests as acute onset of fever, chills, malaise, headache, and myalgias following an average 1–2 days asymptomatic incubation period [9]. Most infections are self-limited resolving within 1–2 weeks. Upper or lower airway complications include otitis media, sinusitis, bronchitis, and pneumonia with or without bacterial coinfection [63, 64, 102]. Risk factors for severe infection include age >65 years or <5 years; pregnancy; preexisting respiratory, cardiac, neurologic, or metabolic conditions; immunosuppression; and obesity. Progressive lethargy and shortness of breath, typically within 5 days of symptom onset, suggest development of lower respiratory tract complications which may rapidly progress to respiratory failure and death in severe cases [64]. Pneumonia due to influenza infection alone versus influenza and bacterial coinfection cannot be reliably distinguished by clinical or radiological grounds, and so a high index of suspicion is needed. Influenza complications outside of the respiratory tract include exacerbation of underlying heart disease including ischemic heart disease and heart failure, myocarditis, encephalopathy, and encephalitis [103].

Measles Illness and Complications

Measles infection manifests by acute onset fever, coryza, conjunctivitis, and cough [10]. Small white papules, Koplik spots, appear on the buccal mucosa within 3 days of fever onset, followed by development of diffuse maculopapular rash 1 or 2 days later. Diarrhea commonly begins shortly following rash onset and may result in dehydration. Symptoms typically resolve within 7 days of fever onset in self-limited illness. Groups at increased risk for measles complications include malnourished infants and those with vitamin A deficiency, adults >20 years old, and immunocompromised individuals [72]. Respiratory complications include otitis media, laryngotracheobronchitis (croup), and pneumonia. Pneumonia, often complicated by bacterial coinfection, is the most common severe complication of measles contributing to respiratory failure and death [72, 104]. Predominant bacterial copathogens include *Streptococcus pneumonia*, *Staphylococcus aureus*, and *Haemophilus influenzae*.

Three rare but severe neurologic complications occur [105]. Acute disseminated encephalomyelitis (ADEM) is a demyelinating autoimmune process that occurs within weeks of acute illness in approximately 1 in 1000 cases. ADEM is characterized by fevers, seizures, and neurologic deficits. Measles inclusion body encephalitis is a progressive lethal brain infection occurring within months of acute illness primarily among individuals with impaired cellular immunity. Subacute sclerosing panencephalitis (SSPE) occurs 5–10 years following initial infection resulting in seizures and cognitive and motor decline resulting in death. SSPE affects an estimated 1 in 10,000 infants under 1 year of age and is attributed to host responses to defective viral particle production in the brain.

SARS and MERS Illness and Complications

Following an average 5-day incubation period, SARS-CoV infection presents with fevers, chills, dry cough, headache, malaise, and dyspnea commonly followed by watery diarrhea [106–108]. Age >60 years and pregnancy are associated with severe disease manifested by progressive respiratory failure within 2 weeks of illness onset [108, 109]. Common laboratory features of SARS included lymphopenia, thrombocytopenia, abnormal coagulation parameters, and elevated lactate dehydrogenase, alanine aminotransferase, and creatine kinase levels [110–112]. Acute kidney injury and proteinuria were observed in 7% and 84% of patients, respectively [113].

Initial symptoms of MERS-CoV infection include fever, chills, cough, shortness of breath, myalgia, and malaise following a mean incubation period of 5 days [114]. Gastrointestinal symptoms, including vomiting and diarrhea, occur in one-third of patients [115–118]. The median times from symptom onset to hospitalization, ICU admission, and death are 4, 5, and 12 days, respectively [118]. MERS patients present with a rapidly progressing pneumonia requiring mechanical ventilation and additional organ support with the first week of illness [109]. Severe disease has been linked to comorbidities including diabetes mellitus (68%), chronic renal disease (49%), hypertension (34%), chronic cardiac disease (28%), chronic pulmonary disease (26%), and obesity (17%) [114]. The median age of those with confirmed MERS is 50 years with a male-to-female ratio of 3.3:1 [114]. Laboratory abnormalities include lymphopenia, leukopenia, thrombocytopenia, elevated serum creatinine levels consistent with acute kidney injury, and elevated liver enzymes [114, 115, 117, 119, 120]. High lactate levels and consumptive coagulopathy have also been reported [119, 121]. Chest radiographic abnormalities are due to viral pneumonitis with or without secondary bacterial pneumonia, and acute kidney injury occurs in up to 43% of patients [114, 119, 120, 122–124].

Smallpox Illness and Complications

As the smallpox disease course was related to the clinical presentation of disease, Rao proposed a clinical classification system [125] that was later adopted by the WHO in 1972 [51]. *Ordinary type smallpox* was the most common clinical type of smallpox. The incubation period was 7–19 days and was followed by fever onset (38.5–40.5 °C), headaches, backaches, vomiting, and diarrhea [51]. Lesions first appeared on mucous membranes (including the tongue, palate, and pharynx) ~1 day prior to macular rash development, where lesions began on the face followed by proximal regions of the extremities, the trunk, and the distal extremities. Lesion development followed a centrifugal dispersion pattern, typically most dense on the face, with papules appearing within 2 days of macular rash development. Papules became vesicular ~2–4 days later followed by a pustular stage (5–7 days postrash) that peaked ~10 days postrash. Pustule resolution quickly followed and was accompanied by lesion flattening, fluid reabsorption, hardening, and scab formation (14–21 days postrash). Rao proposed for ordinary type smallpox to be further subdivided based on the macular rash pattern [125]. These included *discrete ordinary-type smallpox*, characterized by discrete skin lesions; *confluent ordinary-type smallpox*, where pustular skin lesions were confluent on the face and extremities; and *semiconfluent ordinary-type smallpox*, where skin lesions were confluent on the face but disparate over the rest of the body. Modified-type smallpox, where lesions were less numerous than in ordinary-type smallpox, was primarily associated with vaccinated individuals and had an accelerated nonfatal disease course [125]. Flat-type and hemorrhagic-type smallpox were the most lethal forms of the disease but were also very rare (~7% and 3% of patients, respectively) [51]. Flat-type smallpox had high CFRs in both unvaccinated and vaccinated patients (97% and 67%, respectively). Hemorrhagic-type smallpox was nearly 100% fatal in both vaccinated and unvaccinated individuals, and death normally came prior to macular rash development. The clinical symptoms of flat-type smallpox were more severe during the prodromal period and did not subside. Skin lesions were flat and often black or dark purple. Respiratory complications were common and patients were febrile throughout disease. Death typically occurred 8–12 days post-fever onset. Hemorrhagic-type smallpox could be divided into early and late hemorrhagic-type smallpox. *The early form* was characterized by hemorrhage (primarily subconjunctival) early in the disease course. Generalized erythema, petechiae, and ecchymosis within 2 days of fever and flat matter lesions formed across the entire body surface. Lesions turned purple by day 4 with death by day 6 as a result of cardiac and pulmonary complications. In the late form, hemorrhages occurred following rash development and death followed between 8 and 10 days post-fever onset.

Diagnosis

Influenza: Infection Control and Confirmatory Testing

In healthcare settings, patients under evaluation for influenza should be isolated, and standard, droplet, and contact precautions should be implemented [126]. Traditional antigen-based rapid diagnostic assays (RDAs) for influenza lack sensitivity and cannot be relied upon to rule out infection [26]. Newer antigen-based RDAs that employ a digital scan of the test strip, and molecular assays that employ isothermal amplification technology have improved sensitivity and specificity that more closely approximates highly sensitive and specific reverse transcriptase polymerase chain reaction (RT-PCR)-based assays [127]. Acceptable sample types for influenza testing include nasopharyngeal swab or wash and bronchoalveolar lavage specimens. Individuals suspected of zoonotic influenza infection should have case evaluation and specimen testing coordinated through local or state public health authorities.

Measles: Infection Control and Confirmatory Testing

Measles should be considered in patients without preexisting immunity and a compatible febrile rash illness. Travel to a region with ongoing measles transmission or exposure to other individuals with a febrile rash illness should raise suspicion. Patients under evaluation for measles require isolation and implementation of standard, airborne, and contact precautions. Local or state health authorities should be contacted within 24 hours to assist with confirmatory testing, case finding, and infection control. Measles is typically confirmed by measles-specific IgM serology or detection of measles RNA in a nasopharyngeal, throat, or urine specimen by RT-PCR [10]. A fourfold or greater rise in measles IgG titers between acute and convalescent samples tested 2 or more weeks apart can assist with diagnostic uncertainty. Virus can also be cultured from respiratory, blood, and urine specimens in appropriate public health laboratories.

SARS and MERS: Infection Control and Confirmatory Testing

While SARS is no longer circulating, MERS should be suspected in individuals with a compatible febrile illness and an epidemiological risk factor [128]. Risk factors include travel to the Arabian Peninsula or contact with a confirmed or suspected case within 14 days of symptom onset. Patients under evaluation for MERS require isolation and implementation of standard, airborne, and contact precautions.

Confirmatory testing and infection control should be coordinated through local or state health authorities. MERS may be confirmed in designated public health laboratories by RT-PCR testing of lower respiratory tract specimens [129]. Multiple other specimen types including upper respiratory tract samples, serum, and stool should also be collected for testing. Serologic testing can be used to evaluate for suspected infection among individuals no longer shedding virus [129, 130].

Smallpox: Infection Control and Confirmatory Testing

Smallpox has not been observed in over 40 years; however, concerns remain for use as a bioweapon. Major and minor criteria have been established to assist clinicians in recognition of smallpox [131]. Individuals under evaluation should be isolated, and standard, airborne, and contact precautions should be implemented. Local or state health authorities should be contacted to assist with confirmatory testing and public health interventions. PCR identification of variola DNA or isolation of the virus from a clinical specimen is required to confirm a diagnosis in specialized high-containment laboratories.

Clinical Management

Influenza Prevention and Treatment

Annual seasonal influenza vaccination is recommended in the United States for all individuals aged 6 months or older and has been associated with decreased risk of pneumonia and death, particularly among high-risk groups [132–134]. Seasonal influenza vaccination does not provide protection against novel strains. Consequently, efforts are underway to develop a vaccine that would protect against most or all influenza strains [135]. Three classes of drugs are licensed for the treatment of influenza in the United States [136]. Adamantanes, including amantadine and rimantadine, are not currently recommended given resistance of circulating seasonal strains. Baloxavir morboxil, a cap-dependent endonuclease inhibitor, was recently approved for the treatment of uncomplicated influenza [137]. Neuraminidase inhibitors (NAI) include oral oseltamivir, inhaled zanamivir, and intravenous peramivir. Prophylactic use of NAIs is recommended in unvaccinated individuals with risk factors for severe disease and during institutional outbreaks to limit spread. Therapeutic use is recommended for individuals with suspected or confirmed influenza that have developed or are at high risk for influenza complications [26]. Influenza complications, including respiratory and multiorgan failure, are managed with supportive care. Bacterial coinfection should be considered and empirically treated early pending results of microbiologic testing among severe cases.

Measles Prevention and Treatment

Measles can be effectively prevented through vaccination, typically given in combination with vaccines for rubella (MR), mumps (MMR), or varicella (MMR-V). WHO recommends the first dose of measles vaccine be administered at 9 or 12 months of age in high and low prevalence settings, respectively [138]. A second dose should be administered after a minimum of 4-week interval. Nonimmune individuals that have been exposed to measles should receive post-exposure prophylaxis with MMR or immunoglobulin within 72 hours or 6 days, respectively, although not concurrently [139]. Clinical management of patients with measles consists of fluid, electrolyte, and nutritional support and early recognition and treatment of bacterial coinfection [10]. Two doses of vitamin A in children under 2 years have been associated with reduced risk of pneumonia and death [140]. WHO recommends administering 200,000 IU of vitamin A daily for 2 days in children aged 1 year and older, with reduced dosing in younger infants [141].

SARS and MERS Treatment

There are currently no licensed therapeutics or vaccines for SARS or MERS. Consequently, supportive care is the mainstay of treatment [142]. Renal replacement therapy is frequently required in severe illness [119, 143, 144]. Empiric antibiotics are often administered given potential for secondary bacterial infection. Ribavirin and pegylated interferon alpha 2b have been administered to MERS patients, although effectiveness data is lacking [144]. Aerosol-generating procedures including endotracheal intubation are associated with increased risk of healthcare worker infection necessitating strict adherence to infection control measures, including use of eye protection in addition to standard, airborne, and contact precautions [145].

Smallpox Prevention and Treatment

While routine smallpox vaccination ceased at the end of the smallpox eradication program, it is still employed for those at increased risk for exposure. First-generation vaccines comprise a significant proportion of both the US national and global vaccine stockpiles [146]. However, first-generation vaccines carry high risk of adverse events due to use of replication-competent VACV and potential manufacturing contaminants. Second-generation smallpox vaccines have reduced concerns for contaminants and are expected to have similar protective efficacy as first-generation vaccines. ACAM2000® has garnered US Food and Drug Administration licensure for vaccination of those at high risk for *Orthopoxvirus* exposure and is part of the US strategic national stockpile [147]. ACAM2000® and the Lister-derived vaccines

RIVM and Elstree-BN also contribute to the global stockpile. IMVAMUNE (MVA), a third-generation vaccine, is licensed in Europe and Canada and is part of the US national stockpile. Passive immunization with VIG has been employed to treat complications of vaccinations [148, 149]. There has also been increasing interest in the development and licensure of small molecule antivirals for treatment of *Orthopoxvirus* infections. CMX001 (brincidofovir), a DNA synthesis inhibitor, has demonstrated protection against lethal VARV in nonhuman primates [150] and has been granted ophan drug designation while also being included in the US Strategic National Stockpile. ST-246 (tecovirimat), which inhibits viral egress, has potent (IC50 < 0.010 μM) and selective (CC50 > 40 mM) inhibitory activities against multiple orthopoxvirues [151], is the only antipoxvirus therapeutic that has been granted approval in the US and has been added to the Strategic National Stockpile.

References

1. Centers for Disease Control and Prevention. Types of influenza viruses. [cited 2019 March 1]. Available from: https://www.cdc.gov/flu/about/viruses/types.htm.
2. Knipe DM, Howley PM. Fields virology. Philadelphia: Wolters Kluwer/Lippincott Williams & Wilkins Health; 2013.
3. White SK, Ma W, McDaniel CJ, Gray GC, Lednicky JA. Serologic evidence of exposure to influenza D virus among persons with occupational contact with cattle. J Clin Virol. 2016;81:31–3.
4. Hause BM, Collin EA, Liu R, Huang B, Sheng Z, Lu W, Wang D, Nelson EA, Li F. Characterization of a novel influenza virus in cattle and Swine: proposal for a new genus in the Orthomyxoviridae family. MBio. 2014;5:e00031-00014.
5. Krauss S, Webster RG. Avian influenza virus surveillance and wild birds: past and present. Avian Dis. 2010;54:394–8.
6. Tong S, Li Y, Rivailler P, Conrardy C, Castillo DA, Chen LM, Recuenco S, Ellison JA, Davis CT, York IA, Turmelle AS, Moran D, Rogers S, Shi M, Tao Y, Weil MR, Tang K, Rowe LA, Sammons S, Xu X, Frace M, Lindblade KA, Cox NJ, Anderson LJ, Rupprecht CE, Donis RO. A distinct lineage of influenza A virus from bats. Proc Natl Acad Sci U S A. 2012;109:4269–74.
7. Tong S, Zhu X, Li Y, Shi M, Zhang J, Bourgeois M, Yang H, Chen X, Recuenco S, Gomez J, Chen LM, Johnson A, Tao Y, Dreyfus C, Yu W, McBride R, Carney PJ, Gilbert AT, Chang J, Guo Z, Davis CT, Paulson JC, Stevens J, Rupprecht CE, Holmes EC, Wilson IA, Donis RO. New world bats harbor diverse influenza A viruses. PLoS Pathog. 2013;9:e1003657.
8. A revision of the system of nomenclature for influenza viruses: a WHO memorandum. Bull World Health Organ. 1980;58:585–91.
9. Krammer F, Smith GJD, Fouchier RAM, Peiris M, Kedzierska K, Doherty PC, Palese P, Shaw ML, Treanor J, Webster RG, Garcia-Sastre A. Influenza. Nat Rev Dis Primers. 2018;4:3.
10. Moss WJ. Measles. Lancet. 2017;390:2490–502.
11. Horikami SM, Moyer SA. Structure, transcription, and replication of measles virus. Berlin, Heidelberg: Springer; 1995.
12. Fehr AR, Perlman S. Coronaviruses: an overview of their replication and pathogenesis. Methods Mol Biol. 2015;1282:1–23.
13. Jevsnik M, Ursic T, Zigon N, Lusa L, Krivec U, Petrovec M. Coronavirus infections in hospitalized pediatric patients with acute respiratory tract disease. BMC Infect Dis. 2012;12:365.
14. de Wit E, van Doremalen N, Falzarano D, Munster VJ. SARS and MERS: recent insights into emerging coronaviruses. Nat Rev Microbiol. 2016;14:523–34.

15. Graham RL, Donaldson EF, Baric RS. A decade after SARS: strategies for controlling emerging coronaviruses. Nat Rev Microbiol. 2013;11:836–48.
16. Raj VS, Mou H, Smits SL, Dekkers DH, Muller MA, Dijkman R, Muth D, Demmers JA, Zaki A, Fouchier RA, Thiel V, Drosten C, Rottier PJ, Osterhaus AD, Bosch BJ, Haagmans BL. Dipeptidyl peptidase 4 is a functional receptor for the emerging human coronavirus-EMC. Nature. 2013;495:251–4.
17. Li W, Moore MJ, Vasilieva N, Sui J, Wong SK, Berne MA, Somasundaran M, Sullivan JL, Luzuriaga K, Greenough TC, Choe H, Farzan M. Angiotensin-converting enzyme 2 is a functional receptor for the SARS coronavirus. Nature. 2003;426:450–4.
18. Diven DG. An overview of poxviruses. J Am Acad Dermatol. 2001;44:1–16.
19. Buller RM, Palumbo GJ. Poxvirus pathogenesis. Microbiol Rev. 1991;55:80–122.
20. Harrison SC, Alberts B, Ehrenfeld E, Enquist L, Fineberg H, McKnight SL, Moss B, O'Donnell M, Ploegh H, Schmid SL, Walter KP, Theriot J. Discovery of antivirals against smallpox. Proc Natl Acad Sci U S A. 2004;101:11178–92.
21. World Health Organization. Avian influenza: assessing the pandemic threat. [cited 2019 March 11]. Available from: https://apps.who.int/iris/bitstream/handle/10665/68985/WHO_CDS_2005.29.pdf?sequence=1.
22. Lai S, Qin Y, Cowling BJ, Ren X, Wardrop NA, Gilbert M, Tsang TK, Wu P, Feng L, Jiang H, Peng Z, Zheng J, Liao Q, Li S, Horby PW, Farrar JJ, Gao GF, Tatem AJ, Yu H. Global epidemiology of avian influenza A H5N1 virus infection in humans, 1997–2015: a systematic review of individual case data. Lancet Infect Dis. 2016;16:e108–18.
23. Li Q, Zhou L, Zhou M, Chen Z, Li F, Wu H, Xiang N, Chen E, Tang F, Wang D, Meng L, Hong Z, Tu W, Cao Y, Li L, Ding F, Liu B, Wang M, Xie R, Gao R, Li X, Bai T, Zou S, He J, Hu J, Xu Y, Chai C, Wang S, Gao Y, Jin L, Zhang Y, Luo H, Yu H, He J, Li Q, Wang X, Gao L, Pang X, Liu G, Yan Y, Yuan H, Shu Y, Yang W, Wang Y, Wu F, Uyeki TM, Feng Z. Epidemiology of human infections with avian influenza A(H7N9) virus in China. N Engl J Med. 2014;370:520–32.
24. Jhung MA, Nelson DI, Centers for Disease Control and Prevention (CDC). Outbreaks of avian influenza A (H5N2), (H5N8), and (H5N1) among birds--United States, December 2014-January 2015. MMWR Morb Mortal Wkly Rep. 2015;64:111.
25. Centers for Disease Control and Prevention (CDC). Influenza A (H3N2) variant virus-related hospitalizations: Ohio, 2012. MMWR Morb Mortal Wkly Rep. 2012;61:764–7.
26. Paules C, Subbarao K. Influenza. Lancet. 2017;390:697–708.
27. Centers for Disease Control and Prevention. Estimated influenza illnesses, medical visits, hospitalizations, and death in the United States — 2017–2018 influenza season. [cited 2019 March 11]. Available from: https://www.cdc.gov/flu/about/burden/2017-2018.htm#References.
28. Taubenberger JK, Morens DM. 1918 influenza: the mother of all pandemics. Emerg Infect Dis. 2006;12:15–22.
29. World Health Organization. Global influenza surveillance and response system (GISRS). https://www.who.int/influenza/gisrs_laboratory/en/. Accessed 19 Apr 2019.
30. Moss WJ, Strebel P. Biological feasibility of measles eradication. J Infect Dis. 2011;204(Suppl 1):S47–53.
31. Dabbagh A, Laws RL, Steulet C, Dumolard L, Mulders MN, Kretsinger K, Alexander JP, Rota PA, Goodson JL. Progress toward regional measles elimination – worldwide, 2000–2017. MMWR Morb Mortal Wkly Rep. 2018;67:1323–9.
32. Thornton J. Measles cases in Europe tripled from 2017 to 2018. BMJ. 2019;364:l634.
33. Gastanaduy PA, Budd J, Fisher N, Redd SB, Fletcher J, Miller J, DJ MF 3rd, Rota J, Rota PA, Hickman C, Fowler B, Tatham L, Wallace GS, de Fijter S, Parker Fiebelkorn A, DiOrio M. A measles outbreak in an underimmunized Amish Community in Ohio. N Engl J Med. 2016;375:1343–54.
34. Patel MK, Gacic-Dobo M, Strebel PM, Dabbagh A, Mulders MN, Okwo-Bele JM, Dumolard L, Rota PA, Kretsinger K, Goodson JL. Progress toward regional measles elimination – worldwide, 2000–2015. MMWR Morb Mortal Wkly Rep. 2016;65:1228–33.
35. Wallinga J, Heijne JC, Kretzschmar M. A measles epidemic threshold in a highly vaccinated population. PLoS Med. 2005;2:e316.

36. Haagmans BL, Al Dhahiry SH, Reusken CB, Raj VS, Galiano M, Myers R, Godeke GJ, Jonges M, Farag E, Diab A, Ghobashy H, Alhajri F, Al-Thani M, Al-Marri SA, Al Romaihi HE, Al Khal A, Bermingham A, Osterhaus AD, AlHajri MM, Koopmans MP. Middle East respiratory syndrome coronavirus in dromedary camels: an outbreak investigation. Lancet Infect Dis. 2014;14:140–5.

37. Reusken CB, Haagmans BL, Muller MA, Gutierrez C, Godeke GJ, Meyer B, Muth D, Raj VS, Smits-De Vries L, Corman VM, Drexler JF, Smits SL, El Tahir YE, De Sousa R, van Beek J, Nowotny N, van Maanen K, Hidalgo-Hermoso E, Bosch BJ, Rottier P, Osterhaus A, Gortazar-Schmidt C, Drosten C, Koopmans MP. Middle East respiratory syndrome corona- virus neutralising serum antibodies in dromedary camels: a comparative serological study. Lancet Infect Dis. 2013;13:859–66.

38. Azhar EI, El-Kafrawy SA, Farraj SA, Hassan AM, Al-Saeed MS, Hashem AM, Madani TA. Evidence for camel-to-human transmission of MERS coronavirus. N Engl J Med. 2014;370:2499–505.

39. Hemida MG, Chu DK, Poon LL, Perera RA, Alhammadi MA, Ng HY, Siu LY, Guan Y, Alnaeem A, Peiris M. MERS coronavirus in dromedary camel herd, Saudi Arabia. Emerg Infect Dis. 2014;20:1231–4.

40. Raj VS, Farag EA, Reusken CB, Lamers MM, Pas SD, Voermans J, Smits SL, Osterhaus AD, Al-Mawlawi N, Al-Romaihi HE, AlHajri MM, El-Sayed AM, Mohran KA, Ghobashy H, Alhajri F, Al-Thani M, Al-Marri SA, El-Maghraby MM, Koopmans MP, Haagmans BL. Isolation of MERS coronavirus from a dromedary camel, Qatar, 2014. Emerg Infect Dis. 2014;20:1339–42.

41. Ge XY, Li JL, Yang XL, Chmura AA, Zhu G, Epstein JH, Mazet JK, Hu B, Zhang W, Peng C, Zhang YJ, Luo CM, Tan B, Wang N, Zhu Y, Crameri G, Zhang SY, Wang LF, Daszak P, Shi ZL. Isolation and characterization of a bat SARS-like coronavirus that uses the ACE2 recep- tor. Nature. 2013;503:535–8.

42. Li W, Shi Z, Yu M, Ren W, Smith C, Epstein JH, Wang H, Crameri G, Hu Z, Zhang H, Zhang J, McEachern J, Field H, Daszak P, Eaton BT, Zhang S, Wang LF. Bats are natural reservoirs of SARS-like coronaviruses. Science. 2005;310:676–9.

43. Rota PA, Oberste MS, Monroe SS, Nix WA, Campagnoli R, Icenogle JP, Penaranda S, Bankamp B, Maher K, Chen MH, Tong S, Tamin A, Lowe L, Frace M, DeRisi JL, Chen Q, Wang D, Erdman DD, Peret TC, Burns C, Ksiazek TG, Rollin PE, Sanchez A, Liffick S, Holloway B, Limor J, McCaustland K, Olsen-Rasmussen M, Fouchier R, Gunther S, Osterhaus AD, Drosten C, Pallansch MA, Anderson LJ, Bellini WJ. Characterization of a novel coronavirus associated with severe acute respiratory syndrome. Science. 2003;300:1394–9.

44. Alshukairi AN, Zheng J, Zhao J, Nehdi A, Baharoon SA, Layqah L, Bokhari A, Al Johani SM, Samman N, Boudjelal M, Ten Eyck P, Al-Mozaini MA, Zhao J, Perlman S, Alagaili AN. High prevalence of MERS-CoV infection in camel workers in Saudi Arabia. MBio. 2018;9:e01985-18.

45. Skowronski DM, Astell C, Brunham RC, Low DE, Petric M, Roper RL, Talbot PJ, Tam T, Babiuk L. Severe acute respiratory syndrome (SARS): a year in review. Annu Rev Med. 2005;56:357–81.

46. World Health Organization. Middle East respiratory syndrome coronavirus (MERS-CoV). https://www.who.int/emergencies/mers-cov/en/. Accessed 10 Apr 2019.

47. Cho SY, Kang JM, Ha YE, Park GE, Lee JY, Ko JH, Lee JY, Kim JM, Kang CI, Jo IJ, Ryu JG, Choi JR, Kim S, Huh HJ, Ki CS, Kang ES, Peck KR, Dhong HJ, Song JH, Chung DR, Kim YJ. MERS-CoV outbreak following a single patient exposure in an emergency room in South Korea: an epidemiological outbreak study. Lancet. 2016;388:994–1001.

48. Chowell G, Abdirizak F, Lee S, Lee J, Jung E, Nishiura H, Viboud C. Transmission char- acteristics of MERS and SARS in the healthcare setting: a comparative study. BMC Med. 2015;13:210.

49. Hunter JC, Nguyen D, Aden B, Al Bandar Z, Al Dhaheri W, Abu Elkheir K, Khudair A, Al Mulla M, El Saleh F, Imambaccus H, Al Kaabi N, Sheikh FA, Sasse J, Turner A, Abdel Wareth

L, Weber S, Al Ameri A, Abu Amer W, Alami NN, Bunga S, Haynes LM, Hall AJ, Kallen AJ, Kuhar D, Pham H, Pringle K, Tong S, Whitaker BL, Gerber SI, Al Hosani FI. Transmission of Middle East respiratory syndrome coronavirus infections in healthcare settings, Abu Dhabi. Emerg Infect Dis. 2016;22:647–56.

50. Li Y, Carroll DS, Gardner SN, Walsh MC, Vitalis EA, Damon IK. On the origin of smallpox: correlating variola phylogenics with historical smallpox records. Proc Natl Acad Sci U S A. 2007;104:15787–92.

51. Fenner FHD, Isao A, Zdenek J, Ladnyi ID. Smallpox and its eradication. Geneva: World Health Organization; 1988.

52. Koplow DA. Smallpox: the fight to eradicate a global scourge. Berkeley: University of California Press; 2004.

53. Riedel S. Edward Jenner and the history of smallpox and vaccination. Proc (Bayl Univ Med Cent). 2005;18:21–5.

54. Killingley B, Nguyen-Van-Tam J. Routes of influenza transmission. Influenza Other Respir Viruses. 2013;7(Suppl 2):42–51.

55. Bridges CB, Kuehnert MJ, Hall CB. Transmission of influenza: implications for control in health care settings. Clin Infect Dis. 2003;37:1094–101.

56. van Riel D, Munster VJ, de Wit E, Rimmelzwaan GF, Fouchier RA, Osterhaus AD, Kuiken T. Human and avian influenza viruses target different cells in the lower respiratory tract of humans and other mammals. Am J Pathol. 2007;171:1215–23.

57. Shinya K, Kawaoka Y. Influenza virus receptors in the human airway. Uirusu. 2006;56:85–9.

58. Baccam P, Beauchemin C, Macken CA, Hayden FG, Perelson AS. Kinetics of influenza A virus infection in humans. J Virol. 2006;80:7590–9.

59. Ng S, Lopez R, Kuan G, Gresh L, Balmaseda A, Harris E, Gordon A. The timeline of influenza virus shedding in children and adults in a household transmission study of influenza in Managua, Nicaragua. Pediatr Infect Dis J. 2016;35:583–6.

60. Lehners N, Tabatabai J, Prifert C, Wedde M, Puthenparambil J, Weissbrich B, Biere B, Schweiger B, Egerer G, Schnitzler P. Long-term shedding of influenza virus, parainfluenza virus, respiratory syncytial virus and nosocomial epidemiology in patients with hematological disorders. PLoS One. 2016;11:e0148258.

61. Biggerstaff M, Cauchemez S, Reed C, Gambhir M, Finelli L. Estimates of the reproduction number for seasonal, pandemic, and zoonotic influenza: a systematic review of the literature. BMC Infect Dis. 2014;14:480.

62. Herold S, Becker C, Ridge KM, Budinger GR. Influenza virus-induced lung injury: pathogenesis and implications for treatment. Eur Respir J. 2015;45:1463–78.

63. Taubenberger JK, Morens DM. The pathology of influenza virus infections. Annu Rev Pathol. 2008;3:499–522.

64. Chertow DS, Memoli MJ. Bacterial coinfection in influenza: a grand rounds review. JAMA. 2013;309:275–82.

65. Ke C, Mok CKP, Zhu W, Zhou H, He J, Guan W, Wu J, Song W, Wang D, Liu J, Lin Q, Chu DKW, Yang L, Zhong N, Yang Z, Shu Y, Peiris JSM. Human infection with highly pathogenic avian influenza A(H7N9) virus, China. Emerg Infect Dis. 2017;23:1332–40.

66. Luczo JM, Stambas J, Durr PA, Michalski WP, Bingham J. Molecular pathogenesis of H5 highly pathogenic avian influenza: the role of the haemagglutinin cleavage site motif. Rev Med Virol. 2015;25:406–30.

67. Gomez Lorenzo MM, Fenton MJ. Immunobiology of influenza vaccines. Chest. 2013;143:502–10.

68. Remington PL, Hall WN, Davis IH, Herald A, Gunn RA. Airborne transmission of measles in a physician's office. JAMA. 1985;253:1574–7.

69. Laksono BM, de Vries RD, McQuaid S, Duprex WP, de Swart RL. Measles virus host invasion and pathogenesis. Viruses. 2016;8:210.

70. Ludlow M, McQuaid S, Milner D, de Swart RL, Duprex WP. Pathological consequences of systemic measles virus infection. J Pathol. 2015;235:253–65.

71. de Swart RL, Ludlow M, de Witte L, Yanagi Y, van Amerongen G, McQuaid S, Yuksel S, Geijtenbeek TB, Duprex WP, Osterhaus AD. Predominant infection of CD150+ lymphocytes and dendritic cells during measles virus infection of macaques. PLoS Pathog. 2007;3:e178.
72. Perry RT, Halsey NA. The clinical significance of measles: a review. J Infect Dis. 2004;189(Suppl 1):S4–16.
73. Guerra FM, Bolotin S, Lim G, Heffernan J, Deeks SL, Li Y, Crowcroft NS. The basic reproduction number (R0) of measles: a systematic review. Lancet Infect Dis. 2017;17:e420–8.
74. Leuridan E, Hens N, Hutse V, Ieven M, Aerts M, Van Damme P. Early waning of maternal measles antibodies in era of measles elimination: longitudinal study. BMJ. 2010;340:c1626.
75. Griffin DE. Measles virus-induced suppression of immune responses. Immunol Rev. 2010; 236:176–89.
76. Mina MJ, Metcalf CJ, de Swart RL, Osterhaus AD, Grenfell BT. Long-term measles-induced immunomodulation increases overall childhood infectious disease mortality. Science. 2015;348:694–9.
77. Yu IT, Li Y, Wong TW, Tam W, Chan AT, Lee JH, Leung DY, Ho T. Evidence of airborne transmission of the severe acute respiratory syndrome virus. N Engl J Med. 2004;350:1731–9.
78. Chowell G, Castillo-Chavez C, Fenimore PW, Kribs-Zaleta CM, Arriola L, Hyman JM. Model parameters and outbreak control for SARS. Emerg Infect Dis. 2004;10:1258–63.
79. Liu L, Wei Q, Alvarez X, Wang H, Du Y, Zhu H, Jiang H, Zhou J, Lam P, Zhang L, Lackner A, Qin C, Chen Z. Epithelial cells lining salivary gland ducts are early target cells of severe acute respiratory syndrome coronavirus infection in the upper respiratory tracts of rhesus macaques. J Virol. 2011;85:4025–30.
80. Kuba K, Imai Y, Rao S, Gao H, Guo F, Guan B, Huan Y, Yang P, Zhang Y, Deng W, Bao L, Zhang B, Liu G, Wang Z, Chappell M, Liu Y, Zheng D, Leibbrandt A, Wada T, Slutsky AS, Liu D, Qin C, Jiang C, Penninger JM. A crucial role of angiotensin converting enzyme 2 (ACE2) in SARS coronavirus-induced lung injury. Nat Med. 2005;11:875–9.
81. Gu J, Gong E, Zhang B, Zheng J, Gao Z, Zhong Y, Zou W, Zhan J, Wang S, Xie Z, Zhuang H, Wu B, Zhong H, Shao H, Fang W, Gao D, Pei F, Li X, He Z, Xu D, Shi X, Anderson VM, Leong AS. Multiple organ infection and the pathogenesis of SARS. J Exp Med. 2005;202:415–24.
82. Hamming I, Timens W, Bulthuis ML, Lely AT, Navis G, van Goor H. Tissue distribution of ACE2 protein, the functional receptor for SARS coronavirus. A first step in understanding SARS pathogenesis. J Pathol. 2004;203:631–7.
83. Gu J, Korteweg C. Pathology and pathogenesis of severe acute respiratory syndrome. Am J Pathol. 2007;170:1136–47.
84. Middle East Respiratory Syndrome Coronavirus (MERS-CoV). WHO MERS-CoV Global Summary and risk assessment. https://www.who.int/emergencies/mers-cov/mers-summary-2016.pdf. Accessed 19 Apr 2017.
85. Corman VM, Albarrak AM, Omrani AS, Albarrak MM, Farah ME, Almasri M, Muth D, Sieberg A, Meyer B, Assiri AM, Binger T, Steinhagen K, Lattwein E, Al-Tawfiq J, Muller MA, Drosten C, Memish ZA. Viral shedding and antibody response in 37 patients with Middle East respiratory syndrome coronavirus infection. Clin Infect Dis. 2016;62:477–83.
86. Oh MD, Park WB, Choe PG, Choi SJ, Kim JI, Chae J, Park SS, Kim EC, Oh HS, Kim EJ, Nam EY, Na SH, Kim DK, Lee SM, Song KH, Bang JH, Kim ES, Kim HB, Park SW, Kim NJ. Viral load kinetics of MERS coronavirus infection. N Engl J Med. 2016;375:1303–5.
87. Song Z, Xu Y, Bao L, Zhang L, Yu P, Qu Y, Zhu H, Zhao W, Han Y, Qin C. From SARS to MERS, thrusting coronaviruses into the spotlight. Viruses. 2019;11:59.
88. Kim SY, Park SJ, Cho SY, Cha RH, Jee HG, Kim G, Shin HS, Kim Y, Jung YM, Yang JS, Kim SS, Cho SI, Kim MJ, Lee JS, Lee SJ, Seo SH, Park SS, Seong MW. Viral RNA in blood as indicator of severe outcome in Middle East respiratory syndrome coronavirus infection. Emerg Infect Dis. 2016;22:1813–6.
89. Widagdo W, Raj VS, Schipper D, Kolijn K, van Leenders G, Bosch BJ, Bensaid A, Segales J, Baumgartner W, Osterhaus A, Koopmans MP, van den Brand JMA, Haagmans BL. Differential expression of the Middle East respiratory syndrome coronavirus receptor in the upper respiratory tracts of humans and dromedary camels. J Virol. 2016;90:4838–42.

90. Wehrle PF, Posch J, Richter KH, Henderson DA. An airborne outbreak of smallpox in a German hospital and its significance with respect to other recent outbreaks in Europe. Bull World Health Organ. 1970;43:669–79.
91. Eichner M, Dietz K. Transmission potential of smallpox: estimates based on detailed data from an outbreak. Am J Epidemiol. 2003;158:110–7.
92. Breman JG, Henderson DA. Diagnosis and management of smallpox. N Engl J Med. 2002;346:1300–8.
93. Stanford MM, McFadden G, Karupiah G, Chaudhri G. Immunopathogenesis of poxvirus infections: forecasting the impending storm. Immunol Cell Biol. 2007;85:93–102.
94. Martin DB. The cause of death in smallpox: an examination of the pathology record. Mil Med. 2002;167:546–51.
95. Sarkar JK, Mitra AC, Mukherjee MK, De SK, Mazumdar DG. Virus excretion in small-pox. 1. Excretion in the throat, urine, and conjunctiva of patients. Bull World Health Organ. 1973;48:517–22.
96. Guerrant RL, Walker DH, Weller PF. Tropical infectious diseases: principles, pathogens and practice. Saunders/Elsevier: Edinburgh; 2011.
97. Gani R, Leach S. Transmission potential of smallpox in contemporary populations. Nature. 2001;414:748–51.
98. Downie AW, Mc CK, Macdonald A. Viraemia in smallpox. Lancet. 1950;2:513–4.
99. Downie AW, McCarthy K, Macdonald A, Maccallum FO, Macrae AE. Virus and virus anti-gen in the blood of smallpox patients; their significance in early diagnosis and prognosis. Lancet. 1953;265:164–6.
100. Mitra AC, Chatterjee SN, Sarkar JK, Manji P, Das AK. Viraemia in haemorrhagic and other forms of smallpox. J Indian Med Assoc. 1966;47:112–4.
101. Moore ZS, Seward JF, Lane JM. Smallpox. Lancet. 2006;367:425–35.
102. Buchman CA, Doyle WJ, Skoner DP, Post JC, Alper CM, Seroky JT, Anderson K, Preston RA, Hayden FG, Fireman P, et al. Influenza A virus--induced acute otitis media. J Infect Dis. 1995;172:1348–51.
103. Sellers SA, Hagan RS, Hayden FG, Fischer WA 2nd. The hidden burden of influenza: a review of the extra-pulmonary complications of influenza infection. Influenza Other Respir Viruses. 2017;11:372–93.
104. Quiambao BP, Gatchalian SR, Halonen P, Lucero M, Sombrero L, Paladin FJ, Meurman O, Merin J, Ruutu P. Coinfection is common in measles-associated pneumonia. Pediatr Infect Dis J. 1998;17:89–93.
105. Griffin DE. Measles virus and the nervous system. Handb Clin Neurol. 2014;123:577–90.
106. Peiris JS, Lai ST, Poon LL, Guan Y, Yam LY, Lim W, Nicholls J, Yee WK, Yan WW, Cheung MT, Cheng VC, Chan KH, Tsang DN, Yung RW, Ng TK, Yuen KY, SARS Study Group. Coronavirus as a possible cause of severe acute respiratory syndrome. Lancet. 2003;361:1319–25.
107. Leung WK, To KF, Chan PK, Chan HL, Wu AK, Lee N, Yuen KY, Sung JJ. Enteric involvement of severe acute respiratory syndrome-associated coronavirus infection. Gastroenterology. 2003;125:1011–7.
108. Leung GM, Hedley AJ, Ho LM, Chau P, Wong IO, Thach TQ, Ghani AC, Donnelly CA, Fraser C, Riley S, Ferguson NM, Anderson RM, Tsang T, Leung PY, Wong V, Chan JC, Tsui E, Lo SV, Lam TH. The epidemiology of severe acute respiratory syndrome in the 2003 Hong Kong epidemic: an analysis of all 1755 patients. Ann Intern Med. 2004;141:662–73.
109. Hui DS, Memish ZA, Zumla A. Severe acute respiratory syndrome vs. the Middle East respiratory syndrome. Curr Opin Pulm Med. 2014;20:233–41.
110. Hui DS, Sung JJ. Severe acute respiratory syndrome. Chest. 2003;124:12–5.
111. Lee N, Hui D, Wu A, Chan P, Cameron P, Joynt GM, Ahuja A, Yung MY, Leung CB, To KF, Lui SF, Szeto CC, Chung S, Sung JJ. A major outbreak of severe acute respiratory syndrome in Hong Kong. N Engl J Med. 2003;348:1986–94.
112. Wong GW, Hui DS. Severe acute respiratory syndrome (SARS): epidemiology, diagnosis and management. Thorax. 2003;58:558–60.

113. Chu KH, Tsang WK, Tang CS, Lam MF, Lai FM, To KF, Fung KS, Tang HL, Yan WW, Chan HW, Lai TS, Tong KL, Lai KN. Acute renal impairment in coronavirus-associated severe acute respiratory syndrome. Kidney Int. 2005;67:698–705.
114. Assiri A, Al-Tawfiq JA, Al-Rabeeah AA, Al-Rabiah FA, Al-Hajjar S, Al-Barrak A, Flemban H, Al-Nassir WN, Balkhy HH, Al-Hakeem RF, Makhdoom HQ, Zumla AI, Memish ZA. Epidemiological, demographic, and clinical characteristics of 47 cases of Middle East respiratory syndrome coronavirus disease from Saudi Arabia: a descriptive study. Lancet Infect Dis. 2013;13:752–61.
115. Guery B, Poissy J, el Mansouf L, Sejourne C, Ettahar N, Lemaire X, Vuotto F, Goffard A, Behillil S, Enouf V, Caro V, Mailles A, Che D, Manuguerra JC, Mathieu D, Fontanet A, van der Werf S, MERS-CoV Study Group. Clinical features and viral diagnosis of two cases of infection with Middle East respiratory syndrome coronavirus: a report of nosocomial transmission. Lancet. 2013;381:2265–72.
116. Hijawi B, Abdallat M, Sayaydeh A, Alqasrawi S, Haddadin A, Jaarour N, Alsheikh S, Alsanouri T. Novel coronavirus infections in Jordan, April 2012: epidemiological findings from a retrospective investigation. East Mediterr Health J. 2013;19(Suppl 1):S12–8.
117. Memish ZA, Zumla AI, Al-Hakeem RF, Al-Rabeeah AA, Stephens GM. Family cluster of Middle East respiratory syndrome coronavirus infections. N Engl J Med. 2013;368:2487–94.
118. Who Mers-Cov Research Group. State of knowledge and data gaps of Middle East respiratory syndrome coronavirus (MERS-CoV) in humans. PLoS Curr. 2013;5.
119. Arabi YM, Arifi AA, Balkhy HH, Najm H, Aldawood AS, Ghabashi A, Hawa H, Alothman A, Khaldi A, Al Raiy B. Clinical course and outcomes of critically ill patients with Middle East respiratory syndrome coronavirus infection. Ann Intern Med. 2014;160:389–97.
120. Zaki AM, van Boheemen S, Bestebroer TM, Osterhaus AD, Fouchier RA. Isolation of a novel coronavirus from a man with pneumonia in Saudi Arabia. N Engl J Med. 2012;367:1814–20.
121. Al-Tawfiq JA, Hinedi K, Ghandour J, Khairalla H, Musleh S, Ujayli A, Memish ZA. Middle East respiratory syndrome coronavirus: a case-control study of hospitalized patients. Clin Infect Dis. 2014;59:160–5.
122. Ajlan AM, Ahyad RA, Jamjoom LG, Alharthy A, Madani TA. Middle East respiratory syndrome coronavirus (MERS-CoV) infection: chest CT findings. AJR Am J Roentgenol. 2014;203:782–7.
123. Zumla A, Hui DS, Perlman S. Middle East respiratory syndrome. Lancet. 2015;386:995–1007.
124. Saad M, Omrani AS, Baig K, Bahloul A, Elzein F, Matin MA, Selim MA, Al Mutairi M, Al Nakhli D, Al Aidaroos AY, Al Sherbeeni N, Al-Khashan HI, Memish ZA, Albarrak AM. Clinical aspects and outcomes of 70 patients with Middle East respiratory syndrome coronavirus infection: a single-center experience in Saudi Arabia. Int J Infect Dis. 2014;29:301–6.
125. Rao AR. Smallpox. Bombay: The Kothari Book Depot; 1972.
126. Centers for Disease Control and Prevention. Prevention strategies for seasonal influenza in healthcare settings. https://www.cdc.gov/flu/professionals/infectioncontrol/healthcaresettings.htm. Accessed 17 Apr 2019.
127. Merckx J, Wali R, Schiller I, Caya C, Gore GC, Chartrand C, Dendukuri N, Papenburg J. Diagnostic accuracy of novel and traditional rapid tests for influenza infection compared with reverse transcriptase polymerase chain reaction: a systematic review and meta-analysis. Ann Intern Med. 2017;167:394–409.
128. Centers for Disease Control and Prevention. Middle East Respiratory Syndrome (MERS). Interim Patient under Investigation (PUI) guidance and case definitions. https://www.cdc.gov/coronavirus/mers/case-def.html. Accessed 17 Apr 2019.
129. Memish ZA, Al-Tawfiq JA, Makhdoom HQ, Assiri A, Alhakeem RF, Albarrak A, Alsubaie S, Al-Rabeeah AA, Hajomar WH, Hussain R, Kheyami AM, Almutairi A, Azhar EI, Drosten C, Watson SJ, Kellam P, Cotten M, Zumla A. Respiratory tract samples, viral load, and genome fraction yield in patients with Middle East respiratory syndrome. J Infect Dis. 2014;210:1590–4.

130. Woo PC, Yuen KY, Lau SK. Epidemiology of coronavirus-associated respiratory tract infections and the role of rapid diagnostic tests: a prospective study. Hong Kong Med J. 2012;18(Suppl 2):22–4.
131. Centers for Disease Control and Prevention. Evaluating patients for smallpox: acute, generalized vesicular or pustular rash illness protocol. https://www.cdc.gov/smallpox/clinicians/ algorithm-protocol.html. Accessed 17 Apr 2019.
132. Chan TC, Fan-Ngai Hung I, Ka-Hay Luk J, Chu LW, Hon-Wai CF. Effectiveness of influenza vaccination in institutionalized older adults: a systematic review. J Am Med Dir Assoc. 2014;15:226.e1–6.
133. Beck CR, McKenzie BC, Hashim AB, Harris RC, University of Nottingham Influenza and the ImmunoCompromised (UNIIC) Study Group, Nguyen-Van-Tam JS. Influenza vaccination for immunocompromised patients: systematic review and meta-analysis by etiology. J Infect Dis. 2012;206:1250–9.
134. Grohskopf LA, Sokolow LZ, Broder KR, Walter EB, Fry AM, Jernigan DB. Prevention and control of seasonal influenza with vaccines: recommendations of the Advisory Committee on Immunization Practices-United States, 2018-19 influenza season. MMWR Recomm Rep. 2018;67:1–20.
135. Paules CI, Marston HD, Eisinger RW, Baltimore D, Fauci AS. The pathway to a universal influenza vaccine. Immunity. 2017;47:599–603.
136. Centers for Disease Control and Prevention. Influenza antiviral medications: summary for clinicians. https://www.cdc.gov/flu/professionals/antivirals/summary-clinicians.htm. Accessed 19 Apr 2019.
137. Hayden FG, Sugaya N, Hirotsu N, Lee N, de Jong MD, Hurt AC, Ishida T, Sekino H, Yamada K, Portsmouth S, Kawaguchi K, Shishido T, Arai M, Tsuchiya K, Uehara T, Watanabe A, Baloxavir Marboxil Investigators G. Baloxavir marboxil for uncomplicated influenza in adults and adolescents. N Engl J Med. 2018;379:913–23.
138. World Health Organization. Measles vaccines: WHO position paper, April 2017–recommendations. Vaccine. 2019;37:219–22.
139. Centers for Disease Control and Prevention. Measles (Rubeola): for healthcare professionals. https://www.cdc.gov/measles/hcp/index.html. Accessed 19 Apr 2019.
140. Huiming Y, Chaomin W, Meng M. Vitamin A for treating measles in children. Cochrane Database Syst Rev. 2005:CD001479.
141. World Health Organization. Measles and vitamin A. https://www.who.int/wer/2009/wer8435. pdf#page=3. Accessed 19 Apr 2019.
142. Chan JF, Lau SK, To KK, Cheng VC, Woo PC, Yuen KY. Middle East respiratory syndrome coronavirus: another zoonotic betacoronavirus causing SARS-like disease. Clin Microbiol Rev. 2015;28:465–522.
143. Albarrak AM, Stephens GM, Hewson R, Memish ZA. Recovery from severe novel coronavirus infection. Saudi Med J. 2012;33:1265–9.
144. Omrani AS, Saad MM, Baig K, Bahloul A, Abdul-Matin M, Alaidaroos AY, Almakhlafi GA, Albarrak MM, Memish ZA, Albarrak AM. Ribavirin and interferon alfa-2a for severe Middle East respiratory syndrome coronavirus infection: a retrospective cohort study. Lancet Infect Dis. 2014;14:1090–5.
145. Tran K, Cimon K, Severn M, Pessoa-Silva CL, Conly J. Aerosol generating procedures and risk of transmission of acute respiratory infections to healthcare workers: a systematic review. PLoS One. 2012;7:e35797.
146. Arita I. Smallpox vaccine and its stockpile in 2005. Lancet Infect Dis. 2005;5:647–52.
147. Petersen BW, Damon IK, Pertowski CA, Meaney-Delman D, Guarnizo JT, Beigi RH, Edwards KM, Fisher MC, Frey SE, Lynfield R, Willoughby RE. Clinical guidance for smallpox vaccine use in a postevent vaccination program. MMWR Recomm Rep. 2015;64:1–26.
148. Feery BJ. The efficacy of vaccinial immune globulin. A 15-year study. Vox Sang. 1976;31:68–76.

149. Sharp JC, Fletcher WB. Experience of anti-vaccinia immunoglobulin in the United Kingdom. Lancet. 1973;1:656–9.
150. Mucker EM, Goff AJ, Shamblin JD, Grosenbach DW, Damon IK, Mehal JM, Holman RC, Carroll D, Gallardo N, Olson VA, Clemmons CJ, Hudson P, Hruby DE. Efficacy of tecovirimat (ST-246) in nonhuman primates infected with variola virus (smallpox). Antimicrob Agents Chemother. 2013;57:6246–53.
151. Yang G, Pevear DC, Davies MH, Collett MS, Bailey T, Rippen S, Barone L, Burns C, Rhodes G, Tohan S, Huggins JW, Baker RO, Buller RL, Touchette E, Waller K, Schriewer J, Neyts J, DeClercq E, Jones K, Hruby D, Jordan R. An orally bioavailable antipoxvirus compound (ST-246) inhibits extracellular virus formation and protects mice from lethal orthopoxvirus challenge. J Virol. 2005;79:13139–49.

Chapter 6
Zoonotic Infections and Biowarfare Agents in Critical Care: Anthrax, Plague, and Tularemia

Ryan C. Maves and Catherine M. Berjohn

Introduction

There are greater than 1400 identified human pathogens. Of these, more than 60% are of zoonotic origin, infecting humans by means of an animal reservoir [1]. These diseases include ubiquitous viruses like influenza, less common but deadly illnesses like rabies, and neglected parasites such as echinococcosis and cysticercosis. The subset of bacterial zoonoses is similarly varied, with common pathogens in industrialized settings (including *Salmonella* and *Bartonella henselae*, the agent of cat-scratch disease) existing alongside diseases of poverty in the tropics like melioidosis (*Burkholderia pseudomallei*) and leptospirosis.

In this chapter, we will review three key zoonotic bacterial diseases implicated as potential bioweapons. The use of disease as a weapon has long and inglorious history. As early as the fourth century BCE, Herodotus wrote of Scythian archers dipping their arrows into the decomposing cadavers of humans and snakes prior to firing them at their enemies. The intentional use of smallpox as a weapon of war against Native Americans was historically attested during the French and Indian War. Organized biowarfare programs, with full knowledge of Koch's postulates and the germ theory of disease, began on a small scale during the First World War but expanded dramatically during the interwar years and into the Second World War. The Japanese imperial government is known to have released pathogens directly

R. C. Maves (✉) · C. M. Berjohn
Division of Infectious Diseases, Naval Medical Center, San Diego, CA, USA

Uniformed Services University, Bethesda, MD, USA
e-mail: ryan.c.maves.mil@mail.mil; catherine.m.berjohn.mil@mail.mil

© Springer Nature Switzerland AG 2020
J. Hidalgo, L. Woc-Colburn (eds.), *Highly Infectious Diseases in Critical Care*,
https://doi.org/10.1007/978-3-030-33803-9_6

over regions of China, while Nazi Germany performed human experimentation into biowarfare but did not appear to have utilized them in combat [2].

Following the war, both the United States and Soviet Union had large-scale biowarfare programs until the signing in 1972 of the *Convention on the Prohibition of the Development, Production and Stockpiling of Bacteriological (Biological) and Toxin Weapons and on their Destruction* (or *BWC*). Despite the BWC, however, nations continued to conduct research into bioweapons, as demonstrated by the accidental 1979 release of *Bacillus anthracis* in the town of Sverdlovsk in Russia [3]. In more recent years, non-state entities, such as rogue individuals, cults, and terrorist movements, have come to play a larger role in the use of bioterrorism, most notably the intentional mailing of *B. anthracis* spores in the United States in 2001 [4].

Although the three diseases (anthrax, plague, and tularemia) under discussion are considered potential bioweapons, it is important to recognize that naturally occurring cases of these diseases are far more common than cases of bioterrorism. Indeed, only anthrax has been clearly used as a weapon of terror or war against human targets in modern times. (This is distinct from chemical weapons, which have been used many times in many settings.) Despite this, it is critical that all cases of these diseases be promptly reported to regional and national health authorities whenever they are suspected, in order to safeguard patients, clinical staff, bystanders, and public health.

Anthrax (*Bacillus anthracis*)

Bacillus anthracis is an aerobic, gram-positive, spore-forming bacterium which occurs naturally in the soil in many regions of the world. Most commonly a disease of herbivores infected through grazing in contaminated soil, anthrax may be transmitted to humans through exposure to infected animals by consumption, by inhalation of spores from wool or hides, by inoculation of the skin, or more recently by injection of contaminated drugs [5]. Shortly after the September 2001 terrorist attacks in the United States, public fears were again stoked by 22 cases of anthrax due to spores being sent to public figures in the mail, with 5 resulting deaths [6, 7]. Endemic anthrax remains an important public health threat in developing countries as well as an occasional disease of veterinarians, farmers, and injection drug users in industrialized settings.

B. anthracis produces a trio of plasmid-encoded proteins, protective antigen, edema factor, and lethal factor, which cause its virulence and are potential targets for therapy. Protective factor binds to the other two proteins, creating two toxins (edema toxin and lethal toxin) that mediate tissue injury in humans [8]. Edema toxin impairs intracellular water homeostasis, producing cellular edema. Lethal toxin stimulates high-level production of tumor necrosis factor-α and interleukin-1-β, leading to lysis of macrophages, release of additional mediators of inflammation, multisystem organ failure, and death [9].

Clinical manifestations of anthrax The presenting syndromes of anthrax vary depending on the route of exposure. Cutaneous anthrax comprises up to 95% of cases, resulting from direct inoculation of *B. anthracis* spores through skin breaks or injection, followed by germination, soft tissue necrosis, and a black "coal-like" eschar which is painless. (This lesion is the source of anthrax's name, from the Greek word for "coal.") Frequently, a surrounding rim of edema may surround the eschar, which sloughs off within 3 weeks of onset [10]. Fever, lymphangitis, and painful proximal lymphadenopathy typically accompany the lesion. Secondary hematogenous spread of the disease is common, with a mortality of 10–40% in untreated cases [11] (Fig. 6.1).

Gastrointestinal and oropharyngeal anthrax are rare forms of anthrax, most reported in rural parts of the developing world (including sub-Saharan Africa, as well as Eastern, Southern, and Central Asia). Both occur after the ingestion of contaminated and undercooked meat. In oropharyngeal disease, mucosal edema and ulceration are followed by the development of pharyngeal pseudomembranes, with the potential for airway obstruction. Gastrointestinal anthrax is highly lethal, with necrosis developing throughout the entire gastrointestinal tract with resulting pain, fever, nausea, dysentery, visceral perforation, and sepsis. In the oropharyngeal form, pseudomembranes are seen in the oropharynx, and upper airway obstruction can develop. In the gastrointestinal form, a necrotizing infection progresses from the esophagus to the cecum. Fever, nausea, vomiting, abdominal pain, gastrointestinal bleeding, and bloody diarrhea are typical symptoms. Death results from intestinal perforation or sepsis [12, 13].

Inhalational anthrax is the most lethal form of the disease, resulting from the deposition of anthrax spores into the alveoli following inhalation. Following phagocytosis by pulmonary macrophages, *B. anthracis* is transported via lymphatics to the mediastinal lymph nodes. After a period of dormancy which may last between 10 and 60 days, the endospores germinate, release edema and lethal toxin, and produce a fulminant and often lethal illness. The typical clinical course of inhalational

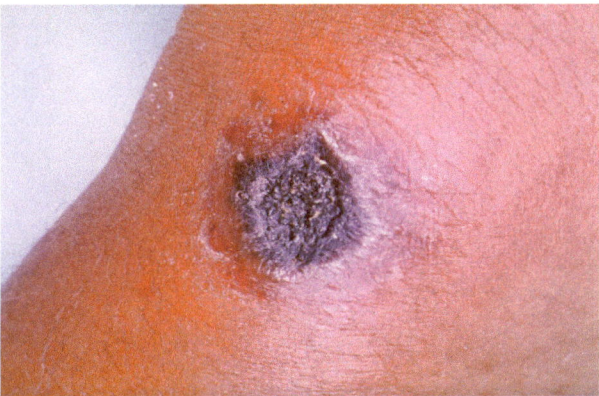

Fig. 6.1 The lesion of cutaneous anthrax, with a black central necrotic lesion surrounded by a rim of edema. (Source: Public Health Information Library, Centers for Disease Control and Prevention. Accessed online on 11 March 2019 at https://phil.cdc.gov/details_linked.aspx?pid=2033)

anthrax is biphasic, with an initial nonspecific syndrome including fever, dry cough, dyspnea, chest pain, and myalgia that may resemble a typical viral respiratory infection. After 2–3 days, severe illness follows, with hemorrhagic mediastinitis, respiratory failure, and shock [14]. Mediastinal widening and large pleural effusions are common findings; airspace opacities on chest radiography are less frequent, although a hemorrhagic necrotizing pneumonitis has been noted on autopsy specimens [15]. Clinically significant pericardial effusions and ascites occurred in 17% and 21% of victims in the Sverdlovsk outbreak, respectively, and may require drainage [16]. Bacteremia is typical and leads to a secondary meningitis in half of cases on inhalational anthrax, requiring aggressive therapy [16] (Fig. 6.2).

The diagnosis of anthrax is complex and requires a high index of suspicion, given the infrequency of this disease in industrialized countries. Typical laboratory findings include a neutrophil-predominant leukocytosis (from normal ranges to 49,600 cells per µL), elevated liver transaminases, hyponatremia, and hypoxemia [17, 18]. Chest radiography demonstrates mediastinal widening and pleural effusions, with consolidation and infiltrates less frequent. Mediastinal widening in particular is strongly suggestive of anthrax in the appropriate clinical syndrome and mandates it consideration as a diagnosis [18, 19].

Close coordination with hospital microbiology laboratories, as well as public health laboratories, is critical for the diagnosis of anthrax. Large gram-positive rods in short chains that are positive on India ink staining are presumptive of *B. anthracis* until confirmatory tests are obtained. Special culture methods are generally not necessary, as *B. anthracis* grows readily from clinical specimens on conventional media. Routine Biosafety Level 2 conditions and biosafety cabinets are adequate for staff safety. In general, most hospital laboratories will not fully characterize a suspected anthrax specimen; confirmatory testing will be performed by public health laboratories via the Centers for Disease Control and Prevention (CDC) Laboratory Response Network in the United States, Public Health England or Health Protection

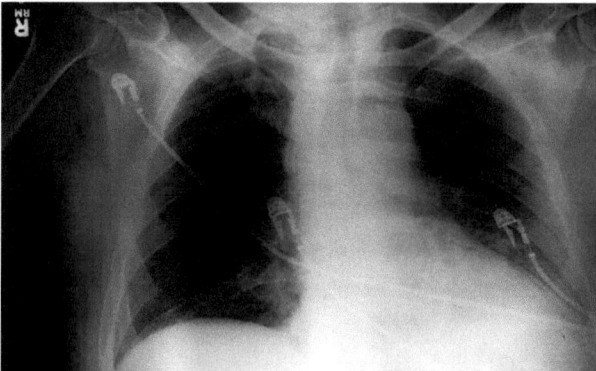

Fig. 6.2 Anteroposterior radiograph of the chest in a patient with inhalational anthrax, with a prominent superior mediastinum and possible small left pleural effusion. (Source: Jernigan JA et al. Emerg Infect Dis 2001;7:933–944)

Scotland in the United Kingdom, or comparable national agencies. In the United States, advanced anthrax diagnostics are available through the CDC, the US Army Medical Research Institute for Infectious Diseases (USAMRIID), and the Naval Medical Research Center (NMRC), including serologic testing, immunohistochemistry, and polymerase chain reaction (PCR) [20]. Recommended clinical specimens for analysis will vary by presenting syndrome and include blood culture, serum for antibody testing, plasma for direct detection of lethal factor, serosal fluid, cerebrospinal fluid, and tissue from biopsy of cutaneous eschars. A complete guide by syndrome is available from the CDC website at https://www.cdc.gov/anthrax/specificgroups/lab-professionals/recommended-specimen.html.

The treatment of anthrax also varies based on clinical syndrome and is divided into meningeal and non-meningeal disease for purposes of antimicrobial therapy. Given the increased severity and intensity of therapy for anthrax meningitis, it is recommended that patients receive either confirmation of the diagnosis via early lumbar puncture or empiric therapy directed against meningitis [21]. It is important to recognize that mortality for inhalational anthrax, with or without meningitis, carries an exceptionally high mortality even with appropriate therapy. Despite this, general critical care principles of respiratory, hemodynamic, and other organ system-based support still apply.

The empiric antimicrobial management of anthrax includes an intravenous fluoroquinolone (ciprofloxacin, levofloxacin, or moxifloxacin) with a carbapenem (meropenem or imipenem) and either a protein synthesis inhibitor or rifampin. Either clindamycin or linezolid is acceptable as a protein synthesis inhibitor; rifampin indirectly blocks protein synthesis through the inhibition of RNA polymerase (and thus messenger RNA synthesis) and appears to have comparable efficacy. Non-meningeal disease may be treated with either a fluoroquinolone or a carbapenem in combination with a protein synthesis inhibitor. Once antimicrobial susceptibility has been determined, intravenous penicillin G or ampicillin may be used in lieu of a carbapenem for susceptible isolates (see Tables 6.1 and 6.2).

Given the high risk of maternal and fetal death in anthrax infections, pregnant women should receive the same therapy as non-pregnant adults [22]. Uncomplicated cutaneous anthrax can be treated with oral ciprofloxacin or doxycycline for 7–10 days. Since concomitant inhalational exposure is difficult to exclude, however, an extended course of 60 days of therapy is usually preferred [23, 24].

In addition to antimicrobial drug therapy, routine intensive care support measures should be provided to critically ill patients with anthrax. Peritoneal effusions and ascites may serve as reservoirs for lethal toxin [25], and serosal drainage has been associated with survival in retrospective cases [18, 26]. Hemodynamic support with vasopressors may be provided as per standard practice for patients in shock; although there is limited data on the use of adjunctive corticosteroids, it is interesting to note that lethal toxin appears to repress the glucocorticoid receptor [27], and corticosteroids may have utility in the treatment of anthrax-associated airway edema in addition to vasopressor-resistant shock [20].

In combination with antibiotics and (if indicated) corticosteroids, immunotherapy is available to be given in combination with antibacterial therapy. Raxibacumab

Table 6.1 Intravenous therapy for anthrax with meningitis or if meningitis has not yet been excluded

Bactericidal agent (fluoroquinolone)
Ciprofloxacin, 400 mg every 8 h
OR
Levofloxacin, 750 mg every 24 h
OR
Moxifloxacin, 400 mg every 24 h
PLUS
Bactericidal agent (β-lactam)
For all strains, regardless of penicillin susceptibility or if susceptibility is unknown
Meropenem, 2 g every 8 h
OR
Imipenem, 1 g every 6 h[a]
Alternatives for penicillin-susceptible strains only
Penicillin G, 4 million units every 4 h
OR
Ampicillin, 3 g every 6 h
PLUS
Protein synthesis inhibitor
Linezolid, 600 mg every 12 h[b]
OR
Clindamycin, 900 mg every 8 h
OR
Rifampin, 600 mg every 12 h[c]
OR
Chloramphenicol, 1 g every 6–8 h[d]

Duration of treatment: ≥2–3 weeks until clinical criteria for stability are met. Patients exposed to aerosolized spores will require prophylaxis to complete an antimicrobial drug course of 60 days from onset of illness. Preferred drugs are indicated in boldface
[a]Increased risk for seizures associated with imipenem/cilastatin treatment
[b]Linezolid should be used with caution in patients with thrombocytopenia. Linezolid use for >14 days has additional hematopoietic toxicity
[c]Rifampin is not a protein synthesis inhibitor. However, it may be used in combination with other antimicrobial drugs on the basis of its in vitro synergy
[d]Should only be used if other options are not available because of toxicity concerns
Recommendations derived from Hendricks et al. [20]

and obiltoxaximab are two distinct monoclonal antibodies directed against protective antigen [28–31]. Anthrax immunoglobulin intravenous (AIGIV) is a purified polyclonal preparation of anti-anthrax immunoglobulin derived from vaccinated donors [32]. All three are either approved or have orphan drug status in the United States and the European Union, but none are commercially available and must be obtained from the CDC's Strategic National Stockpile. In the absence of comparative human trials, all three are reasonable options to be administered to suspected or confirmed anthrax victims.

Table 6.2 Intravenous therapy for anthrax when meningitis has been excluded

Bactericidal drug
For all strains, regardless of penicillin susceptibility or if susceptibility is unknown
Ciprofloxacin, 400 mg every 8 h
OR
Levofloxacin, 750 mg every 24 h
OR
Moxifloxacin, 400 mg every 24 h
OR
Meropenem, 2 g every 8 h
OR
Imipenem, 1 g every 6 h[a]
OR
Vancomycin, 60 mg/kg/d intravenous divided every 8 h (maintain serum trough concentrations of 15–20 μg/mL)
Alternatives for penicillin-susceptible strains
Penicillin G, 4 million units every 4 h
OR
Ampicillin, 3 g every 6 h
PLUS
Protein synthesis inhibitor
Clindamycin, 900 mg every 8 h
OR
Linezolid, 600 mg every 12 h[b]
OR
Doxycycline, 200 mg initially, then 100 mg every 12 h[c]
OR
Rifampin, 600 mg every 12 h[d]

Duration of treatment: for 2 weeks until clinical criteria for stability are met. Patients exposed to aerosolized spores will require prophylaxis to complete an antimicrobial drug course of 60 days from onset of illness. Preferred drugs are indicated in boldface
[a]Increased risk for seizures associated with imipenem/cilastatin treatment
[b]Linezolid should be used with caution in patients with thrombocytopenia because it might exacerbate it. Linezolid use for >14 days has additional hematopoietic toxicity
[c]A single 10–14-day course of doxycycline is not routinely associated with tooth staining
[d]Rifampin is not a protein synthesis inhibitor. However, it may be used in combination with other antimicrobials drugs on the basis of its in vitro synergy
Recommendations derived from Hendricks et al [20]

Prophylaxis for patients exposed to anthrax should include either oral ciprofloxacin (500 mg twice daily), levofloxacin (750 mg daily), or doxycycline (100 mg twice daily) for 60 days, regardless of laboratory test results. Nasal swab testing (by culture or PCR) can confirm exposure to anthrax in large groupings, but a negative swab does not exclude exposure in an individual. Persons exposed to penicillin-susceptible strains may receive prophylaxis with high-dose oral penicillin or amoxicillin in limited circumstances, but fluoroquinolones or doxycycline is preferred [20].

The anthrax vaccine (AVA-Biothrax, BioPort Corporation, Lansing, Michigan, USA) is the only licensed human anthrax vaccine in the United States and has received licensure in Italy, Germany, the United Kingdom, France, the Netherlands, Poland, and Singapore as of 2018. The vaccine is derived from supernatant material from cultures of a toxigenic, nonencapsulated strain of *B. anthracis*. Approximately 95% of individuals seroconvert after the third dose of vaccine; the US military currently uses a six-dose series. Headache and other systemic symptoms have been reported in 1% (101/10,722) of US military recipients, with injection site reactions in 3.6% [24].

Plague (*Yersinia pestis*)

Plague is caused by *Yersinia pestis*, a gram-negative bacillus and a relative of common pathogens including *Escherichia coli* and *Klebsiella*. *Y. pestis* is most often transmitted to humans from a rodent or rabbit reservoir via flea vectors, principally the species *Xenopsylla cheopis* worldwide [33] and *Oropsylla montana* in North America [34]. Other potential routes of transmission include direct contact with infected body fluids and the inhalation of infected respiratory droplets [35, 36]. Similar to other gram-negative infections, the lipopolysaccharide (LPS) endotoxin associated with its outer cell membrane is a major drive of virulence, implicated in the systemic inflammatory response, acute respiratory distress syndrome, and multiorgan failure associated with fatal plague [37, 38].

Other than malaria and possibly the modern human immunodeficiency virus (HIV) epidemic, few infections have had as profound effect on human history as plague. The "Justinian Plague" of the sixth century CE took the lives of an estimated 100 million people, including a Roman emperor; the better-known "Black Death" of the fourteenth century CE was responsible for over 40 million deaths, or a third of the population of Europe. In modern times, outbreaks of plague have struck China in the late nineteenth century and Vietnam during the 1960s [39]. Contemporary plague remains endemic in sub-Saharan Africa and Madagascar, where over 90% of current cases occur. In Madagascar alone, there were over 13,000 suspected cases between 1998 and 2016 [40], with a new outbreak in 2017 leading to 2400 additional cases and over 200 deaths [41].

Like anthrax, the CDC classifies plague as a Category A threat agent and potential bioweapon. An aerosolized release of 50 kg of *Yersinia pestis* over a population of five million people is estimated to be capable of causing 150,000 infections and 36,000 deaths [42]. Intentional dispersion of *Yersinia pestis* as an aerosol will lead to outbreaks of pneumonic plague, while the release of infected fleas will typically result in bubonic or septicemic plague outbreaks [36, 42, 43]. Historically, plague was described as a bioweapon in 1346 when the Tartars besieging the city of Kaffa catapulted the corpses of plague victims in the city. Plague has been used as a bioweapon by the military forces of Russia against Sweden and of Japan against China.

The biowarfare program of the United States had plague in its arsenal before the destruction of the US biological weapon stockpile in the early 1970s.

The clinical manifestations of plague vary depending on the route of exposure. Similar to anthrax, plague exists in a primarily cutaneous and lymphatic form, *bubonic plague*, and a respiratory form, *pneumonic plague*. Both modes of plague can be complicated by a third systemic form, *septicemic plague*. The incubation period and clinical manifestations vary according to mode of transmission. Eighty-five percent of plague cases diagnosed in the United States are bubonic, 10–12% are primary septicemic, and roughly 3% are primary pneumonic plague [43]. Bubonic plague may progress to septicemic or pneumonic plague in 23% and 9% of cases, respectively. Data on plague in pregnancy is limited [36, 44–47]. Less common forms of plague, such as pharyngeal plague and plague meningitis, occur less frequently.

Bubonic plague is the most common form of naturally occurring plague. After entering the body through a fleabite, bacteria migrate via cutaneous lymphatics to the regional lymph nodes. After evading host defenses, *Y. pestis* replicates within lymph nodes, with the resulting lymphadenitis producing the signature lesion known as the "bubo." Most buboes develop in the groin, axilla, or neck. These enlarged lymph nodes are necrotic and contain dense concentrations of bacteria [48, 49]. Endotoxin and other virulence factors subsequently contribute to disease progression, bacteremia, sepsis, and often death [35–37, 50–54]. Patients with suspected bubonic plague should be managed with strict contact precautions, including the use of gowns, gloves, and surgical masks by clinical staff (Fig 6.3).

Plague is highly contagious by the airborne route. Inhalation of aerosolized droplets of *Y. pestis* from an infected host, including particles from a draining bubo,

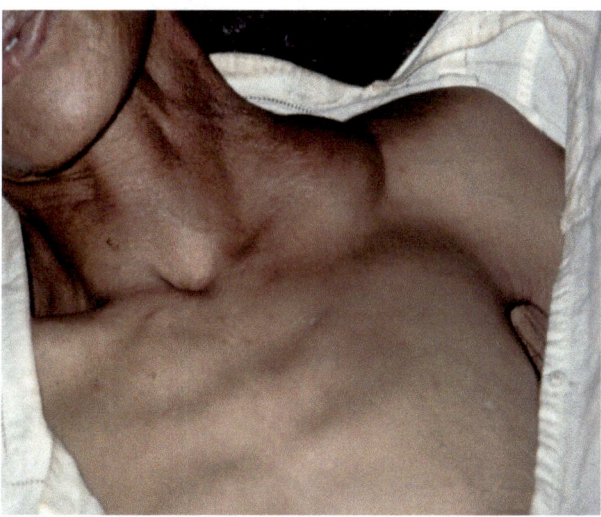

Fig. 6.3 A cervical bubo in a patient in Madagascar with bubonic plague. (Source: Prentice MB, Rahalison L. Lancet 2007; 369:1196–1207)

results in primary **pneumonic plague,** a rapidly progressive pneumonia with sepsis that is rapidly fatal without prompt treatment. Secondary pneumonic plague may occur in up to 12% of individuals with bubonic or primary septicemic plague following the hematogenous spread of *Y. pestis* to the lungs. After 1–6 days of incubation, there is a rapid onset of fever, dyspnea, chest pain, and a productive cough. Acute hypoxemic respiratory failure is common and often requires mechanical ventilation. Bilateral alveolar opacities, pleural effusions, and occasional cavitation are common features on chest radiography. Secondary pneumonic plague may have a nodular, miliary appearance associated with hematogenous spread. Hilar node enlargement is often present [55].

Because of the high risk of transmission, the strict use of droplet precautions by clinical staff is mandatory, in addition to gowns and glove use, until effective antimicrobial therapy has been received by the patient for at least 48 hours. Chemoprophylaxis should be given to potentially exposed personnel. Although N95 respirators are not strictly necessary for protection against plague, other high-consequence pathogens presenting with fulminant respiratory disease do require such protection. Given the rarity of plague in most settings, strong consideration for N95 respirator use should be made in the initial phases of evaluation of suspected plague [56–58]. The untreated mortality rate of primary pneumonic plague is 100% [59] (Fig. 6.4).

Primary **septicemic plague** results from the direct inoculation of *Y. pestis* bacilli into the bloodstream, presenting as a febrile sepsis syndrome similar to other gram-negative bacteremias with delirium, hypotension, and nausea. Secondary septicemic plague occurs as a result of progression of either bubonic or pneumonic

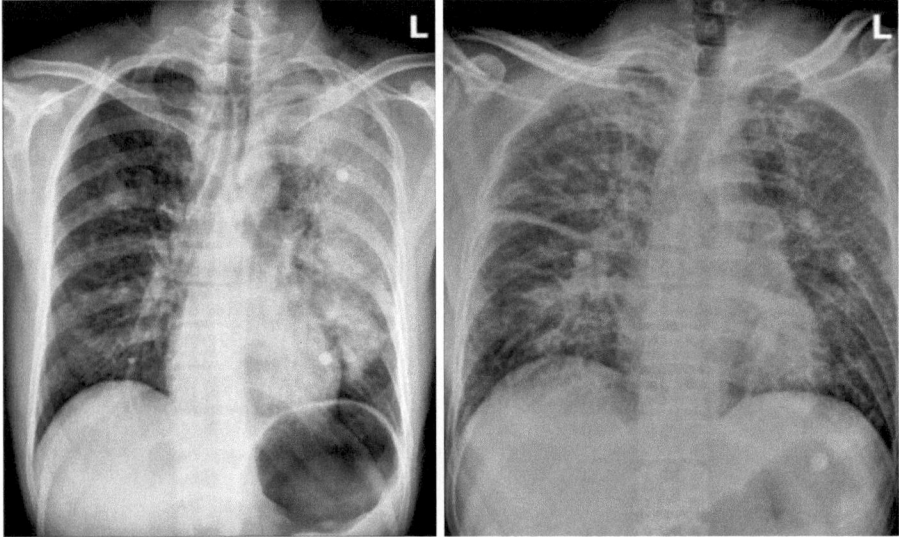

Fig. 6.4 Posteroanterior chest radiographs of patients with pneumonic plague (Source: Lin YF et al., BMC Infect Dis 2016;16:85)

infections with resulting bacteremia. Meningitis infrequently occurs after hematogenous spread [35, 36]. Abdominal pain, hepatosplenomegaly, disseminated intravascular coagulation, digital gangrene, and purpura fulminans are common features. Similar to pneumonic plague, untreated mortality rate of septicemic plague is 100%, with a high mortality even with rapid critical care intervention [36, 40, 60, 61].

The **laboratory diagnosis of plague** is based on general hematologic and chemical parameters, culture, serology, and molecular assays. A leukocytosis with neutrophilic predominance and band forms is typical, with coagulopathy, increased levels of liver transaminases, and elevated creatinine occurring in more severe illness. Gram stains of lymph node aspirates, sputum, or blood may demonstrate gram-negative bacilli with bipolar staining, similar to other *Enterobacteriaceae*. Cultures may be positive for *Y. pestis* within 24–48 hours. Although some automated bacterial identification systems may misidentify *Y. pestis*, newer mass spectrometry systems based on matrix-assisted laser desorption/ionization time of flight (MALDI-TOF) can identify *Y. pestis* rapidly and reliably following culture growth [62]. Additional tests for detection and confirmation include detection of the *Y. pestis* F1 antigen, IgM immunoassays, PCR, and immunohistochemistry on formalin-fixed tissues [63]; these tests are most often available at regional and national reference laboratories, such as the CDC and Laboratory Response Network in the United States or the Emerging and Vector-borne Diseases Programme in the European Union.

Plague should be suspected in persons with fever and lymphadenopathy if they reside in, or have recently traveled to, a plague-endemic area and if bipolar-staining, gram-negative bacilli are seen in affected tissues. The diagnosis of plague should be presumed if immunofluorescence staining of smear or material is positive for the presence of *Y. pestis* F1 antigen or if a single serum specimen shows levels of antibody to the F1 antigen at a titer of 1:10 or greater. Confirmation of plague may be based on a single anti-F1 antibody titer of more than 1:128 dilution or a fourfold rise in paired anti-F1 antibody titers [64]. Multiple cases of pneumonic plague in a nonendemic area should raise concern for bioterrorism. Treatment of suspected plague should not be delayed while awaiting diagnostic confirmation, although pre-antibiotic cultures and specimens should be obtained as best possible.

The recommended antimicrobial drugs for the **treatment of plague** are streptomycin or, more commonly, gentamicin. Current US recommendations are listed on Table 6.2. Doxycycline has shown efficacy comparable to gentamicin in a small randomized trial in patients with principally bubonic plague [65]. Fluoroquinolones and chloramphenicol are alternative agents with acceptable efficacy [66–69]. Methylprednisolone and imipenem have shown evidence of efficacy in murine models of plague but lack supporting human data at this time [70, 71]. Treatment should last for 10–14 days. Oral therapy may be initiated once a patient demonstrates clinical stabilization and improvement.

The intentional release of plague, with exposure of large numbers of patients through a presumably respiratory route, may require alternative approaches to therapy. Symptomatic patients should ideally receive treatment with a parenteral aminoglycoside as described above, but oral ciprofloxacin (taken as 500 mg twice daily) and doxycycline (100 mg twice daily) are appropriate options for treatment and for post-exposure prophylaxis, including for persons who come within 2 meters of an infected patient with pneumonic plague [72].

In addition to appropriate post-exposure prophylaxis, the prevention of plague relies on careful infection prevention practices. There is presently no commercially available vaccine against plague. Patients suspected of plague should be placed immediately into droplet precautions, with access to the patient room restricted to essential staff. Gowns, gloves, surgical masks, and eye protection should be worn by all staff. Aerosolizing procedures should be kept to an absolute minimum and avoided if possible. As noted before, negative pressure isolation with N95 masks is not necessary for plague, although infections that may present similarly to pneumonic plague (e.g., severe coronavirus infections such as SARS or MERS) may require negative pressure rooms or PAPRs, thus requiring a higher level of protection while diagnostic testing is underway. Following 48 hours of therapy with appropriate antibiotics and with clear clinical improvement, patients with both nonpneumonic plague and pneumonic plague may be removed from isolation [73] (Table 6.3).

Table 6.3 Antimicrobial therapy guidelines for the treatment of plague

	Antibiotic	Dose	Route of administration	Notes
Adults	Streptomycin	1 g twice daily	IM	Not widely available in the United States
	Gentamicin	5 mg/kg once daily, or 2 mg/kg loading dose followed by 1.7 mg/kg every 8 hours	IM or IV	Not FDA approved but considered an effective alternative to streptomycin[1] Due to poor abscess penetration, consider alternative or dual therapy for patients with bubonic disease
	Levofloxacin	500 mg once daily	IV or PO	Bactericidal. FDA approved based on animal studies but limited clinical experience treating human plague. A higher dose (750 mg) may be used if clinically indicated
	Ciprofloxacin	400 mg every 8–12 hours	IV	Bactericidal. FDA approved based on animal studies but limited clinical experience treating human plague
		500–750 mg twice daily	PO	
	Doxycycline	100 mg twice daily or 200 mg once daily	IV or PO	Bacteriostatic but effective in a randomized trial when compared to gentamicin[2]
	Moxifloxacin	400 mg once daily	IV or PO	
	Chloramphenicol	25 mg/kg every 6 hours	IV	Not widely available in the United States

Table 6.3 (continued)

	Antibiotic	Dose	Route of administration	Notes
Children[3]	Streptomycin	15 mg/kg twice daily (maximum 2 g/day)	IM	Not widely available in the United States
	Gentamicin	2.5 mg/kg/dose every 8 hours	IM or IV	Not FDA approved but considered an effective alternative to streptomycin.[1] Due to poor abscess penetration, consider alternative or dual therapy for patients with bubonic disease
	Levofloxacin	10 mg/kg/dose (maximum 500 mg/dose)	IV or PO	Bactericidal. FDA approved based on animal studies but limited clinical experience treating human plague
	>Ciprofloxacin	15 mg/kg/dose every 12 hours (maximum 400 mg/dose)	IV	Bactericidal. FDA approved based on animal studies but limited clinical experience treating human plague
		20 mg/kg/dose every 12 hours (maximum 500 mg/dose)	PO	
	Doxycycline	Weight <45 kg: 2.2 mg/kg twice daily (maximum 100 mg/dose) Weight ≥45 kg: same as adult dose	IV or PO	Bacteriostatic, but FDA approved and effective in a randomized trial when compared to gentamicin.[2] No tooth staining after multiple short courses[4]
	Chloramphenicol (for children >2 years)	25 mg/kg every 6 h (maximum daily dose, 4 g)	IV	Not widely available in the United States
Pregnant women[3]	Gentamicin	Same as adult dose	IM or IV	See notes above
	Doxycycline	Same as adult dose	IV	See notes above
	Ciprofloxacin	Same as adult dose	IV	See notes above

IV intravenous; *IM* intramuscular; *PO* by mouth
[1]Boulanger et al. [88]
[2]Mwengee et al. [65]
[3]All recommended antibiotics for plague have relative contraindications for use in children and pregnant women; however, use is justified in life-threatening situations
[4]Todd et al. [87]
Source: Centers for Disease Control and Prevention. Accessed online on 11 March 2019 at https://www.cdc.gov/plague/healthcare/clinicians.html

Tularemia (*Francisella tularensis*)

Tularemia is caused by *Francisella tularensis*, an intracellular, aerobic gram-negative coccobacillus. Similar to plague, it has a natural small-mammal reservoir of rabbits and rodents. Also similar to plague and anthrax, tularemia occurs in a primarily respiratory form (pneumonic tularemia) and in a primarily cutaneous and lymphatic form (ulceroglandular tularemia). The United States and the former Soviet Union developed biological weapons that could disperse *F. tularensis* in the mid-twentieth century [42], and there remains a concern that *F. tularensis* could be used as an agent of bioterrorism.

F. tularensis can survive in soil, water, and animal carcasses for many weeks. Chlorination of water prevents its spread through water contamination. As few as ten organisms may be sufficient to cause human disease [74]. Human transmission most often results from tick and flea bites, animal handling, ingestion of contaminated food and water, and inhalation of aerosols. Unlike plague, there is no direct human-to-human transmission. Deliberate aerosolized dispersion of *F. tularensis* is hypothesized to cause large-scale outbreaks of severe respiratory disease [9, 75].

Tularemia is endemic throughout the northern hemisphere. Approximately 80–150 cases per year occur in the United States, with the highest incidence in south-central and western states. The predominant mode of transmission to humans in the United States is·by tick bites, most often in spring and summer, with hunting and similar outdoor activities associated with an increased risk of exposure [76]. In Europe, the incidence of tularemia is considerably higher, with over 1000 cases per year in Hungary and the Czech Republic and over 4000 cases per year in Sweden and Finland. Mosquito-borne transmission or consumption of contaminated water predominates as a mode of exposure in parts of Europe, although these vary by country [77].

F. tularensis infected humans via the conjunctiva, respiratory tract, gut, or breaks in the skin. Organisms are taken up by and replicate within macrophages, leading to apoptosis of the macrophage and release into local lymph nodes as well as bacteremia [74]. This bacteremia leads to secondary seeding of the lungs, pleura, spleen, liver, and kidney. Pathologic examination of infected tissue may show granulomatous inflammation with necrosis. Following inhalational exposure, hemorrhagic airway inflammation may progress to pneumonia, pleuritis, and pleural effusion. Human immunity is principally cell-mediated, with antibody responses playing a role in diagnosis but having an uncertain contribution to host defense.

The clinical manifestations of tularemia depend on the site of entry, exposure dose, and host immune factors. Based on the site of initial infection and presenting syndrome, tularemia may be described as primary pneumonic, typhoidal, ulceroglandular, oculoglandular, oropharyngeal, or septic. Ulceroglandular tularemia is the most common form of the infection, typically following with a week of a vector bite or animal contact. A majority of patients present with fever (85%), with chills (52%), headache (45%), cough (38%), and myalgias (31%) occurring in many. Other nonspecific constitutional symptoms occur with variable frequency, such as chest and abdominal pain, nausea, vomiting, and diarrhea. The hallmark lesion is a tender papule at the site of initial inoculation which subsequently ulcerates, with painful enlarged lymphadenopathy proximal to the ulcer. This lesion may clinically resemble a plague bubo, and plague must be considered in the differential diagnosis. A purely "glandular" form, with lymphadenopathy but no visible ulcer, can occur as well. In cases of ingestion of contaminated material, an exudative pharyngitis and tonsillitis may develop, with subsequent pharyngeal ulceration and cervical lymphadenopathy. Inoculation of the eye will lead to oculoglandular tularemia, also with accompanying cervical lymphadenopathy. Cases of systemic tularemia without clinically apparent lymphadenopathy are known as typhoidal tularemia. Fever, diarrhea, shock, and meningeal signs are typical (Figs. 6.5 and 6.6).

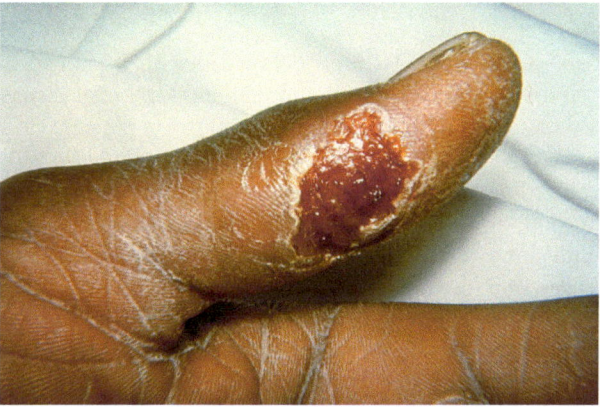

Fig. 6.5 Cutaneous ulcer due to ulceroglandular tularemia. (Source: Public Health Information Library, Centers for Disease Control and Prevention. Accessed online on 11 March 2019 at https://phil.cdc.gov/Details.aspx?pid=1344)

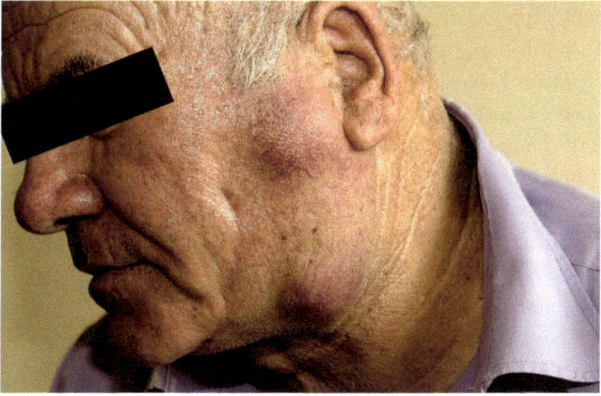

Fig. 6.6 Typical clinical presentation of oculoglandular tularemia with ocular congestion and pre-auricular and cervical lymphadenitis. (Source: Ulu-Kilic A, Doganay M, Travel Med Infect Dis 2014; 12:609–616)

Pneumonic tularemia results from the inhalation of aerosolized organisms or from hematogenous spread from other sites of infection. Following the inhalation of the organism, patients may suffer initially from nonspecific fever and chills, followed by a dry or minimally productive cough, pleurisy, dyspnea, and subsequently hemoptysis. Respiratory symptoms were absent in nearly half of patients in a recent series from Finland, however [78]. Pleural effusions are common and may be unilateral or bilateral. Pneumonic tularemia can progress rapidly to acute hypoxemic respiratory failure, disseminated intravascular coagulation, rhabdomyolysis, and eventually multiorgan failure [9, 74]. Virtually any organ may be involved in severe tularemia, including peritonitis, pericarditis, appendicitis, osteomyelitis, and meningitis, although such presentations are less frequent than the more "classic" forms. The mortality rate of untreated pneumonic tularemia is 60%, but rapid institution of antimicrobial therapy reduces the morality rate to 2.5% or less [74, 79].

The diagnosis of tularemia is often delayed due to its nonspecific presenting signs and symptoms, in the case of pneumonic and typhoidal disease, and may be confounded by clinical similarity to plague or anthrax in the case of ulceroglandular disease. Delayed or absent response to routine treatment for skin ulcers or community-acquired pneumonia may serve as diagnostic clues, as may be a history of animal, arthropod, or outdoor freshwater exposure. Routine laboratory tests usually lack distinguishing features and may include a mild lymphocytosis, elevated liver transaminases, and markers of rhabdomyolysis such as elevated serum creatine kinase concentration and urine myoglobin [74, 79].

Chest radiographs most often show unilateral or bilateral airspace opacities, with hilar adenopathy and pleural effusion in approximately 30% each. Cavitation occurs in approximately 15% of cases [80]. Chest radiographs may be normal in 7% of patients, although computed tomography reveals thoracic pathology in the great majority [78].

Although *F. tularensis* may be cultivated from blood, tissue, or sputum in the clinical microbiology laboratory, it requires specialized media (usually cysteine-enriched) to grow. Special precautions must be taken for the protection of laboratory staff, similar to plague and anthrax; like the other pathogens of interest, clinicians must notify the microbiology laboratory in the event of a suspected case. Routine microbiology procedures can be performed in Biosafety Level 2 conditions with a biological safety cabinet, but aerosolizing procedures must occur under Biosafety Level 3 conditions [79].

Serologic diagnosis may be utilized given the challenges involved in culturing *Francisella*. Serum testing by enzyme-linked immunosorbent assay (ELISA) may be negative early in illness but typically produces a fourfold rise in titer over the course of the disease; a single anti-*F. tularensis* IgG titer of 1:160 is sufficient to support the diagnosis, however [81]. As the ELISA detects antibodies against the bacterial endotoxin, false-positive tests may arise in cases of infections with bacteria that have structurally similar endotoxin, including *Brucella*, *Proteus*, and *Yersinia* species. Confirmatory testing with Western blot, immunofluorescence, or microagglutination titer testing will improve the specificity of ELISA testing [81–83]. Antigen detection methods, such as direct fluorescent antibodies or immunochemical stains, may be performed on tissue specimens, along with PCR-based testing which may be valuable in outbreak settings [84, 85].

The standard treatment for tularemia in adults is streptomycin, 10–15 mg per kg, given intramuscularly (IM) or intravenously (IV) twice daily, but gentamicin, 5 mg per kg, given IM or IV once daily, is equivalent in efficacy and is the standard therapy nowadays. Milder cases of ulceroglandular disease may be treated with doxycycline (IV or oral). Fluoroquinolones or chloramphenicol may be given in selected cases when available; beta-lactams and macrolides are not recommended. Treatment with streptomycin, gentamicin, or ciprofloxacin should be continued for 10 days. Treatment with doxycycline or chloramphenicol should be continued for 14–21 days. Patients beginning treatment with doxycycline, chloramphenicol, or ciprofloxacin can be switched to oral antibiotics when clinically improving and tolerating oral medications. Complete medication recommendations may be seen on Table 6.4.

Chemoprophylactic regimens for the prevention of tularemia are similar to those used for plague. Individuals exposed to *F. tularensis* may be protected against systemic infection if they receive prophylactic antibiotics during the incubation period. For post-exposure prophylaxis, either doxycycline or ciprofloxacin, taken orally twice daily for 14 days, is a recommended regimen. Ciprofloxacin is generally preferred over doxycycline in pregnancy, but either are acceptable given the risk of serious disease and the low risk of skeletal abnormalities in the fetus with such relatively brief tetracycline exposure [79].

A live attenuated vaccine, first developed in Russia, is not generally available but has been given in the United States by the US Army Medical Research Institute of Infectious Diseases (USAMRIID) as an investigational new drug. The vaccine is administered via scarification, similar to smallpox vaccines. Due to dwindling stocks of the original vaccine strain, a newer attenuated strain was tested in a recent phase 2 trial, with the novel vaccine showing high rates of seroconversion among recipients [86].

Disclaimer

Table 6.4 Recommended antimicrobial drugs for the treatment of tularemia

	Preferred choices	Alternative choices	Choices for mass casualty settings or post-exposure prophylaxis
Adults	Streptomycin 1 g IM twice daily × 10 days	Doxycycline 100 mg IV twice daily × 14–21 days	Doxycycline 100 mg orally twice daily × 14 days
	Gentamicin 5 mg/kg IM or IV once daily × 10 days	Chloramphenicol 15 mg/kg IV 4 times daily × 14–21 days Ciprofloxacin 400 mg IV twice daily × 14–21 days	Ciprofloxacin 500 mg orally twice daily × 14 days
Children	Streptomycin 15 mg/ kg IM twice daily × 10 days	Doxycycline × 14–21 days: 100 mg IV twice daily if = or >45 kg 2.2 mg/kg IV twice daily if <45 kg	Doxycycline × 14 days 100 mg orally twice daily if = or >45 kg Give 2.2 mg/kg orally twice daily if <45 kg
	Gentamicin 2.5 mg/kg IM or IV three times daily × 10 days	Chloramphenicol 15 mg/kg IV 4 times daily × 14–21 days Ciprofloxacin 15 mg/kg mg IV twice daily × 10 days	Ciprofloxacin 15 mg/kg mg orally twice daily × 14 days
Pregnant women	Streptomycin 1 g IM twice daily × 10 days	Doxycycline 100 mg IV twice daily × 14–21 days	Ciprofloxacin 500 mg orally twice daily × 14 days
	Gentamicin 5 mg/kg IM or IV once daily × 10 days	Ciprofloxacin 400 mg IV twice daily × 10 days	Doxycycline 100 mg orally twice daily × 14 days

Adapted from Dennis et al. [36]

References

1. Taylor LH, Latham SM, Woolhouse ME. Risk factors for human disease emergence. Philos Trans R Soc Lond Ser B Biol Sci. 2001;356:983–9.
2. Barras V, Greub G. History of biological warfare and bioterrorism. Clin Microbiol Infect. 2014;20:497–502.
3. Meselson M, Guillemin J, Hugh-Jones M, et al. The Sverdlovsk anthrax outbreak of 1979. Science. 1994;266:1202–8.
4. Jaton K, Greub G. Clinical microbiologists facing an anthrax alert. Clin Microbiol Infect. 2014;20:503–6.
5. Vieira AR, Salzer JS, Traxler RM, et al. Enhancing surveillance and diagnostics in anthrax-endemic countries. Emerg Infect Dis. 2017;23.
6. Bush LM, Abrams BH, Beall A, Johnson CC. Index case of fatal inhalational anthrax due to bioterrorism in the United States. N Engl J Med. 2001;345:1607–10.
7. Hughes JM, Gerberding JL. Anthrax bioterrorism: lessons learned and future directions. Emerg Infect Dis. 2002;8:1013–4.
8. Friebe S, van der Goot FG, Burgi J. The ins and outs of anthrax toxin. Toxins (Basel). 2016;8.
9. Adalja AA, Toner E, Inglesby TV. Clinical management of potential bioterrorism-related conditions. N Engl J Med. 2015;372:954–62.
10. Shafazand S. When bioterrorism strikes: diagnosis and management of inhalational anthrax. Semin Respir Infect. 2003;18:134–45.

11. Doganay M, Metan G, Alp E. A review of cutaneous anthrax and its outcome. J Infect Public Health. 2010;3:98–105.
12. Sirisanthana T, Brown AE. Anthrax of the gastrointestinal tract. Emerg Infect Dis. 2002;8:649–51.
13. Purcell B, Worsham P, Friedlander A. Anthrax. In: Dembek ZS, editor. Medical aspects of biological warfare. Falls Church, VA: Borden Institute and US Army Office of the Surgeon General; 2007.
14. Barakat LA, Quentzel HL, Jernigan JA, et al. Fatal inhalational anthrax in a 94-year-old Connecticut woman. JAMA. 2002;287:863–8.
15. Abramova FA, Grinberg LM, Yampolskaya OV, Walker DH. Pathology of inhalational anthrax in 42 cases from the Sverdlovsk outbreak of 1979. Proc Natl Acad Sci U S A. 1993;90:2291–4.
16. Bower WA, Hendricks K, Pillai S, et al. Clinical framework and medical countermeasure use during an anthrax mass-casualty incident. MMWR Recomm Rep. 2015;64:1–22.
17. Mayer TA, Bersoff-Matcha S, Murphy C, et al. Clinical presentation of inhalational anthrax following bioterrorism exposure: report of 2 surviving patients. JAMA. 2001;286:2549–53.
18. Holty JE, Bravata DM, Liu H, Olshen RA, McDonald KM, Owens DK. Systematic review: a century of inhalational anthrax cases from 1900 to 2005. Ann Intern Med. 2006;144:270–80.
19. Holty JE, Kim RY, Bravata DM. Anthrax: a systematic review of atypical presentations. Ann Emerg Med. 2006;48:200–11.
20. Hendricks KA, Wright ME, Shadomy SV, et al. Centers for disease control and prevention expert panel meetings on prevention and treatment of anthrax in adults. Emerg Infect Dis. 2014;20:e130687.
21. Katharios-Lanwermeyer S, Holty JE, Person M, et al. Identifying meningitis during an anthrax mass casualty incident: systematic review of systemic anthrax since 1880. Clinical Infect Dis. 2016;62:1537–45.
22. Meaney-Delman D, Zotti ME, Creanga AA, et al. Special considerations for prophylaxis for and treatment of anthrax in pregnant and postpartum women. Emerg Infect Dis. 2014;20.
23. Bartlett JG, Inglesby TV Jr, Borio L. Management of anthrax. Clin Infect Dis. 2002;35:851–8.
24. Inglesby TV, O'Toole T, Henderson DA, et al. Anthrax as a biological weapon, 2002: updated recommendations for management. JAMA. 2002;287:2236–52.
25. Walsh JJ, Pesik N, Quinn CP, et al. A case of naturally acquired inhalation anthrax: clinical care and analyses of anti-protective antigen immunoglobulin G and lethal factor. Clin Infect Dis. 2007;44:968–71.
26. Klempner MS, Talbot EA, Lee SI, Zaki S, Ferraro MJ. Case records of the Massachusetts General Hospital. Case 25-2010. A 24-year-old woman with abdominal pain and shock. N Engl J Med. 2010;363:766–77.
27. Webster JI, Moayeri M, Sternberg EM. Novel repression of the glucocorticoid receptor by anthrax lethal toxin. Ann N Y Acad Sci. 2004;1024:9–23.
28. Yamamoto BJ, Shadiack AM, Carpenter S, et al. Efficacy projection of obiltoxaximab for treatment of inhalational anthrax across a range of disease severity. Antimicrob Agents Chemother. 2016;60:5787–95.
29. Yamamoto BJ, Shadiack AM, Carpenter S, et al. Obiltoxaximab prevents disseminated Bacillus anthracis infection and improves survival during pre- and postexposure prophylaxis in animal models of inhalational anthrax. Antimicrob Agents Chemother. 2016;60:5796–805.
30. Migone TS, Bolmer S, Zhong J, et al. Added benefit of raxibacumab to antibiotic treatment of inhalational anthrax. Antimicrob Agents Chemother. 2015;59:1145–51.
31. Kummerfeldt CE. Raxibacumab: potential role in the treatment of inhalational anthrax. Infect Drug Resist. 2014;7:101–9.
32. Kammanadiminti S, Patnaikuni RK, Comer J, Meister G, Sinclair C, Kodihalli S. Combination therapy with antibiotics and anthrax immune globulin intravenous (AIGIV) is potentially more effective than antibiotics alone in rabbit model of inhalational anthrax. PLoS One. 2014;9:e106393.

33. Andrianaivoarimanana V, Kreppel K, Elissa N, et al. Understanding the persistence of plague foci in Madagascar. PLoS Negl Trop Dis. 2013;7:e2382.
34. Hinnebusch BJ, Bland DM, Bosio CF, Jarrett CO. Comparative ability of Oropsylla montana and Xenopsylla cheopis fleas to transmit Yersinia pestis by two different mechanisms. PLoS Negl Trop Dis. 2017;11:e0005276.
35. Smego RA, Frean J, Koornhof HJ. Yersiniosis I: microbiological and clinicoepidemiological aspects of plague and non-plague Yersinia infections. Eur J Clin Microbiol Infect Dis. 1999;18:1–15.
36. Inglesby TV, Dennis DT, Henderson DA, et al. Plague as a biological weapon: medical and public health managemen. Working Group on Civilian Biodefense t. JAMA. 2000;283:2281–90.
37. Atkinson S, Williams P. Yersinia virulence factors – a sophisticated arsenal for combating host defences. F1000Res. 2016;5.
38. Knirel YA, Anisimov AP. Lipopolysaccharide of Yersinia pestis, the cause of plague: structure, genetics, biological properties. Acta Nat. 2012;4:46–58.
39. Khan IA. Plague: the dreadful visitation occupying the human mind for centuries. Trans R Soc Trop Med Hyg. 2004;98:270–7.
40. Andrianaivoarimanana V, Piola P, Wagner DM, et al. Trends of human plague, Madagascar, 1998–2016. Emerg Infect Dis. 2019;25:220–8.
41. Mead PS. Plague in Madagascar – a tragic opportunity for improving public health. N Engl J Med. 2018;378:106–8.
42. Christopher GW, Cieslak TJ, Pavlin JA, Eitzen EM Jr. Biological warfare. A historical perspective. JAMA. 1997;278:412–7.
43. Kwit N, Nelson C, Kugeler K, et al. Human plague - United States, 2015. MMWR Morb Mortal Wkly Rep. 2015;64:918–9.
44. Crook LD, Tempest B. Plague. A clinical review of 27 cases. Arch Intern Med. 1992;152:1253–6.
45. Watson AK, Ellington S, Nelson C, Treadwell T, Jamieson DJ, Meaney-Delman DM. Preparing for biological threats: addressing the needs of pregnant women. Birth Defects Res. 2017;109:391–8.
46. Wong TW. Plague in a pregnant patient. Trop Dr. 1986;16:187–9.
47. Welty TK, Grabman J, Kompare E, et al. Nineteen cases of plague in Arizona. A spectrum including ecthyma gangrenosum due to plague and plague in pregnancy. West J Med. 1985;142:641–6.
48. Guinet F, Ave P, Filali S, et al. Dissociation of tissue destruction and bacterial expansion during bubonic plague. PLoS Pathog. 2015;11:e1005222.
49. Guinet F, Ave P, Jones L, Huerre M, Carniel E. Defective innate cell response and lymph node infiltration specify Yersinia pestis infection. PLoS One. 2008;3:e1688.
50. Sodeinde OA, Subrahmanyam YV, Stark K, Quan T, Bao Y, Goguen JD. A surface protease and the invasive character of plague. Science. 1992;258:1004–7.
51. Straley SC. The plasmid-encoded outer-membrane proteins of Yersinia pestis. Rev Infect Dis. 1988;10 Suppl 2:S323–6.
52. Straley SC, Skrzypek E, Plano GV, Bliska JB. Yops of Yersinia spp. pathogenic for humans. Infect Immun. 1993;61:3105–10.
53. Lemaitre N, Sebbane F, Long D, Hinnebusch BJ. Yersinia pestis YopJ suppresses tumor necrosis factor alpha induction and contributes to apoptosis of immune cells in the lymph node but is not required for virulence in a rat model of bubonic plague. Infect Immun. 2006;74:5126–31.
54. Zhou D, Han Y, Yang R. Molecular and physiological insights into plague transmission, virulence and etiology. Microbes Infect. 2006;8:273–84.
55. Ketai L, Tchoyoson Lim CC. Radiology of biological weapons--old and the new? Semin Roentgenol. 2007;42:49–59.
56. Siegel JD, Rhinehart E, Jackson M, Chiarello L; the Healthcare Infection Control Practices Advisory Committee. 2007 Guideline for Isolation Precautions: Preventing Transmission of Infectious Agents in Healthcare Settings. Updated September 2018. Accessed online on 11 March 2019 at https://www.cdc.gov/infectioncontrol/guidelines/isolation/index.html.

57. Pechous RD, Sivaraman V, Stasulli NM, Goldman WE. Pneumonic plague: the darker side of Yersinia pestis. Trends Microbiol. 2016;24:190–7.
58. Silver S. Laboratory-acquired lethal infections by potential bioweapons pathogens including Ebola in 2014. FEMS Microbiol Lett. 2015;362:1–6.
59. Kugeler KJ, Staples JE, Hinckley AF, Gage KL, Mead PS. Epidemiology of human plague in the United States, 1900–2012. Emerg Infect Dis. 2015;21:16–22.
60. Forrester JD, Apangu T, Griffith K, et al. Patterns of human plague in Uganda, 2008–2016. Emerg Infect Dis. 2017;23:1517–21.
61. Hull HF, Montes JM, Mann JM. Septicemic plague in New Mexico. J Infect Dis. 1987;155:113–8.
62. Tourdjman M, Ibraheem M, Brett M, et al. Misidentification of Yersinia pestis by automated systems, resulting in delayed diagnoses of human plague infections--Oregon and New Mexico, 2010–2011. Clin Infect Dis. 2012;55:e58–60.
63. Demeure CE, Dussurget O, Mas Fiol G, Le Guern AS, Savin C, Pizarro-Cerda J. Yersinia pestis and plague: an updated view on evolution, virulence determinants, immune subversion, vaccination, and diagnostics. Genes Immun. 2019;20:357.
64. Koirala J. Plague: disease, management, and recognition of act of terrorism. Infect Dis Clin N Am. 2006;20:273–87, viii.
65. Mwengee W, Butler T, Mgema S, Mhina G, Almasi Y, Bradley C, Formanik JB, Rochester CG. Treatment of plague with gentamicin or doxycycline in a randomized clinical trial in Tanzania. Clin Infect Dis. 2006;42(5):614–21.
66. Russell P, Eley SM, Green M, et al. Efficacy of doxycycline and ciprofloxacin against experimental Yersinia pestis infection. J Antimicrob Chemother. 1998;41:301–5.
67. Steward J, Lever MS, Russell P, et al. Efficacy of the latest fluoroquinolones against experimental Yersinia pestis. Int J Antimicrob Agents. 2004;24:609–12.
68. Heine HS, Hershfield J, Marchand C, et al. In vitro antibiotic susceptibilities of Yersinia pestis determined by broth microdilution following CLSI methods. Antimicrob Agents Chemother. 2015;59:1919–21.
69. Wendte JM, Ponnusamy D, Reiber D, Blair JL, Clinkenbeard KD. In vitro efficacy of antibiotics commonly used to treat human plague against intracellular Yersinia pestis. Antimicrob Agents Chemother. 2011;55:3752–7.
70. Levy Y, Vagima Y, Tidhar A, et al. Adjunctive corticosteroid treatment against Yersinia pestis improves bacterial clearance, immunopathology, and survival in the mouse model of bubonic plague. J Infect Dis. 2016;214:970–7.
71. Heine HS, Louie A, Adamovicz JJ, et al. Evaluation of imipenem for prophylaxis and therapy of Yersinia pestis delivered by aerosol in a mouse model of pneumonic plague. Antimicrob Agents Chemother. 2014;58:3276–84.
72. Inglesby TV, Henderson DA, O'Toole T, Dennis DT. Safety precautions to limit exposure from plague-infected patients. JAMA. 2000;284:1648–9.
73. Siegel JD, Rhinehart E, Jackson M, Chiarello L, the Healthcare infection Control Practices Advisory Committee. 2007 Guideline for isolation precautions: preventing transmission of infectious agents in healthcare settings. Atlanta: Centers for Disease Control and Prevention; 2007.
74. Hepburn MJ, Simpson AJ. Tularemia: current diagnosis and treatment options. Expert Rev Anti-Infect Ther. 2008;6:231–40.
75. Balali-Mood M, Moshiri M, Etemad L. Medical aspects of bio-terrorism. Toxicon. 2013;69:131–42.
76. Centers for Disease C, Prevention. Tularemia – United States, 2001–2010. MMWR Morb Mortal Wkly Rep. 2013;62:963–6.
77. Maurin M, Gyuranecz M. Tularaemia: clinical aspects in Europe. Lancet Infect Dis. 2016; 16:113–24.
78. Vayrynen SA, Saarela E, Henry J, Lahti S, Harju T, Kauma H. Pneumonic tularaemia: experience of 58 cases from 2000 to 2012 in Northern Finland. Infect Dis (Lond). 2017;49:758–64.

79. Dennis DT, Inglesby TV, Henderson DA, et al. Tularemia as a biological weapon: medical and public health management. JAMA. 2001;285:2763–73.
80. Rubin SA. Radiographic spectrum of pleuropulmonary tularemia. AJR Am J Roentgenol. 1978;131:277–81.
81. Yanes H, Hennebique A, Pelloux I, et al. Evaluation of in-house and commercial serological tests for diagnosis of human tularemia. J Clin Microbiol. 2018;56.
82. Chaignat V, Djordjevic-Spasic M, Ruettger A, et al. Performance of seven serological assays for diagnosing tularemia. BMC Infect Dis. 2014;14:234.
83. Kilic S, Celebi B, Yesilyurt M. Evaluation of a commercial immunochromatographic assay for the serologic diagnosis of tularemia. Diagn Microbiol Infect Dis. 2012;74:1–5.
84. Gunnell MK, Lovelace CD, Satterfield BA, Moore EA, O'Neill KL, Robison RA. A multiplex real-time PCR assay for the detection and differentiation of Francisella tularensis subspecies. J Med Microbiol. 2012;61:1525–31.
85. Yapar D, Erenler AK, Terzi O, Akdogan O, Ece Y, Baykam N. Predicting tularemia with clinical, laboratory and demographical findings in the ED. Am J Emerg Med. 2016;34:218–21.
86. Mulligan MJ, Stapleton JT, Keitel WA, et al. Tularemia vaccine: safety, reactogenicity, "Take" skin reactions, and antibody responses following vaccination with a new lot of the Francisella tularensis live vaccine strain – a phase 2 randomized clinical Trial. Vaccine. 2017;35:4730–7.
87. Todd SR, Dahlgren FS, Traeger MS, Beltrán-Aguilar ED, Marianos DW, Hamilton C, McQuiston JH, Regan JJ. No visible dental staining in children treated with doxycycline for suspected Rocky Mountain spotted fever. J Pediatr. 2015;16e(5):1246–51.
88. Boulanger LL, Ettestad P, Fogarty JD, Dennis DT, Romig D, Mertz G. Gentamicin and tetracyclines for the treatment of human plague: review of 75 cases in New Mexico, 1985–1999. Clin Infect Dis. 2004;38(5):663–9.

Chapter 7
Hemorrhagic Fevers

James Sullivan and Stephen Brannan

Introduction

Hemorrhagic fevers, for the most part, are viral in origin and are related to five viral families: *Arenaviridae*, *Filoviridae*, *Bunyaviridae*, *Flaviviridae*, and *Rhabdoviridae*. None of these families find humans as the primary natural reservoir, and thus a vector is the primary cause of dissemination of the organism initially. Vectors identified include ticks, mosquitoes, bats, and rodents [1]. Human-to-human transmission can take place in some cases leading to widespread epidemics and the possibility of pandemics. One such pandemic initiated in Western Africa during 2014–2016. Ebola virus disease (EVD) led to death in approximately 75% of laboratory-confirmed Ebola cases, throughout ten countries, during this time frame (11325/15261) [2]. All of these viruses lead to a common path to pathogenesis leading to microvascular destruction, capillary leak, multiorgan dysfunction, and death. While the vast majority of these cases involved three countries in Western Africa, three European countries had confirmed cases of Ebola virus disease as well as four cases confirmed in the United States. The cost was especially high in Liberian healthcare workers as 8% of physicians, nurses, and midwives contracted the disease and died during the outbreak. This devastating effect led to holes in the treatment of other more common and more controllable diseases such as malaria, tuberculosis, and HIV causing further morbidity and mortality due to reduced access to treatment [3].

All of these viruses are RNA viruses. As a result, all are obligate intracellular parasites in humans and thus need a vector to transmit disease initially. However, once active infection takes place, human-to-human transmission can take place in some cases. For most of these microorganisms, humans are dead-end hosts. That is, they are incidental to the natural cycle and do not participate in perpetuation of disease transmission. However, in the setting of yellow fever, Phlebotomus fever,

J. Sullivan (✉) · S. Brannan
Department of Anesthesiology, University of Nebraska Medical Center, Omaha, NE, USA
e-mail: Jsulliva@unmc.edu; Stephen.Brannan@unmc.edu

© Springer Nature Switzerland AG 2020   119
J. Hidalgo, L. Woc-Colburn (eds.), *Highly Infectious Diseases in Critical Care*,
https://doi.org/10.1007/978-3-030-33803-9_7

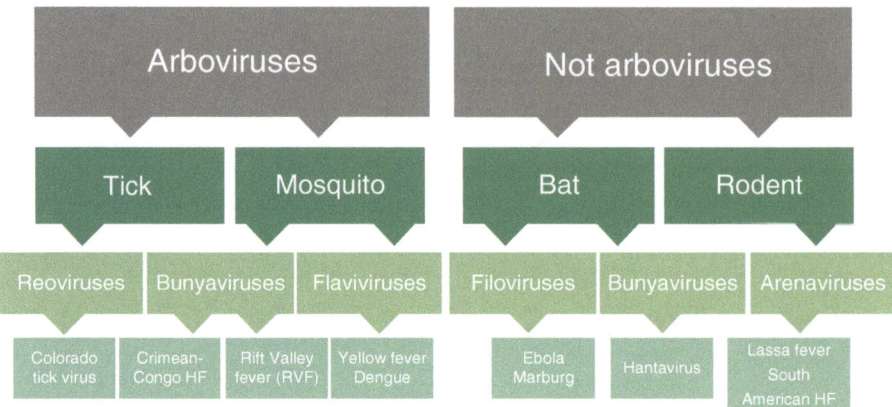

Fig. 7.1 Viral hemorrhagic fevers

chikungunya, Zika, and dengue, humans are definitive hosts, i.e., they participate and are necessary for viral propagation [4]. Most viral hemorrhagic fevers present initially in the same way. Fever and malaise are common and may appear the same as other more common illnesses such as malaria or influenza leading to confusion and delay in diagnosis (Fig. 7.1).

Filoviridae: Ebola Virus and Marburg Virus

Transmission

Human-to-human transmission of EVD is known to occur via inoculation. Injection of the virus directly into the bloodstream, for instance, through contaminated medical equipment, or by direct contact with broken skin or mucous membranes, is the primary known route. The virus is known to stay in body fluids (e.g., urine, saliva, sweat, feces, vomit, breast milk, and semen) for up to 7 days. On inanimate surfaces such as needles and syringes, the virus can stay viable at room temperature for days to weeks. The 1976 Ebola epidemic was associated primarily with hospital transmission [5] although subsequent epidemics such as the 2014 outbreak in Sierra Leone have seen an increased rate of non-hospital human-to-human transmission, especially intimate contact through caregiving or burial preparation [6]. Importantly, most experts agree the virus does not spread unless the host is exhibiting signs and symptoms of the disease.

Whereas human-to-human transmission of EVD is established, zoonotic spread from animal vectors is somewhat less clear. Although bats have been commonly implicated as reservoirs, like the hammer-headed fruit bat *Hypsignathus monstrosus* and the little collared bat *Myonycteris torquata* in the 2014–2016 outbreak [7], EV antibodies and seropositive rates in bats before, during, and after outbreaks have exhibited low prevalence rates or even been absent [8]. Moreover, evidence of EV in some tissues of rodents and shrews suggests the virus persists in natural vectors but serologic and antigenic confirmatory testing have yet to confirm this [9]. Animal models such as bats have shown high titers of EV replication without illness [10]. Thus the ecological mechanism through which Ebola virus circulates in nature and is transmitted to humans requires further investigation and understanding.

Unlike its familial relative Ebola, Marburg virus zoonotic transmission is better understood. Several species of bats are known vectors, and transmission can also occur from spillover hosts like nonhuman primates. Like Ebola, postmortem exposure to humans or animals is associated with high risk of transmission. Furthermore, human-to-human transmission of Marburg virus is like that of Ebola virus, that is, direct inoculation of the bloodstream by injection or exposure to bodily fluids via mucus membranes. Marburg virus is also found in semen weeks to months following the onset of symptoms.

Virology

Ebolavirus is a genus of the *Filoviridae* family of enveloped, non-segmented negative-strand RNA viruses. Five known subtypes or species are named for the country or region in which they were first discovered: Zaire (now the Democratic Republic of Congo), Sudan, Bundibugyo, Tai Forest (formerly Cote d'Ivoire), and Reston. Since the discovery in 1976, the Zaire, Sudan, and Bundibugyo subtypes were associated with large outbreaks in Africa. The Reston subtype found in the Western Pacific causes highly pathogenic disease in nonhuman primates but is not known to cause human illness.

The Ebola virus genome is approximately 19 kb in size and encodes seven proteins. The nucleoprotein (NP) functions to protect the viral genomic nucleic acids from host cell nucleases and other host proteins involved with cellular innate immunity [11]. Glycoproteins (GPs) are encoded by the viral genome to serve several important purposes. First, GP1 is the receptor-binding subunit and facilitates viral entry into host cells. Second, the GP2 subunit helps the viral lipid bilayer fuse with the host cell. Third, the GPs function later in the infective timeline to downregulate expression of multiple host cell surface molecules responsible for host immune surveillance and cell adhesion while also neutralizing humoral immunity [12]. An RNA-dependent RNA polymerase (L) uses the viral RNA strands to generate nucleotide templates which subsequently hijacks the host intracellular translation to produce the viral proteins. Four structural proteins are also encoded in Ebola virus genomes. VP24 blocks the interferon signaling pathway by inhibition of its nuclear localization such that interferon genes are not transcribed. VP30 activates primary transcription along the RNA strand and helps with RNA editing. VP35 binds and stabilizes NP [13] while also inhibiting several host immune mechanisms (such as the upregulation of CD4, CD80, CD86, and MHC class II antigens). Finally, VP 40 plays a primary role in viral assembly and budding.

As another genus of the *Filoviridae* family of enveloped, non-segmented negative-strand RNA viruses, *Marburgvirus* exhibits many similarities to *Ebolavirus*. It also contains a genome of approximately 19 kb encoding seven proteins. Its outer surface GP facilitates binding to host cell membranes and fuses with the host lipid bilayer, thus releasing the viral NP into the host cytosol. However, unlike Ebola virus, the Marburg virus has a single GP. The L protein generates positive-strand RNA from the negative-strand RNA viral genome which then undergo translation via the host cell apparatus to generate viral proteins. Once a critical level of viral proteins is present in the host cell, the L protein transitions to formation of the viral genome for progeny viral particles [14]. The Marburg viral proteins are named and function similarly to those detailed above for *Ebolavirus* including VP24 which is unique to the Filoviridae family of viruses [15].

Clinical Presentation

Clinical diagnosis of filovirus hemorrhagic fever is challenging because the early, nonspecific signs and symptoms often resemble much more common illnesses to endemic areas such as typhoid fever and malaria. Furthermore, because of the similarities between Ebola and Marburg viral structure and pathogenesis, the clinical presentation for both are indistinguishable. While fever, chills, myalgias, weakness, abdominal pain, diarrhea, vomiting, and headache demonstrate an acute onset, the characteristic bruising or hemorrhage is a later finding. The incubation periods for these two viruses are similar ranging from 2 to 21 days after virus exposure with an average of 8–10 days [2]. Fevers can begin as high as 39–40 degrees Celsius. Some reports show an inverse relationship between heart rate and temperature early in the disease [16, 17]. Progression is associated with tachycardia, and higher pulse rates were documented in fatal cases. Aside from fatally ill patients experiencing hypotension and shock, blood pressure fluctuations throughout the disease course are not well documented in case reports. Nearly every case of filovirus hemorrhagic fever includes a rash of varying characteristics, although commonly nonpruritic, erythematous, and maculopapular with initial localization progressing to more diffuse.

Diagnosis

Diagnosis of EBV is difficult initially due to the commonality of physical symptoms with more common disease states. Non-descript symptoms of fever, headache, myalgias, and the like all have similarities with malaria, influenza, and typhoid to name a few. All of these infectious processes are far and away more prevalent in the communities shared with Ebola and often lead to misdiagnosis initially. A high level of suspicion should be kept in those areas where Ebola is endemic and when travel from these areas is suspected or known. Anyone who presents with these symptoms and has a possible exposure should undergo RT-PCR testing during the initial workup. RT-PCR in a patient who has been symptomatic for less than 72 hours has a low sensitivity, and thus those patients with a negative test should be rechecked once the 72-hour threshold of symptoms has been met to ensure diagnosis [18]. The diagnostic process leads to difficulty as RT-PCR testing is cumbersome, takes time, and is expensive. For this reason, qualitative antigen detection testing has been developed and adopted by the WHO in some cases. This testing gives results in approximately a half hour from samples of whole blood, serum, or plasma by detection of the Ebola VP 40 antigen. The VP 40 antigen is the most abundant protein in the filovirus and is necessary for viral budding. Qualitative antigen testing, though less accurate, is less expensive, gives more rapid results, does not require electricity, and is easier to perform, all of which are important given the economic and logistical constraints of the countries where Ebola is endemic [19].

Treatment

Treatment for EVD centers on three main aspects: supportive care, prevention, and intervention. During the Western African epidemic of Ebola virus disease from 2013 to 2015, there were more than 28,600 cases with greater than 11,300 fatalities from 2013 to 2015. These cases had a 37–74% mortality rate in those diagnosed in Ebola treatment centers in Western Africa [20]. Of these known cases, a total of 27 patients were transferred to centers in Europe or the United States or were diagnosed locally. Of these 27 cases of patients treated in centers where all supportive measures were used, 82% survived.

The gastrointestinal system was involved in all of the patients treated. Ubiquitous in these patients was severe diarrhea, but abdominal distention or ileus was present in around a third. Hypoxemia was found in at least half of the cases treated in these centers, most of which was thought due to non-cardiogenic pulmonary edema. Most of these patients needed at least supplemental oxygen (70%) with a significant number suffering progression and needing some form of mechanical support (41%). Renal replacement therapy was needed in approximately 20% of the cases and was utilized in over half of the cases where oliguria was present. Thirty percent needed intravenous hemodynamic support thought primarily related to a distributive picture. Encephalopathy was present in a third of the cases with frank coma present in around a tenth of the cases.

Due to the variety of clinical findings, the first part of care centers around supportive care. Judicious use of intravenous fluids is necessary to offset the volume loss from the gastrointestinal tract. This pathway proved difficult in light of ongoing hypoxemia and pulmonary infiltrates. Electrolyte replacement was provided via the intravenous route due to severe stomatitis and gastrointestinal involvement. Parenteral nutrition was also utilized due to the severe gastrointestinal disruption found in all cases. Renal replacement therapy should be considered in all patients who develop oliguria or severe metabolic derangement unresponsive to the less intensive therapy.

Therapeutic options are limited in the care of patients with Ebola virus disease, and during the pandemic of 2013–2015, attempts at treatment were tried. Medications such as ZMapp, TKM-Ebola, and brincidofovir were utilized during this outbreak with mixed results. Each had its own complications.

TKM-Ebola was a medication developed to combat viral replication. It consisted of small interfering RNA particles which became imbedded into the replication process and disrupted the genetic code. Kraft et al. treated two separate patients at the University of Nebraska Medical and Emory University Hospital. Both these patients suffered systemic effects from the medication including a concern for worsening pulmonary edema, fever, and rigors. While both patients survived, there were questions regarding the safety of the medication [20]. A randomized control trial was undertaken by Dunning et al. which showed no benefit to human subjects with this medication and with fears of possible systemic toxicity [21]. Currently, it has been removed from production.

Brincidofovir is an oral medication and is a prodrug of cidofovir which is conjugated to lipid to allow for intracellular delivery of the medication. It was used in two patients in the United States during the epidemic, one in Dallas, Texas, and one at the University of Nebraska. It is a nucleotide analog which prevents the incorporation of deoxycytidine, thereby stopping viral chain elongation. Dunning et al. conducted a phase 2 trial in Western Africa where four patients were enrolled in the study. Unfortunately, all four died of illness consistent with Ebola virus disease. The study was terminated early with the withdrawal of support from the manufacturer for production of the drug to treat EVD [22]. Favipiravir, a different nucleotide analog, is currently being studied and in one study had some benefit in reduction of viral load, lower infectivity, and extended survival in nonhuman primates [23]. It has been used clinically to treat two patients, one from France and one from Spain, though its mechanism has not been clearly established [24].

Antibody-based therapy can be used via two distinct mechanisms: convalescent sera or whole blood (plasma/blood collected from survivors) and monoclonal antibodies. Convalescent sera was first used in EVD patients in 1976 when a lab worker was treated with two separate doses of convalescent plasma. Again in 1995, eight workers were then treated with convalescent whole blood which was transfused into eight patients, and seven of them survived; however, one study on nonhuman primates showed no benefit to plasma therapy [25–27]. The largest study evaluating the use of passive immunity to date was a non-randomized control trial which examined the use of anti-Ebola IgG which showed no survival benefit compared to historical survival data [28]. While the clinical utility of blood products remains in question, there are benefits to this type of therapy which make it likely to be used in the future. Blood taken from survivors is easily available and is a ready source of specific antibodies even in resource-limited conditions, while production of monoclonal antibodies takes months and is expensive. While whole blood treatment may be beneficial, it has complications associated with it such as transfusion reactions. Plasma on the other hand, while still needing ABO compatibility in this setting, does not need a crossmatch, thereby making the risk of reaction less. Plasma can be stored longer than whole blood and given over a shorter period of time [29].

The second method of antibody treatment is through monoclonal antibody production. Many different antibodies have been developed against Ebola though few have been studied in humans. The benefit of these products is that they may combine multiple antibodies which target multiple areas of the virus. Two of the most studied are ZMapp and ZMab. Both these medications bind to proteins on the viral particle which foster attachment and uptake into the host cells, thus preventing infection from taking place [30]. ZMapp is a cocktail comprised of three chimeric anti-Ebola IgG monoclonal antibodies formed from tobacco plants. Initial studies on rhesus macaque monkeys showed a rescue rate of 100% when given up to 5 days post-live virus exposure with reversal of even advanced symptoms of the disease and have even showed cross-reactivity among different strains of Ebola [31]. Beginning in 2015, a clinical trial of ZMapp in combination with favipiravir was undertaken during the Ebola outbreak in Western Africa. This trial was terminated early due to inability to enroll but did show a non-statistically significant benefit to those treated. Hospital stays were shorter in this population, and the mortalities in the treatment arm all came before the completion of therapy [32]. Two patients were treated with ZMapp under compassionate use at Emory University during 2014. Both patients also received the full gambit of high level of care including intravenous fluids, electrolyte replacement, and convalescent plasma throughout their care. However, in both cases, the individuals had clinical improvement within 24 h after receiving the first dose [33]. ZMapp has also been shown in mice airways to perform as a topical barrier against Ebola, decreasing mobility of the virus as well as facilitating elimination [34].

ZMab is a combination monoclonal antibody produced from a murine model. After multiple studies in nonhuman primates, it has been used twice in compassionate use models. Schibler. et al. describe the addition of ZMab to plasma and favipiravir in a physician who contracted the disease in 2014 with a rapid decrease in viral load after therapy. Petrosillo et al. describe the treatment of a physician with viral induced interstitial pneumonia who was treated with the same therapy which points to a temporal relationship between a decrease in viral load in bronchial secretions and the dosing of ZMab.

The downsides to these medications are that they are quite expensive, take a long time to make, are not readily available at the outset of an outbreak, appear to have a decrease in effectiveness when given later in the course, and need technology not available in Ebola endemic regions. The certitude of effectiveness is also limited by the lack of randomized controlled trials, but there does seem to be good clinical data to support their use.

Crimean-Congo Fever

Transmission

Crimean-Congo hemorrhagic fever (CCHF) is an important arbovirus due to its wide geographic presence. Case reports and outbreaks have occurred from Southeastern Europe to Africa, across the Middle East, and into Western China. The disease was first described in 1944 when a group of soldiers from the former Soviet Union reclaiming part of Crimea from German control exhibited an illness characterized by fever and hemorrhage. A decade later, similar symptoms were observed in the Congo, and the same virus was isolated, thus giving rise to its name [35]. More recently genetic sequencing has revealed diversity greater than any other arthropod-borne virus. While studies thus far have shown CCHF virus is maintained exclusively in *ixodid* tick species native to the particular geographic area (most prominently in Europe, the *Hyalomma marginatum*), the lack of illness in its vectors has proved challenging over the years [36]. Vertical transmission occurs as the ticks support viral replication throughout all aspects of their life cycle and passage of the virus between mates. Horizontal transmission from ticks to mammals happens when a tick consumes a blood meal and either allows the virus to enter the host primarily through its saliva or when the virus passes from an infected host into the tick. Human-to-human transmission is possible when coming in contact with virus-containing body fluids, though standard barrier methods prevent transmission [37].

Virology

Crimean-Congo virus is a member of the *Nairovirus* genus within the family *Bunyaviridae*, with other genera including *Orthobunyavirus*, *Hantavirus*, *Phlebovirus*, and *Tospovirus*. CCHF virus is one of seven nairoviral serotypes consisting of a negative-sense, single-stranded RNA genome divided into three circular segments [38]. Each segment is named for its size, with the small (S) segment encoding the nucleocapsid protein, the medium (M) segment encoding the envelope proteins, and the large (L) segment encoding the RNA polymerase [39]. The M segment polyprotein undergoes cotranslational cleavage and posttranslational processing in the endoplasmic reticulum to produce the G_N and G_C transmembrane glycoproteins. While studies to identify specific cellular receptors used by CCHF virus to gain entry to host cells, recent work suggests G_C may bind to nucleolin as an essential step [40]. Once inside the host cell, the viral RNA-dependent RNA polymerase produces positive-sense complementary RNA used to generate new viral genomic strands, while messenger RNA is produced from the viral genome. Transcription, translation, and modification of viral proteins through the host endoplasmic reticulum and Golgi apparatus produce virion particles that uptake the genome and exit the cell completing the viral replication cycle [41].

Clinical Presentation

Clinical illness from CCHF virus infection most often causes subclinical infection, in one study estimated at 88% [42]. Like other hemorrhagic fevers previously discussed, symptoms are often nonspecific, most commonly sudden onset of fever, fatigue, myalgia, and headaches, with others including nausea, vomiting, abdominal pain, diarrhea, and hemorrhage [43]. Hoogstraal classically described the four primary phases of clinical disease: incubation, prehemorrhagic period, hemorrhagic period, and convalescent period [35]. The incubation period can vary depending on the viral load, mode of transmission, and other factors but in general ranges from 3 to 7 days with a maximal period of 13 days [44]. The onset of symptoms heralds the beginning of the prehemorrhagic phase which can last 4–5 days. Between day 3 and 5 of the disease is when the hemorrhagic period begins for those unfortunate to develop the less common, severe form of the disease. Bleeding can occur in virtually any organ but most commonly along mucus membranes (gastrointestinal tract, respiratory tract, urinary tract, etc.). The convalescent period for those who survive the hemorrhagic period is 10–20 days into the disease process and is characterized by memory, hearing, and vision loss, tachycardia, dyspnea, and polyneuritis. Laboratory changes seen in the first 5 days predicting fatal outcomes in 90% of patients were studied by Swanepoel and colleagues [45]. These include elevated white blood cell count, thrombocytopenia, transaminitis, prolonged partial thromboplastin time, and hypofibrinogenemia.

Diagnosis

Diagnosis includes having a high index of suspicion in those at risk for contracting the disease, including agricultural workers, animal husbandry, veterinarians, campers, hikers, soldiers, healthcare workers, and anyone traveling to endemic areas, as the initial symptoms are nonspecific. Enzyme-linked immunosorbent assay detection of specific IgM and IgG antibodies is possible starting 5 days after the onset of symptoms, but often serial surveillance demonstrating increased antibody levels is needed to confirm recent subclinical infection. Reverse transcriptase polymerase chain reaction (RT-PCR) provides rapid and accurate detection of the virus and is useful for confirming early disease [44].

Treatment

Treatment of CCHF, like other hemorrhagic fevers, is mainly supportive in nature. This includes hemodynamic support via fluids, vasopressors, and inotropes; respiratory support which can include need for intubation and mechanical support of ventilation; and hemorrhage control including transfusion of blood components to maintain adequate oxygen-carrying capacity and correction of coagulopathy and, in severe cases, disseminated intravascular coagulation. Meta-analysis of the use of ribavirin for treatment of CCHF demonstrated insufficient evidence due to a large portion of non-randomized studies with high risk of bias [46].

Lassa Fever

Transmission

Lassa virus is a segmented negative-strand RNA virus belonging to the family *Arenaviridae*. This family comprises a total of 23 species divided into 2 major categories: the Old World complex (Africa, Europe, and Asia) and the New World complex (North and South America) [72]. Lassa virus belongs to the Old World complex and is endemic to sub-Saharan Africa, particularly the Western African countries of Sierra Leone, Guinea, Liberia, and Nigeria. It was first described in 1970 in a case report of three missionary nurses in the northern Nigerian city of Lassa [73]. The natural vectors for Lassa virus are rodents belonging to the *Mastomys* genus [74].

Transmission occurs from both rodent contact and person to person. In the case of rodent contact, this occurs by direct contact with rodent excrement or consumption of infected rodents. Poor housing and lack of hygiene are associated with increased incidence of *Mastomys* habitation which increases the risk of Lassa virus [75] and is unfortunately commonplace for most inhabitants of endemic areas. Periods of cooler weather are associated with higher risk of transmission as the rodents tend to congregate around human settlements. Interpersonal transmission of the virus happens with exposure to the live virus in human secretions including blood, urine, and feces of an infected individual [51]. Nosocomial infection resulting in a seropositive status was associated primarily with history of injection and living with a person displaying hemorrhage in the past 12 months [76]. Among healthcare workers utilizing standard protective barriers, the risk is significantly reduced. Importantly, Lassa virus is excreted in the urine for 3–9 weeks from the time of infection and up to 3 months in semen [77].

Virology

Arenaviruses contain single-stranded, bisegmented, ambisense-coding RNA genomes contained within two segments: a small (S) segment approximately 3400 nucleotides in length and a large (L) segment approximately 7100 nucleotides [47]. Each segment encodes two proteins in opposite polarity. The S segment generates the nucleoprotein (NP) from the 3′ end and the glycoprotein precursor (GPC) from the 5′ end, with the latter undergoing posttranslational modification producing the GP1 and GP2 proteins. The L segment, meanwhile, produced the L protein (RNA-dependent RNA polymerase) at its 3′ end and the zinc-binding (Z) protein at its 5′ end [48]. GP1 atop viral spikes facilitates entry into the cell via binding to host cell receptors, with recent studies demonstrating alpha dystroglycan as an essential target [49] and G2P aiding with fusion of the host cell membrane with the viral envelope. This released ribonucleoprotein structures into the cytosol where the lower pH triggers initiation of viral genomic replication and production of messenger RNA from both genomic and antisense RNA templates [50]. Virion proteins then localize to the endoplasmic reticulum where packaging of new virial particles and eventual exocytosis occurs through mechanisms not yet fully understood, just as the extent of the Z protein and NP protein functions [51].

Pathogenesis and Clinical Presentation

Lassa virus usually invades humans through the nasopharyngeal mucosa with rapid infection of immune cells. It then travels through the lymphatic tissue until it reaches the bloodstream and spreads to every organ and tissue in the body. Hepatocellular, adrenal, and splenic necrosis with adrenal cytoplasmic inclusions were most commonly found in postmortem examinations, though not fully accounting for cause of death in those patients [52]. Stimulation of macrophages and dendritic cells by the virus results in release of mediators causing endothelial dysfunction which, combined with impaired hepatocytes and inhibition of platelet aggregation, contributes to hypovolemic shock in severe cases [53]. These also contribute to swelling seen in several organ systems, including pleural effusions, pericardial effusions, and cerebral edema though usually not significant enough to fatal on their own. The precise mechanistic explanation for Lassa fever fatality is incompletely understood with various theories ranging from derangement of proinflammatory cytokines similar to sepsis to inhibition by the virus of host immune responses [54]. Pregnant patients, particularly those in the third trimester, are at an elevated risk of death.

The incubation period for Lassa virus varies from 3 to 21 days [55]. Like many other viral hemorrhagic fevers, the illness presents with nonspecific, flu-like symptoms of fever, generalized weakness, malaise, and in some cases headache and sore throat which makes it difficult to distinguish early on from other endemic febrile diseases. Due to its initial spread via the nasopharynx and lymphatics, pharyngitis and cervical lymphadenopathy are commonly seen in those diagnosed with the virus, along with facial edema. Until symptoms begin, infected persons are considered to be noncontagious with the vast majority of patients (approaching 80%) exhibiting only mild symptoms and illness, while the remaining 20% can progress along a more severe clinical course [56]. Of these, the most useful diagnostic features for Lassa virus are fever (often >38 °C), pharyngitis, retrosternal pain, and proteinuria with fever, sore throat, and emesis predicting outcomes [55]. Sensorineural deafness occurs in up to one-third of patients regardless of disease severity with most eventually recovering [57]. More serious central nervous dysfunctions such as altered mental status, seizures, and coma are often seen in those critically ill with the disease prior to death.

As Swanepoel and colleagues had found with Congo-Crimean virus, Johnson and colleagues found laboratory values predictive of worse outcomes. Specifically, viremia of less than 10^3 median tissue culture infectious dose when hospitalized had 3.7 times greater survival chance; patients with serum titers greater than 10^3 and AST > 150 IU/L were 21 times more likely to suffer a fatal outcome than patients not meeting these criteria [58]. Other common laboratory findings include thrombocytopenia, elevated transaminases and amylase, leukopenia early, normal prothrombin and partial thromboplastic times with no evidence of disseminated intravascular coagulation, and renal insufficiency including proteinuria.

Diagnosis

As with all febrile illnesses, a high index of suspicion for Lassa fever based on a good history, physical exam, and laboratory data is helpful in guiding testing, but due to the high overlap of clinical presentations, often broad testing is required to arrive rapidly at the specific causative agent. Serum reverse transcriptase polymerase chain reaction (RT-PCR) is the gold standard for rapid identification of Lassa virus but unfortunately is not regularly employed in endemic areas due to the high cost associated with its necessary equipment. Therefore serum enzyme-linked immunosorbent assays are more commonly used with IgM and IgG antibodies detectable in about half of patients during the first 3 days. However, only about 15% of patients are IgM positive as it takes IgM 10–21 days and IgG 21 days after symptom onset to be fully detectable. Therefore a significant time lag often occurs between diagnoses during which time severe patients will progress rapidly. That is why empiric treatment is often started prior to definitive diagnosis. Viral cultures from bodily fluids are not routinely done, and immunohistochemical staining at autopsy is another method for definitive diagnosis [51].

Treatment

Treatment of Lassa fever includes immediate isolation and preventive measures to minimize risk of nosocomial infection and healthcare worker exposure. Supportive treatment including intravenous fluids, blood product administration, intubation for mechanical support of ventilation in the case of respiratory failure or airway protection for severe neurological symptoms, renal replacement therapy for severe renal insufficiency, and infusion of vasoactive medications for support of blood pressure and hemodynamics in the face of shock are all important measures. Ribavirin is almost twice as effective when given intravenously versus orally and when given within 6 days of illness onset can reduce mortality by 90% [57]. Ribavirin for post-exposure prophylaxis for those with a definitive high-risk exposure is also recommended [59].

Yellow Fever

Transmission

Yellow fever is an arthropod-borne virus, often referred to as an arbovirus, of the *Flavivirus* genus from the *Flaviviridae* family. Other viruses in this family include Zika, dengue, chikungunya, Japanese encephalitis, and West Nile. It is endemic to sub-Saharan Africa and tropical South America with intermittent epidemics. In nature, sylvatic or jungle transmission occurs between nonhuman primates and mosquitoes, while urban transmission occurs between humans and mosquitoes. In Africa, some intermediate transmission between humans and nonhuman primates happens. The primary vector in Africa is *Aedes* species mosquitoes with transmission occurring seasonally, though with an elevated risk in July through October when the rainy season transitions to the dry season. The *Haemagogus* mosquito species is the primary vector in South America where increased transmission risk falls in January through May during their rainy season [60]. When cycling through the population, infants and children are at risk as immunity tends to build with exposure as people age. The incidence is estimated at 200,000 cases per year globally with 30,000 deaths for an estimated case fatality ratio of 15%, though locally it trends higher for endemic and epidemic areas [61].

Virology

Yellow fever virus is an enveloped virus approximately 50–60 nm consisting of a genome comprised of single-stranded, positive-sense RNA encoding three structural proteins and seven non-structural (NS) proteins (NS2A, NS2B, NS3, NS4A, 2K, NS4B, and NS5). Structural proteins include the capsid (C), premembrane/membrane (prM/M), and envelope (E). The virus obtains entry into the cell by endocytosis and endosomal fusion. Its genome is then translated into a polyprotein which undergoes protease posttranslational modifications resulting in the mature structural and nonstructural proteins allowing for further replication and maturation of new virions. Genomic replication occurs on the host cell's rough endoplasmic reticulum with assembly of the virus particle in the Golgi apparatus, where it undergoes transport out of the cell through exocytosis as well as via cell lysis on some occasions [62].

Though all virus proteins play important roles in its life cycle, a few warrant highlighting for their function in host immune response. NS1 and NS3 proteins are targets for immune elimination of the virus. Specifically, NS1 stimulates cytotoxic antibodies resulting in activation of the complement cascade culminating in immune-mediated lysis of infected cells. NS3 causes host cytotoxic T cell stimulation and is helpful in clearing infected cells during host recovery from acute illness.

The E protein responsible for initial entry into host cells remains on the host cell surface following endocytosis of the virus components and stimulates production of neutralizing antibodies responsible for protecting the host from reinfection [63].

Pathogenesis

Yellow fever infection produces both neurotropic and viscerotropic patterns in vertebrate hosts. While neurological involvement is seen in many animal models, the incidence in humans is very low, usually affecting infants. In all cases, encephalitis is rarely a cause of death for a host animal. Major organs affected in humans include the liver, spleen, heart, and kidneys due to being sites of viral replication. Hepatic injury occurs by eosinophilic degeneration with condensed nuclear chromatin (Councilman bodies) signifying apoptosis mediated by lymphocyte infiltration rather than ballooning and rarefaction necrosis observed in other forms of viral hepatitis resulting in preservation of the liver reticular architecture on histology [64]. Decreased synthesis of vitamin K-dependent coagulation factors, along with platelet dysfunction and disseminated intravascular coagulation, contributes to hemorrhagic processes. As with the liver, eosinophilic damage also occurs in the kidneys resulting in fatty change to the renal tubular endothelium without inflammation due to direct viral injury and other factors like hypotension secondary to hepatorenal syndrome [65]. Viral replication in host myocardial cells results in myocardial degeneration and fatty change.

Clinical Presentation

Clinically, yellow fever infections exhibit a spectrum from subclinical infection to life-threatening disease with older adults more severely afflicted. After inoculation by an infected mosquito, the abrupt onset of symptoms typically occurs 3–6 days later with a median onset of 4.3 days [66]. Classically infected persons progress through a period of infection, a period of remission, and a period of intoxication. Nonspecific symptoms like fever, malaise, myalgias, nausea, and emesis coincide with viremia causing flushed skin, reddening of mucosal sites, and hepatic enlargement with tenderness during the period of infection. Not surprisingly, characteristic laboratory findings include elevation of transaminase levels, the degree to which may predict the severity of hepatic dysfunction as the disease progresses [67], with aspartate aminotransferase (AST) levels higher than alanine aminotransferase (ALT) due to concomitant myocardial and skeletal muscle injury. Leukopenia with neutropenia is also observed. As the disease enters the period of remission, the symptoms subside, and those with abortive disease recover. However, for approximately 15% of infected individuals, after about 48 hours, they progress to the period of intoxication on the third to sixth day after onset of symptoms. This period is marked by worsening of initial symptoms with the addition of jaundice from worsening hepatic injury, oliguria with profound azotemia from worsening renal injury, and hemorrhagic diathesis secondary to the liver's inability to synthesize vitamin K-dependent clotting factors and the development of disseminated intravascular coagulation. Bradycardia and conduction defects noted on electrocardiogram result from myocardial injury. Onset of shock with multiorgan dysfunction is mediated by proinflammatory cytokines and is described as being similar to the pathogenesis of bacterial sepsis and the systemic immune response syndrome [68].

Diagnosis and Treatment

Diagnosis of yellow fever is difficult to make early on like other viral hemorrhagic fevers. Serologic testing employing enzyme-linked immunosorbent assay (ELISA) for IgM provides a presumptive diagnosis for a single sample. Trending the titer counts to correlate with expected increases and falls as a patient's course progresses is needed for confirmation. Drawbacks to this method include cross-reactivity with other flaviviruses and presence of antibodies from prior receipt of the live-attenuated vaccine. The most rapid method of detection is polymerase chain reaction to amplify RNA from blood samples. This also allows for identification of the specific viral strain which is helpful for epidemiological purposes [69]. Viral isolation occurs either postmortem from liver tissues or inoculation of mosquito or mammalian cell cultures. Unfortunately, there is no antiviral medication available for treatment, so care is purely supportive. Ribavirin was studied in rodent models with some promise, but nonhuman primate trials proved discouraging without major benefit. However, given its efficacy in other viral illness, further investigation is warranted with potentially higher doses and/or in combination with synergistic medications [70]. The yellow fever live-attenuated 17D vaccine was first developed in 1937, and since then, over 600 million doses have been administered with remarkable consistency in regard to both safety and efficacy over the years. Rare complications include neurotropic and viscerotropic effects as the native disease would. Despite its longevity, specific mechanisms of its clinical effect remain incompletely understood [71].

Conclusion

Viral hemorrhagic fevers have made a resurgence in curiosity among the scientific community and the public at large due to recent major outbreaks in endemic areas, primarily Western Africa, along with occasional outbreaks beyond the normal geographic distribution due to increase globalization and migration. Although discovered many decades ago, most remain incompletely understood in terms of pathogenesis, and they remain frustrating for clinicians due to the homogenous clinical presentations despite very different causative agents. Despite new research promising better diagnostic and therapeutic options for acute illness, the vast majority of those impacted in endemic areas remain underserved as gold standards of care remain out of reach due to economic situations. As developed countries continue to lead the way in scientific inquiry in response to local and distant outbreaks alike, mobilization of resources to help those continually affected by these horrendous diseases requires ongoing attention and multidisciplinary approaches.

References

1. Hidalgo J, Richards GA, Jimenez JIS, Baker T, Amin P. Viral hemorrhagic fever in the tropics: report from the task force on tropical diseases by the World Federation of Societies of Intensive and Critical Care Medicine. J Crit Care. 2017;42:366–72.
2. Center for Disease Control. Ebola Virus. 2019; Available at: https://www.cdc.gov/vhf/ebola/index.html. Accessed 1 Feb 2019.
3. Parpia AS, Ndeffo-Mbah ML, Wenzel NS, Galvani AP. Effects of response to 2014-2015 Ebola outbreak on deaths from malaria, HIV/AIDS, and tuberculosis, West Africa. Emerg Infect Dis. 2016;22(3):433–41.
4. Wang RY, Li K. Host factors in the replication of positive-strand RNA viruses. Chang Gung Med J. 2012;35(2):111–24.
5. Ebola haemorrhagic fever in Zaire, 1976. Bull World Health Organ. 1978;56(2):271–93.
6. Ajelli M, Parlamento S, Bome D, Kebbi A, Atzori A, Frasson C, et al. The 2014 Ebola virus disease outbreak in Pujehun, Sierra Leone: epidemiology and impact of interventions; Emergence of Zaire Ebola Virus Disease in Guinea; Ebola viral disease outbreak--West Africa, 2014; Ebola virus disease in West Africa--the first 9Â months of the epidemic and forward projections; Camacho A, Kucharski A, Aki-Sawyerr Y, White MA, Flasche S, Baguelin M, et al. Temporal changes in ebola transmission in Sierra Leone and implications for control requirements: a real-time modelling study. PLoS Curr. 2015;7. doi:https://doi.org/10.1371/currents.outbreaks.406ae55e83ec0b5193e30856b9235ed2; Dynamics and control of Ebola virus transmission in Montserrado, Liberia: a mathematical modelling analysis; Strategies for containing Ebola in West Africa; Spatiotemporal spread of the 2014 outbreak of Ebola virus disease in Liberia and the effectiveness of non-pharmaceutical interventions: a computational modelling analysis; Characterizing the transmission dynamics and control of ebola virus disease; West African Ebola epidemic after one year--slowing but not yet under control; The role of different social contexts in shaping influenza transmission during the 2009 pandemic; Determinants of the spatiotemporal dynamics of the 2009 H1N1 pandemic in Europe: implications for real-time modelling; Chains of transmission and control of Ebola virus disease in Conakry, Guinea, in 2014: an observational study; Transmission dynamics and control of Ebola virus disease (EVD): a review; Early transmission dynamics of Ebola virus disease (EVD), West Africa, March to August 2014; Althaus CL. Estimating the Reproduction Number of Ebola Virus (EBOV) During the 2014 Outbreak in West Africa. PLoS Currents. 2014;6. doi:https://doi.org/10.1371/currents.outbreaks.91afb5e0f279e7f29e7056095255b288; Gomes MFC, Pastore Y Piontti A, Rossi L, Chao D, Longini I, Halloran ME, et al. Assessing the international spreading risk associated with the 2014 West African Ebola outbreak. PLoS Currents. 2014;6. doi:https://doi.org/10.1371/currents.outbreaks.cd818f63d40e24aef769dda7df9e0da5; Transmission potential and design of adequate control measures for Marburg hemorrhagic fever; Superspreading and

the effect of individual variation on disease emergence; Strategies for containing an emerging influenza pandemic in Southeast Asia; Dietz PM, Jambai A, Paweska JT, Yoti Z, Ksaizek TG. Epidemiology and risk factors for Ebola virus disease in Sierra Leoneâ€"23 May 2014 to 31 January 2015. Clin Infec Dis. 2015. Ahead of print; Efficacy and effectiveness of an rVSV-vectored vaccine expressing Ebola surface glycoprotein: interim results from the Guinea ring vaccination cluster-randomised trial.

7. Ansari AA. Clinical features and pathobiology of Ebolavirus infection. J Autoimmun. 2014;55:1–9.
8. Baseler L, Chertow DS, Johnson KM, Feldmann H, Morens DM. The pathogenesis of Ebola virus disease. Annu Rev Pathol. 2017;12:387–418.
9. Feldmann H, Wahl-Jensen V, Jones SM, Stroher U. Ebola virus ecology: a continuing mystery. Trends Microbiol. 2004;12(10):433–7.
10. Swanepoel R, Leman PA, Burt FJ, Zachariades NA, Braack LE, Ksiazek TG, et al. Experimental inoculation of plants and animals with Ebola virus. Emerg Infect Dis. 1996;2(4):321–5.
11. Kirchdoerfer RN, Abelson DM, Li S, Wood MR, Saphire EO. Assembly of the Ebola virus nucleoprotein from a chaperoned VP35 complex. Cell Rep. 2015;12(1):140–9.
12. Vande Burgt NH, Kaletsky RL, Bates P. Requirements within the Ebola viral glycoprotein for Tetherin antagonism. Viruses. 2015;7(10):5587–602.
13. Huang Y, Xu L, Sun Y, Nabel GJ. The assembly of Ebola virus nucleocapsid requires virion-associated proteins 35 and 24 and posttranslational modification of nucleoprotein. Mol Cell. 2002;10(2):307–16.
14. Brauburger K, Hume AJ, Muhlberger E, Olejnik J. Forty-five years of Marburg virus research. Viruses. 2012;4(10):1878–927.
15. Bamberg S, Kolesnikova L, Moller P, Klenk HD, Becker S. VP24 of Marburg virus influences formation of infectious particles. J Virol. 2005;79(21):13421–33.
16. Martini G. Clinical syndrome. In: Martini G, Sieger R, editors. Marburg virus disease. Berlin/Heidelberg: Springer; 1971. p. 1971.
17. Bonnet MJ, Akamituna P, Mazaya A. Unrecognized Ebola hemorrhagic fever at Mosango Hospital during the 1995 epidemic in Kikwit, Democratic Republic of the Congo. Emerg Infect Dis. 1998;4(3):508–10.
18. Hewlett AL, Varkey JB, Smith PW, Ribner BS. Ebola virus disease: preparedness and infection control lessons learned from two biocontainment units. Curr Opin Infect Dis. 2015;28(4):343–8.
19. Stamm LV. Ebola virus disease: rapid diagnosis and timely case reporting are critical to the early response for outbreak control. Am J Trop Med Hyg. 2015;93(3):438–40.
20. Kraft CS, Hewlett AL, Koepsell S, Winkler AM, Kratochvil CJ, Larson L, et al. The use of TKM-100802 and convalescent plasma in 2 patients with Ebola virus disease in the United States. Clin Infect Dis. 2015;61(4):496–502.
21. Dunning J, Sahr F, Rojek A, Gannon F, Carson G, Idriss B, et al. Experimental treatment of Ebola virus disease with TKM-130803: a single-arm phase 2 clinical trial. PLoS Med. 2016;13(4):e1001997.
22. Dunning J, Kennedy SB, Antierens A, Whitehead J, Ciglenecki I, Carson G, et al. Experimental treatment of Ebola virus disease with Brincidofovir. PLoS One. 2016;11(9):e0162199.
23. Guedj J, Piorkowski G, Jacquot F, Madelain V, Nguyen THT, Rodallec A, et al. Antiviral efficacy of favipiravir against Ebola virus: a translational study in cynomolgus macaques. PLoS Med. 2018;15(3):e1002535.
24. Zhang T, Zhai M, Ji J, Zhang J, Tian Y, Liu X. Recent progress on the treatment of Ebola virus disease with Favipiravir and other related strategies. Bioorg Med Chem Lett. 2017;27(11):2364–8.
25. Emond RT, Evans B, Bowen ET, Lloyd G. A case of Ebola virus infection. Br Med J. 1977;2(6086):541–4.
26. Mupapa K, Massamba M, Kibadi K, Kuvula K, Bwaka A, Kipasa M, et al. Treatment of Ebola hemorrhagic fever with blood transfusions from convalescent patients. International Scientific and Technical Committee. J Infect Dis. 1999;179(Suppl 1):S18–23.

27. Jahrling PB, Geisbert JB, Swearengen JR, Larsen T, Geisbert TW. Ebola hemorrhagic fever: evaluation of passive immunotherapy in nonhuman primates. J Infect Dis. 2007;196(Suppl 2):S400–3.
28. van Griensven J, Edwards T, Baize S, Ebola-Tx Consortium. Efficacy of convalescent plasma in relation to dose of Ebola virus antibodies. N Engl J Med. 2016;375(23):2307–9.
29. van Griensven J, De Weiggheleire A, Delamou A, Smith PG, Edwards T, Vandekerckhove P, et al. The use of Ebola convalescent plasma to treat Ebola virus disease in resource-constrained settings: a perspective from the field. Clin Infect Dis. 2016;62(1):69–74.
30. Moekotte AL, Huson MA, van der Ende AJ, Agnandji ST, Huizenga E, Goorhuis A, et al. Monoclonal antibodies for the treatment of Ebola virus disease. Expert Opin Investig Drugs. 2016;25(11):1325–35.
31. Qiu X, Wong G, Audet J, Bello A, Fernando L, Alimonti JB, et al. Reversion of advanced Ebola virus disease in nonhuman primates with ZMapp. Nature. 2014;514(7520):47–53.
32. PREVAIL II Writing Group, Multi-National PREVAIL II Study Team, Davey RT Jr, Dodd L, Proschan MA, Neaton J, et al. A randomized, controlled trial of ZMapp for Ebola virus infection. N Engl J Med. 2016;375(15):1448–56.
33. Lyon GM, Mehta AK, Varkey JB, Brantly K, Plyler L, McElroy AK, et al. Clinical care of two patients with Ebola virus disease in the United States. N Engl J Med. 2014;371(25):2402–9.
34. Yang B, Schaefer A, Wang YY, McCallen J, Lee P, Newby JM, et al. ZMapp reinforces the airway mucosal barrier against Ebola virus. J Infect Dis. 2018;218(6):901–10.
35. Hoogstraal H. The epidemiology of tick-Bourne Crimean-Congo hemorrhagic fever in Asia, Europe, and Africa. J Med Entomol. 1979;15(4):307.
36. Dreshaj S, Ahmeti S, Ramadani N, Dreshaj G, Humolli I, Dedushaj I. Current situation of Crimean-Congo hemorrhagic fever in Southeastern Europe and neighboring countries: a public health risk for the European Union? Travel Med Infect Dis. 2016;14(2):81–91.
37. Athar MN, Khalid MA, Ahmad AM, Bashir N, Baqai HZ, Ahmad M, et al. Crimean-Congo hemorrhagic fever outbreak in Rawalpindi, Pakistan, February 2002: contact tracing and risk assessment. Am J Trop Med Hyg. 2005;72(4):471–3.
38. Bajpai S, Nadkar MY. Crimean Congo hemorrhagic fever: requires vigilance and not panic. J Assoc Physicians India. 2011;59:164–7.
39. Hewson R, Chamberlain J, Mioulet V, Lloyd G, Jamil B, Hasan R, et al. Crimean-Congo haemorrhagic fever virus: sequence analysis of the small RNA segments from a collection of viruses world wide. Virus Res. 2004;102(2):185–9.
40. Xiao X, Feng Y, Zhu Z, Dimitrov DS. Identification of a putative Crimean-Congo hemorrhagic fever virus entry factor. Biochem Biophys Res Commun. 2011;411(2):253–8.
41. Bente DA, Forrester NL, Watts DM, McAuley AJ, Whitehouse CA, Bray M. Crimean-Congo hemorrhagic fever: history, epidemiology, pathogenesis, clinical syndrome and genetic diversity. Antivir Res. 2013;100(1):159–89.
42. Bodur H, Akinci E, Ascioglu S, Onguru P, Uyar Y. Subclinical infections with Crimean-Congo hemorrhagic fever virus, Turkey. Emerg Infect Dis. 2012;18(4):640–2.
43. Yilmaz GR, Buzgan T, Irmak H, Safran A, Uzun R, Cevik MA, et al. The epidemiology of Crimean-Congo hemorrhagic fever in Turkey, 2002-2007. Int J Infect Dis. 2009;13(3):380–6.
44. Ergonul O. Crimean-Congo haemorrhagic fever. Lancet Infect Dis. 2006;6(4):203–14.
45. Swanepoel R, Gill DE, Shepherd AJ, Leman PA, Mynhardt JH, Harvey S. The clinical pathology of Crimean-Congo hemorrhagic fever. Rev Infect Dis. 1989;11(Suppl 4):S794–800.
46. Johnson S, Henschke N, Maayan N, Mills I, Buckley BS, Kakourou A, et al. Ribavirin for treating Crimean Congo haemorrhagic fever. Cochrane Database Syst Rev. 2018;6:CD012713.
47. Archer AM, Rico-Hesse R. High genetic divergence and recombination in Arenaviruses from the Americas. Virology. 2002;304(2):274–81.
48. Bowen MD, Rollin PE, Ksiazek TG, Hustad HL, Bausch DG, Demby AH, et al. Genetic diversity among Lassa virus strains. J Virol. 2000;74(15):6992–7004.
49. Cao W, Henry MD, Borrow P, Yamada H, Elder JH, Ravkov EV, et al. Identification of alpha-dystroglycan as a receptor for lymphocytic choriomeningitis virus and Lassa fever virus. Science. 1998;282(5396):2079–81.

50. Rojek JM, Kunz S. Cell entry by human pathogenic arenaviruses. Cell Microbiol. 2008; 10(4):828–35.
51. Gunther S, Lenz O. Lassa virus. Crit Rev Clin Lab Sci. 2004;41(4):339–90.
52. Walker DH, McCormick JB, Johnson KM, Webb PA, Komba-Kono G, Elliott LH, et al. Pathologic and virologic study of fatal Lassa fever in man. Am J Pathol. 1982;107(3): 349–56.
53. Roberts PJ, Cummins D, Bainton AL, Walshe KJ, Fisher-Hoch SP, McCormick JB, et al. Plasma from patients with severe Lassa fever profoundly modulates f-met-leu-phe induced superoxide generation in neutrophils. Br J Haematol. 1989;73(2):152–7.
54. Yun NE, Walker DH. Pathogenesis of Lassa fever. Viruses. 2012;4(10):2031–48.
55. McCormick JB, King IJ, Webb PA, Johnson KM, O'Sullivan R, Smith ES, et al. A case-control study of the clinical diagnosis and course of Lassa fever. J Infect Dis. 1987;155(3):445–55.
56. World Health Organization. Lassa Fever. 2917; Available at: https://www.who.int/emergencies/diseases/lassa-fever/en/. Accessed 15 Jan 2019.
57. Richmond JK, Baglole DJ. Lassa fever: epidemiology, clinical features, and social consequences. BMJ. 2003;327(7426):1271–5.
58. Johnson KM, McCormick JB, Webb PA, Smith ES, Elliott LH, King IJ. Clinical virology of Lassa fever in hospitalized patients. J Infect Dis. 1987;155(3):456–64.
59. Bausch DG, Hadi CM, Khan SH, Lertora JJ. Review of the literature and proposed guidelines for the use of oral ribavirin as postexposure prophylaxis for Lassa fever. Clin Infect Dis. 2010;51(12):1435–41.
60. Center for Disease Control. Yellow Fever. 2019; Available at: https://www.cdc.gov/yellowfever/index.html. Accessed 1 Feb 2019.
61. Pan American Health Organization. Yellow Fever. 2019; Available at: https://www.paho.org/hq/index.php?option=com_topics&view=article&id=69&Itemid=40784&lang=en. Accessed 1 Feb 2019.
62. Monath TP, Vasconcelos PF. Yellow fever. J Clin Virol. 2015;64:160–73.
63. Monath TP. Yellow fever: an update. Lancet Infect Dis. 2001;1(1):11–20.
64. Monath TP, Ballinger ME, Miller BR, Salaun JJ. Detection of yellow fever viral RNA by nucleic acid hybridization and viral antigen by immunocytochemistry in fixed human liver. Am J Trop Med Hyg. 1989;40(6):663–8.
65. Monath TP, Brinker KR, Chandler FW, Kemp GE, Cropp CB. Pathophysiologic correlations in a rhesus monkey model of yellow fever with special observations on the acute necrosis of B cell areas of lymphoid tissues. Am J Trop Med Hyg. 1981;30(2):431–43.
66. Johansson MA, Arana-Vizcarrondo N, Biggerstaff BJ, Staples JE. Incubation periods of Yellow fever virus. Am J Trop Med Hyg. 2010 Jul;83(1):183–8.
67. Tuboi SH, Costa ZG, da Costa Vasconcelos PF, Hatch D. Clinical and epidemiological characteristics of yellow fever in Brazil: analysis of reported cases 1998-2002. Trans R Soc Trop Med Hyg. 2007;101(2):169–75.
68. Centers for Disease Control and Prevention (CDC). Fatal yellow fever in a traveler returning from Venezuela, 1999. MMWR Morb Mortal Wkly Rep. 2000;49(14):303–5.
69. Nunes MR, Vianez JL Jr, Nunes KN, da Silva SP, Lima CP, Guzman H, et al. Analysis of a reverse transcription loop-mediated isothermal amplification (RT-LAMP) for yellow fever diagnostic. J Virol Methods. 2015;226:40–51.
70. Monath TP. Treatment of yellow fever. Antivir Res. 2008;78(1):116–24.
71. Beck AS, Barrett AD. Current status and future prospects of yellow fever vaccines. Expert Rev Vaccines. 2015;14(11):1479–92.
72. Charrel RN, de Lamballerie X. Arenaviruses other than Lassa virus. Antiviral Res. 2003;57(1–2):89–100.
73. Frame JD, Gocke DJ, Baldwin JM, Troup JM. Lassa fever, a new virus disease of man from west africa. Am J Trop Med Hyg. 1970;19(4):670–6.
74. Salazar-Bravo J, Ruedas LA, Yates TL. Mammalian reservoirs of arenaviruses. Curr Top Microbiol Immunol. 2002;262:25–63.

75. Bonner PC, Schmidt WP, Belmain SR, Oshin B, Baglole D, Borchert M. Poor housing quality increases risk of rodent infestation and Lassa fever in refugee camps of Sierra Leone. Am J Trop Med Hyg. 2007;77(1):169–75.
76. Kernéis S, Koivogui L, Magassouba N'F, Koulemou K, Lewis R, Aplogan A, Grais RF, Guerin PJ, Fichet-Calvet E, Aksoy S. Prevalence and risk factors of Lassa seropositivity in inhabitants of the forest region of Guinea: a cross-sectional study. PLoS Negl Trop Dis. 2009;3(11):e548.
77. Richmond JK. Lassa fever: epidemiology, clinical features, and social consequences. BMJ. 2003;327(7426):1271–5.

Chapter 8
Multidrug Resistance Bacterial Infection

Laila Woc-Colburn and Denise Marie A. Francisco

Introduction

Antibiotics have drastically changed the medical landscape when they were first introduced in the 1940s. But, as long as antibiotics have been used, resistant bacteria have emerged. In fact, resistant strains have even been identified prior to antibiotic introduction showing that while antibiotic overuse and misuse along with a decreasing number of new antibiotics in the past couple of years certainly can be a cause behind the increasing resistance patterns, some bacteria have already been carrying resistance genes by themselves, which further add to the growing problem of multidrug resistance organisms.

The figure below (Fig. 8.1) shows how quickly antibiotic resistance can be identified after a certain antibiotic has been introduced to the public.

The causes behind antibiotic resistance can be multifactorial. They can be linked to inappropriate antibiotic usage from the prescriber's side (overuse, inappropriateness), the usage of antibiotics in other areas other than health care (antibiotic use in agriculture and livestock), and the lack of development of new antibiotics in the past couple of years [4].

Unfortunately, the development of these new drug-resistant strains of bacteria is causing the health-care system money and, most importantly, lives. In a study in the United States, it was estimated that antimicrobial resistant infections resulted in a death rate that was twofold higher than those without resistant infections, and patients stayed an excess of 6.4–12.7 days in the hospital. In terms of medical costs attributable to the resistant infection, this ranged from \$18,588 to \$29,069 per patient [3].

L. Woc-Colburn
Section Infectious Diseases, Department of Medicine, National School of Tropical Medicine, Baylor College of Medicine, Houston, TX, USA

D. M. A. Francisco (✉)
Infectious Diseases, Baylor College of Medicine, Houston, TX, USA
e-mail: denise.francisco@bcm.edu

© Springer Nature Switzerland AG 2020
J. Hidalgo, L. Woc-Colburn (eds.), *Highly Infectious Diseases in Critical Care*,
https://doi.org/10.1007/978-3-030-33803-9_8

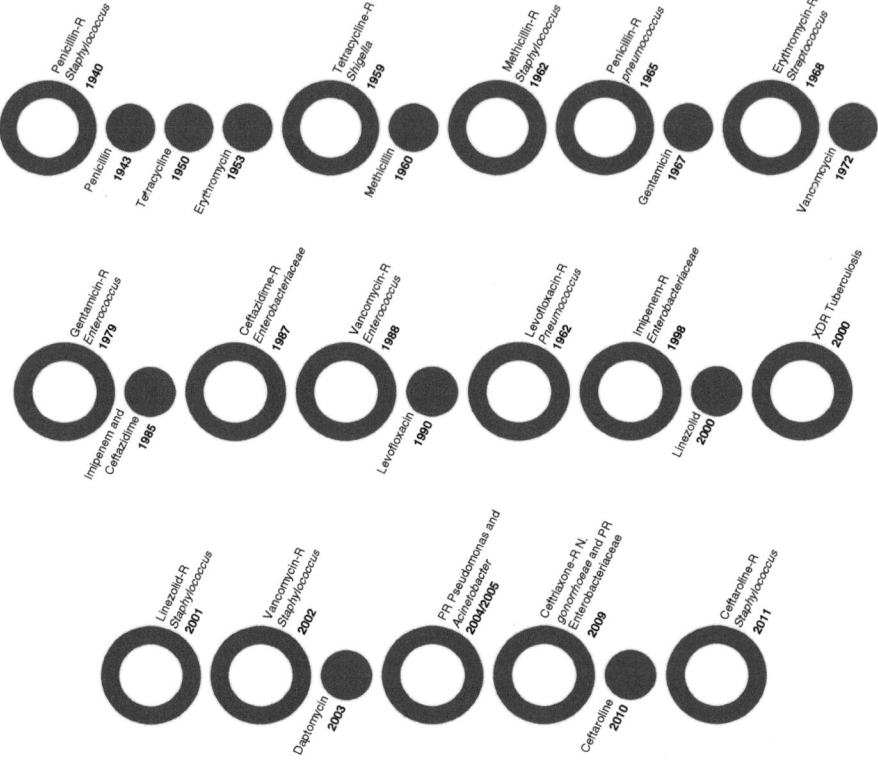

Fig. 8.1 A timeline of key events in antibiotic resistance in chronological order. R Resistant, PR Pan-drug Resistant, XDR Extensively Drug Resistant, Large Circles – Antibiotic Resistance Identified, Small Circles – Antibiotic Introduced (Modified from CDC [1]. Dates are based upon early reports of resistance in the literature. Penicillin was also in limited use before its widespread usage in 1943)

In the United States, the Centers for Disease Control and Prevention (CDC) was able to categorize these antibiotic resistance threats as "Urgent," "Serious," and "Concerning" as seen in Table 8.1.

Enterococcus

Enterococci are gram-positive cocci that usually occur in either pairs (diplococci) or short chains. The species that are of greatest medical importance are *Enterococcus faecalis* and *Enterococcus faecium*.

Enterococci are generally intrinsically resistant to many commonly used antibacterial agents, and this is the most common difference when they are compared to the streptococci, which are also gram-positive cocci. All enterococci intrinsically have increased resistance to penicillin and ampicillin, as well as high-level resistance to most cephalosporins and other semi-synthetic penicillins. This is

Table 8.1 Antibiotic resistance infections ranked by threat level [1]

Urgent threats
Clostridium difficile
Carbapenem-resistant *Enterobacteriaceae* (CRE)
Drug-resistant *Neisseria gonorrhoeae*
Serious threats
Multidrug-resistant *Acinetobacter*
Drug-resistant *Campylobacter*
Fluconazole-resistant *Candida* (a fungus)
Extended-spectrum β-lactamase-producing *Enterobacteriaceae* (ESBLs)
Vancomycin-resistant *Enterococcus* (VRE)
Multidrug-resistant *Pseudomonas aeruginosa*
Drug-resistant non-typhoidal *Salmonella*
Drug-resistant *Salmonella typhi*
Drug-resistant *Shigella*
Methicillin-resistant *Staphylococcus aureus* (MRSA)
Drug-resistant *Streptococcus pneumoniae*
Drug-resistant tuberculosis
Concerning threats
Vancomycin-resistant *Staphylococcus aureus* (VRSA)
Erythromycin-resistant Group A *Streptococcus*
Clindamycin-resistant Group B *Streptococcus*

because of low-affinity penicillin-binding proteins. They are also resistant to clindamycin (through the lsa gene), trimethoprim-sulfamethoxazole (since they can absorb folate), and aminoglycosides (as a single agent, but they can be used for synergistic activity) [2].

Because of its intrinsic reduced susceptibility and growing resistance to usual empiric antibiotics like ampicillin and vancomycin, it has been increasingly difficult to treat *Enterococcus* infections. Below is a table (Table 8.2) that compares and contrasts treatment options for *Enterococcus faecalis* and *Enterococcus faecium*.

Staphylococcus aureus

Staphylococcus aureus infections are clinically important and range from skin and soft tissue infections to widespread bacteremia. Due to the prevalence of these infections and its subsequent treatment, there is a spectrum of antimicrobial resistance with regard to these bacteria.

Methicillin-Resistant Staphylococcus aureus *(MRSA)*

Shortly after the introduction of methicillin in 1960, there was already evidence of methicillin-resistant *Staphylococcus aureus* (MRSA). The gene that confers this resistance is the *mecA* gene.

Table 8.2 Treatment for *Enterococcus faecalis* and *Enterococcus faecium* based on susceptibility patterns [2]

	Enterococcus faecalis	*Enterococcus faecium*
Information		More resistant to penicillin Resistant to synergism with tobramycin
Penicillin-susceptible strains	*Monotherapy* Ampicillin 1–2 g IV every 4–6 hours Penicillin G 18–30 million units IV every 24 hours (continuously or in 6 divided doses) Vancomycin 15 mg/kg/dose IV every 12 hours *Combination therapy* Ampicillin 2 g IV every 4 hours + ceftriaxone 2 g IV every 12 hours Ampicillin OR penicillin G OR vancomycin (doses as above) + gentamicin 1 mg/kg every 8 hours OR streptomycin 5 mg/kg IV every 12 hours	
High-level penicillin resistance	*Monotherapy* Vancomycin 15 mg/kg/dose IV every 12 hours Ampicillin-sulbactam 3 g IV every 6 hours High-dose ampicillin 3–4 g every 4 hours *Combination therapy* Vancomycin OR ampicillin-sulbactam OR high-dose ampicillin (doses as above) + gentamicin 1 mg/kg every 8 hours OR streptomycin 5 mg/kg IV every 12 hours	
High-level aminoglycoside resistance	*Combination therapy* Ampicillin 1–2 g IV every 4–6 hours PLUS Ceftriaxone OR Imipenem + vancomycin OR Fluoroquinolones OR High-dose daptomycin	
Vancomycin resistance	Usually are susceptible to beta-lactams and ampicillin-based regimens are preferred	Often are resistant to beta-lactams and aminoglycosides *Monotherapy* High-dose daptomycin 8–12 mg/kg every 24 hours Linezolid 600 mg every 12 hours Tigecycline 100 mg loading dose followed by maintenance of 50 mg every 12 hours (for intraabdominal infections)

Epidemiologically, there are two major subdivisions of MRSA, one is health-care-associated MRSA (HA-MRSA) and the other one is community-acquired MRSA (CA-MRSA) infection. As the years went on, however, these two classifications are no longer distinct, and with regard to treatment, there is no difference between the HA-MRSA and CA-MRSA.

Table 8.3 Antibiotics for treatment of systemic MRSA infections

Antibiotic	Usual dosage (normal renal function)	Pros	Cons
Antibiotics of choice			
Vancomycin	15–20 mg/kg/dose IV every 8–12 hours, not to exceed 2 g per dose		Needs careful monitoring of levels and renal function
Daptomycin	6–10 mg/kg IV once daily		Cannot be used in pneumonia (surfactant deactivates the antibiotic) Needs weekly creatinine phosphokinase (CPK) monitoring
Teicoplanin	6–12 mg/kg IV once daily	Can be given intramuscularly	
Alternative agents			
Ceftaroline	600 mg IV every 12 hours		
Linezolid	600 mg IV (or orally) twice daily	There is an oral option with good bioavailability	Cannot be used in bloodstream infections Can induce serotonin syndrome if used with other serotonergic agents
Telavancin	10 mg/kg IV once daily		Can cause increased rates of nephrotoxicity

Antibiotics for treatment of systemic MRSA infections include vancomycin, daptomycin, and teicoplanin (when available) as antibiotics of choice, while alternative agents include ceftaroline, linezolid, and telavancin. The treatment options for MRSA infections are summarized in the table below (Table 8.3).

Vancomycin-Intermediate **Staphylococcus aureus** *(VISA)* *and Vancomycin-Resistant* **Staphylococcus aureus** *(VRSA)*

Staphylococcus aureus have now developed increasing resistances against vancomycin, the drug of choice against MRSA. Because of reports of vancomycin treatment failure that were associated with elevated minimal inhibitory concentrations (MICs), the Clinical and Laboratory Standards Institute and the US Food and Drug Administration have actually decreased their MICs for vancomycin as follows:

- Vancomycin susceptible   - ≤ 2 mcg/mL
- Vancomycin intermediate   - 4–8 mcg/mL
- Vancomycin resistant   - ≥ 16 mcg/mL

In patients with VISA or VRSA, it has been suggested to change the patient from vancomycin to daptomycin. It is recommended to repeat susceptibility testing in the intermediate *S. aureus* to make sure that daptomycin continues to be susceptible.

If the patient is not tolerant of daptomycin, there is a choice of either monotherapy or combination therapy. For monotherapy, we can use telavancin, ceftaroline, or linezolid (taking into account the limitations some of these antibiotics can have). For combination therapy, the favored choice is daptomycin (with a higher dose of 8–10 mg/kg daily) with ceftaroline [6].

Enterobacteriaceae

Extended Spectrum β-Lactamase Producing Enterobacteriaceae

Gram-negative pathogens are an important pathogen in the clinical world, with the sources ranging from urinary tract infections to catheter-related ones. The most commonly used antibiotics against the gram negatives include cephalosporins, B-lactam, and B-lactamase inhibitor combinations, but we have seen an increasing number of gram-negative bacteria developing resistance against these common antibiotics.

Extended spectrum β-lactamase (ESBLs) are enzymes produced by bacteria that can hydrolyze one or more oxyimino-B-lactams, thereby reducing the susceptibility to the following antibiotics: ceftazidime, cefotaxime, ceftriaxone, cefpodoxime, or aztreonam [5]. Unfortunately, we are seeing a steady increase of the incidence of these ESBL producing organisms.

With regard to treatment of choice, multiple studies have shown that even with a pathogen that is in vitro susceptible to piperacillin-tazobactam, the treatment of choice remains to be a carbapenem (imipenem, meropenem, doripenem, ertapenem). Summarized in the table below (Table 8.4) is a comparison of the most commonly used carbapenems.

With regard to cephalosporins, there has been evidence that the newer cephalosporin-beta-lactamase inhibitor combinations can be effective. These include ceftolozane-tazobactam and ceftazidime-avibactam.

In light of severe beta-lactam allergies, the choices are unfortunately limited. There is an option of carbapenem desensitization, but other drugs that may be used (with limited evidence) include fluoroquinolones, tigecycline, and eravacycline. For non-severe cystitis caused by ESBL *E. coli*, fosfomycin continues to be an option.

Beta-lactamases and Inducibility: The "SPACE" Organisms

Classically, the bacteria that are commonly associated with ESBL are *Escherichia coli* and *Klebsiella* spp. But there are certain bacteria wherein the genes encoding for these B-lactamases (AmpC) are inducible (increased resistance to antibiotics

Table 8.4 Comparison of the commonly used carbapenems

Carbapenem	Usual dosage (normal renal function)	Pros	Cons
Meropenem	1.5–6 g daily divided every 8 hours	Favored in the setting of seizures or pregnancies Used in meningitis Slightly more active against other gram-negative organisms	
Imipenem	500 mg every 6 hours OR 1000 mg every 8 hours	Slightly more active against gram-positive organisms	Possible central nervous system (CNS) toxicity with the highest risk for seizures Unknown pregnancy profile
Doripenem	500 mg every 8 hours	Equivalent efficacy with meropenem and imipenem	New drug; hence there is limited clinical data
Ertapenem	1000 mg every 24 hours	Once daily dosing	There are reports of ESBL producing organisms that are resistant to ertapenem Resistance may develop with therapy Not used in severe sepsis Limited activity against *Enterococcus* spp. and *Pseudomonas aeruginosa*

can form with exposure to certain antibiotic types). These bacteria are as follows, *Serratia* spp., *Pseudomonas* spp., *Acinetobacter* spp., *Citrobacter* spp., and *Enterobacter*, commonly known as the "SPACE" organisms.

The use of antibiotics that are considered "strong inducers of (AmpC)" in infections caused by the "SPACE organisms" can lead to increased antibiotic resistance in the future. Examples of strong inducers of (AmpC) are ampicillin, first-generation cephalosporins, cefoxitin, and cefotetan, while weak inducers make antibiotic resistance less likely to form – examples of these types of antibiotics are ceftazidime, ceftriaxone, cefotaxime, piperacillin, ticarcillin, aztreonam, and cefepime.

Carbapenem-Resistant Enterobacteriaceae (CRE)

In the extending spectrum of drug resistance, a step above ESBL would be the carbapenem-resistant *Enterobacteriaceae* (CRE). Carbapenemases are beta-lactamases that hydrolyze carbapenem, thereby increasing the pathogen's resistance against not only beta-lactam substrates but carbapenems also. Due to this, if a bacterium is found to have carbapenamase, it is important that additional antibiotic susceptibility testing should be requested (since other resistance genes are frequently present alongside the carbapenamase). It is prudent to ask for aminoglycosides (gentamicin and plazomicin if available), colistin (or polymyxin B), aztreonam, tigecycline, fosfomycin (in cystitis), ceftazidime-avibactam, ceftolozane-tazobactam, and eravacycline (if available).

Due to the limitation in available clinical studies, optimal treatment is still uncertain, and our antibiotic choices are limited. For the most part, the choice of therapy eventually hinges on the in vitro susceptibility patterns of the specific bacteria that one is trying to treat.

For infections caused by *Klebsiella pneumoniae*-carbapenamase producing organisms, the favored antibiotic is ceftazidime-avibactam. For higher MICs (but still susceptible), there is an option of adding a second agent – most commonly a carbapenem for synergistic activity. Another treatment option is meropenem-vaborbactam.

If these newer antibiotics are not available or if the organisms are producing a metallo-beta-lactamase (MBL), there is still an option of combined polymyxin plus a second antibacterial agent.

Polymyxins are a class of antibiotics where there are only two known clinically useful compounds – polymyxin B and colistin. They have a very narrow spectrum of activity and are mostly used in multidrug-resistant infections. Unfortunately, there is a known severe side effect profile, most importantly – nephrotoxicity; hence renal function should be closely monitored with its use.

For options with regard to the second agent, tigecycline is a consideration, especially in infections located in the gastrointestinal (GI) and respiratory tract. Eravacycline is another newer option that can be used in combination with the polymixins. Another possible second agent is meropenem, especially if the MIC is ≤8 mcg/mL.

If the strain is highly resistant, there is an option of a combined ceftazidime-avibactam plus aztreonam since MBLs give resistance to all beta-lactam-type antibiotics except aztreonam.

Newer drug options include plazomicin, an aminoglycoside antibiotic which has shown activity against CRE. In the United States, plazomicin has already been approved for complicated urinary tract infections (UTI), but there is limited data with regard to treating systemic infections.

References

1. CDC. Antibiotic resistance threats in the United States. Atlanta: Department of Health and Human Services Centers for Disease Control and Prevention; 2013. www.cdc.gov/drugresis-tance/biggest_threats.html. Accessed 12 Dec 2018.
2. Kristich CJ. Enterococcal infection—treatment and antibiotic resistance. In: Gilmore MS, editor. Enterococci from commensals to leading causes of drug resistant infection. Boston: Massachusetts Eye and Ear Infirmary; 2014. p. 123–84.
3. Roberts RH. Hospital and societal costs of antimicrobial-resistant infections in a Chicago teaching hospital: implications for antibiotic stewardship. Clin Infect Dis. 2009;49:1175–84.
4. Ventola C. The antibiotic resistance crisis: part 1: causes and threats. P T. 2015;40:277–83.
5. Doi Y. The ecology of extended-spectrum b-lactamases (ESBLs) in the developed world. J Travel Med. 2016;24:S44–51.
6. Sakoulas G. Antimicrobial salvage therapy for persistent staphylococcal bacteremia using daptomycin plus ceftaroline. Clin Ther. 36:1317.

Chapter 9
Central Nervous System Infection

Ahmed Reda Taha

Meningitis

From the first description of meningococcemia and meningococcal meningitis, before identification of the etiologic organism (by Vieusseux in 1806), until the early twentieth century, bacterial meningitis was considered a nearly uniformly fatal disease, although some patients with meningococcal meningitis survived without antimicrobial therapy. The advent of various experimental procedures followed by antisera therapy directed against meningococci reduced mortality rates during World War I, but the introduction of sulfonamides and penicillins along with other antimicrobial agents heralded the reduction in morbidity and survival possible with modern antimicrobial therapy. Despite these achievements and the introduction of several new antimicrobial agents with in vitro activity against the major meningeal pathogens plus some limited improvement in diagnostic assays, bacterial meningitis remains associated with unacceptably high morbidity and mortality [1].

The classic triad of meningitis is fever, neck stiffness, and altered mental status. The full triad is present in only about 46% of adults with bacterial meningitis. However, almost all patients with bacterial meningitis have at least one of these features, so the absence of all three makes bacterial meningitis unlikely. Patients may also complain of headache, nausea, vomiting, and photophobia. It is difficult, if not impossible, to exclude bacterial meningitis based on the physical examination. Findings may include nuchal rigidity (pain on passive flexion of the neck), Kernig sign, and Brudzinski sign. Kernig sign is elicited with the patient in the supine position. The thigh is flexed on the abdomen with the knee flexed. Attempts to passively extend the leg cause pain when meningeal irritation is present.

A. R. Taha (✉)
Sheikh Khalifa Medical City, Critical Care Department, Abu Dhabi, United Arab Emirates

© Springer Nature Switzerland AG 2020

J. Hidalgo, L. Woc-Colburn (eds.), *Highly Infectious Diseases in Critical Care*,
https://doi.org/10.1007/978-3-030-33803-9_9

Brudzinski sign is elicited with the patient in the supine position and is positive when passive flexion of the neck results in flexion of the hips and knees. Unfortunately, nuchal rigidity is only 30% sensitive in meningitis, and the sensitivity of Kernig and Brudzinski signs may be as low as 5%. A more recently described putative sign of meningitis is "jolt accentuation": headache aggravated by shaking the head quickly back and forth in the horizontal plane, The diagnostic value of this maneuver was evaluated in a study of 34 patients presenting to an outpatient clinic or emergency department with headache and fever [2–4]. Patients with bacterial meningitis may also have focal neurologic deficits or seizures. Less than 50% of children with bacterial meningitis have nuchal rigidity. The possibility of bacterial meningitis should be considered in every child with fever, vomiting, photophobia, lethargy, or altered mental status [5]. Many cases of bacterial meningitis in children are preceded by upper respiratory tract infections or otitis media. Signs of meningitis in the neonate are nonspecific and include irritability, lethargy, poor feeding, vomiting, diarrhea, temperature instability (fever or hypothermia), respiratory distress, apnea, seizures, and a bulging fontanel. Patients with viral meningitis complain of fever, headache, stiff neck, photophobia, nausea, and vomiting, but are awake and alert [6].

Tuberculous meningitis presents as either a slowly progressive illness with a persistent and intractable headache that has been present for weeks followed by confusion, lethargy, meningismus, focal neurologic deficits, and cranial nerve deficits or an acute meningoencephalitis characterized by coma, raised intracranial pressure, seizures, and focal neurologic deficits. The basilar meninges are predominantly involved. Fungal meningitis clinically resembles tuberculous meningitis. Patients complain of headache, fever, and malaise, followed by meningeal signs, altered mental status, and cranial nerve palsies [7].

Pathogens causing meningitis depend upon age and predisposing or associated conditions. *Streptococcus pneumoniae* is the most common cause of meningitis in adults older than 20 (45–50% of cases). Infection may begin with pneumonia, otitis media, or sinusitis, *Neisseria meningitidis* is the leading cause of meningococcal meningitis, and meningococcal septicemia are directly spread by large droplet respiratory secretions and tend to infect adolescents who share cigarettes, cokes, and kisses. *Listeria monocytogenes* (about 8% of cases) is a food-borne infection, found in sources as processed meats and unpasteurized cheeses. Neonatal bacterial meningitis infections are acquired from the maternal genitourinary tract; the meningococcal disease occurs primarily in children aged under 5 years, with a peak incidence in those under 1 year [8].

Listeria may cause a rhombencephalitis, or brainstem encephalitis, often with a prodrome of several days of headache, vomiting, and fever, followed by cranial nerve palsies and cerebellar and long-tract motor and sensory deficits. Brainstem abscess, a devastating complication, may arise. Meningitis may also be present. While most patients with *Listeria* infection are immunosuppressed, those with *Listeria* rhombencephalitis are often immunocompetent [9].

Epidemiology of Bacterial Meningitis

For the past 10 years in the United States, the incidence of bacterial meningitis has 31%, largely due to lower rates of *H. influenzae* type B (Hib) and *S. pneumoniae* meningitis in children following the widespread utilization of *S. pneumoniae* and Hib conjugate vaccines.

Another disturbing epidemiologic trend is the emergence of antimicrobial resistance among meningeal pathogens. At present, the most serious is the emergence of penicillin resistance (along with resistance to other antimicrobial agents) among *S. pneumoniae*. Antimicrobial usage, particularly β-lactams in low concentrations for prolonged periods, leads to selection for resistance among pneumococci in children and adults—both the carrier state and invasive disease; nevertheless, penicillin resistance varies widely among developed countries [10]. In addition to this selective pressure, other factors contribute to the development and spread of resistant pathogens, including an extension of their spectrum of resistance and resistance genes among diverse microorganisms and mutations in common genes [11].

Resistance to penicillin involves mutations in one or more penicillin-binding proteins (PBP) in *S. pneumoniae* reducing the affinity for penicillin and related antibiotics. These mutations are usually present in the transpeptidase/penicillin-binding domain. Multiple mutations are required to result in high-level resistance among PBP variants [17]. The genes that encode for the altered PBP are called "mosaics," since they consist of native pneumococcal DNA mixed with fragments of foreign DNA, presumably derived from streptococci normally resident in the healthy human nasopharynx. This foreign DNA has been incorporated by the pneumococci into the chromosome. The worldwide spread of penicillin resistance among *S. pneumoniae* appears to be due to the dissemination of several clones carrying altered PBP genes. In addition, chloramphenicol resistance has appeared among meningococci. If this trend continues on a worldwide basis, the consequences will be devastating as chloramphenicol is widely used as the antimicrobial of choice in resource-limited settings, especially in the sub-Saharan African meningitis belt. Penicillin resistance among meningococci is also spreading, but the impact on therapeutic strategies is not known [12].

The clinical outcome of acute bacterial meningitis depends on multiple factors including the socioeconomic status of the patient (developed vs developing countries), age, pathogen, and clinical characteristics and laboratory manifestations of the acute infection. For example, the case fatality rate for *H. influenzae* type B meningitis in recent reviews has been about 5% [13], a figure similar to that of meningococcal meningitis in the same report. Conversely, the mortality rate associated with pneumococcal meningitis is about 20% versus 15–30% for *Listeria monocytogenes* in recent years [13]. About 30% of the survivors of pneumococcal meningitis develop long-term sequelae such as hearing loss, neuropsychologic impairment, and neurologic deficits [18].

The case fatality rate of *S. pneumoniae* meningitis varies dramatically by age—with a case fatality rate of <10% in children but about 40% in those ⩾50 years old. These results apply only to developed countries. In developing regions, 60–80% of children and adults with pneumococcal meningitis still succumb to the infection [14, 15]. The risk of death is greatest for those with neurologic complications during the acute illness (e.g., cerebrovascular insults, hydrocephalus, brain edema, and involvement of large intracranial blood vessels). Brain infarction with severe irreversible cerebral damage and an increase of intracranial pressure result from cerebrovascular involvement of both arteries and veins. These complications may be diagnosed by computerized tomography, magnetic resonance imaging or angiography, or transcranial Doppler sonography, but these modalities are not widely available in resource-limited settings.

Pathophysiology of Bacterial Meningitis

Various bacteria including the major meningeal pathogens (e.g., *S. pneumoniae*) undergo autolysis under harsh conditions such as exposure to antimicrobial agents and growth to stationary phase. Autolysis consists of self-digestion of the cell wall by peptidoglycan hydrolases termed autolysins. At least three autolysins are recognized in pneumococci, but the major autolysin is the N-acetyl-muramoyl-l-alanine amidase (LytA) [16]. Activation of LytA and autolysis result in the release in subcapsular bacterial components including peptidoglycan, lipoteichoic acid, bacterial DNA, and pneumolysin.

Mechanisms of immune activation Various cell wall products of meningeal pathogens are well-known inducers of the inflammatory host response. The inflammatory response in the subarachnoid space characteristic of acute purulent meningitis can be reproduced by the intracisternal challenge with whole heat-killed unencapsulated pneumococci, their isolated cell walls, lipoteichoic acid, or peptidoglycan, but not by the injection of heat-killed encapsulated strains or isolated capsular polysaccharide [17, 18]. Exact mechanisms of immune activation by pneumococcal cell wall products remain poorly understood, but recent in vitro studies suggest that the first step in immune activation is binding of peptidoglycan and lipoteichoic acid to the pattern recognition receptor membrane CD14 (mCD14). mCD14 is not a transmembrane molecule and thus by itself cannot transmit the activating signal into the cell.

The second step in immune activation is necessary, and this potentially occurs through the toll-like receptor-2 (TLR-2). Coexpression of CD14 and TLR-2 in Chinese hamster ovary fibroblasts confers responsiveness to pneumococcal peptidoglycan and heat-killed *S. pneumoniae* as evidenced by inducible translocation of the nuclear transcription factor NF-κB [19]. It appears that both TLR-2-dependent and TLR-2-independent (pneumolysin) pathways are sufficient to cause inflammation in the absence of the other, but in vivo, both are likely activated.

TLR-2-independent immune activation may be mediated at least in part by the pneumococcal toxin pneumolysin. Pneumolysin stimulates the production of inflammatory mediators in vitro including tumor necrosis factor (TNF)-α, interleukin (IL)-1β, and IL-6 [20]. Pneumolysin is also an inducer and activator of enzymes such as phospholipase A2, COX-2, and inducible nitric oxide synthase (iNOS). However, in a rabbit meningitis model, a pneumolysin-deficient pneumococcal strain resulted in an inflammatory response similar to that induced by injection of the wild-type strain, suggesting that pneumolysin is not essential for the induction of meningeal inflammation [21].

Another potential trigger of immune activation during acute meningitis is bacterial DNA released during bacterial autolysis. Bacterial DNA has substantial immune stimulatory effects on B, NK, and dendritic cells and on monocytes and macrophages [22, 23]. The activity of bacterial DNA is mediated by unmethylated CpG motifs, in particular, base contexts. In fact, when mice or rats are injected intracisternally with bacterial DNA or unmethylated CpG oligonucleotides, meningitis developed within 12 h. Bacterial DNA appears to initiate CNS inflammation by stimulation of macrophages and proinflammatory products such as TNF-α [24].

Intracellular signal transduction pathways For meningeal pathogens, the major inflammatory stimuli are lipopolysaccharide (LPS) and peptidoglycan for gram-negative and gram-positive organisms, respectively. These inflammatory stimuli activate I-κB kinase NF-κB pathways and three mitogen-activated protein kinase (MAPK) pathways: extracellular signal-regulated kinases (ERK) 1 and 2, c-Jun N-terminal kinase (JNK), and p38 [25, 26]. As a result of activation of these signaling pathways, a variety of transcription factors are activated, NF-κB (p50/p65) and activator protein-1 (cFos/cJun), which coordinate the induction of many genes encoding a variety of inflammatory mediators [27].

LPS strongly activates different kinds of kinases, suggesting a similar but not identical activation of signal transduction pathways by these major inflammatory mediators of meningeal pathogens [28].

The vicious cycle of pathophysiologic alterations (Fig. 9.1) shows that the combination of lipid peroxidation and cellular energy depletion process may contribute substantially to endothelial cell injury during bacterial meningitis. Once endothelial dysfunction occurs, the consequences include cerebrovascular autoregulation loss, loss of CO_2 reactivity of cerebral vessels, and increased permeability of the BBB. BBB permeability disruption allows plasma constituents to enter the brain, resulting in vasogenic cerebral edema and an increase in intracranial pressure [29, 30].

Intracranial pressure is a multifactorial process in meningitis and is related not only to vasogenic edema but also cytotoxic edema resulting from leukocyte infiltration, interstitial edema resulting from blockade of normal CSF pathways, and increased blood volume in the brain [31, 32]. Marked increases in intracranial pressure can be deleterious in patients with bacterial meningitis by causing cerebral herniation or decreasing cerebral perfusion (a reduction in cerebral perfusion pressure and loss of cerebrovascular autoregulation) and can ultimately lead to irreversible brain injury or death.

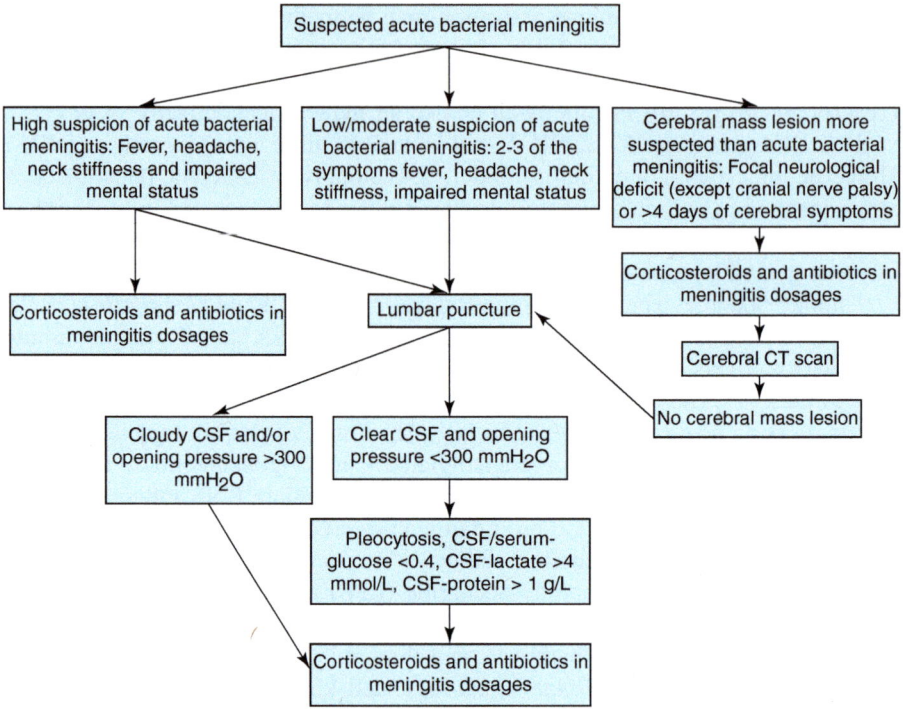

Fig. 9.1 Algorithm for diagnostic and treatment management on admission in patients with suspected community-acquired acute bacterial meningitis. CSF cerebrospinal fluid

Laboratory Studies

Routine blood work is often unrevealing. The white blood cell count is usually elevated, with a shift toward immature forms; however, severe infection can be associated with leukopenia. The platelet count may also be reduced. Leukopenia and thrombocytopenia have correlated with a poor outcome in patients with bacterial meningitis [6, 33].

Coagulation studies may be consistent with disseminated intravascular coagulation. Results of serum chemistry tests are usually commensurate with the severity of the overall process and may reveal an anion gap metabolic acidosis or hyponatremia; in one series, hyponatremia was present in 30% of patients but was usually mild and did not require specific treatment [34].

Blood cultures Two sets of blood cultures should be obtained from all patients prior to the initiation of antimicrobial therapy. Blood cultures are often positive and can be useful in the event that cerebrospinal fluid cannot be obtained before the administration of antimicrobials. Approximately 50–90% of patients with bacterial meningitis have positive blood cultures [35, 36, 44]; lower yields have been reported in some studies in patients with meningococcal infection. Cultures obtained after antimicrobial therapy are much less likely to be positive, particularly for meningococcus [38].

Tests of serum and urine for bacterial antigens, as well as cultures of mucosal surfaces for the causative pathogen, are not generally helpful.

Lumbar puncture Examination of the cerebrospinal fluid (CSF) is crucial for establishing the diagnosis of bacterial meningitis, identifying the causative organism, and performing in vitro susceptibility testing [39].

Indications for CT scan before LP Every patient with suspected meningitis should have CSF obtained unless lumbar puncture (LP) is contraindicated.

Computed tomographic (CT) scan is performed to exclude a mass lesion or increased intracranial pressure; these abnormalities might rarely lead to cerebral herniation during removal of large amounts of CSF, and cerebral herniation could have devastating consequences.

Based upon these risks and in agreement with the 2004 Infectious Diseases Society of America (IDSA) guidelines for the management of bacterial meningitis, a CT scan of the head before LP should be performed in adult patients with suspected bacterial meningitis who have one or more of the following risk factors [8, 40]:

- Immunocompromised state (e.g., HIV infection, immunosuppressive therapy, solid organ or hematopoietic cell transplantation)
- History of central nervous system (CNS) disease (mass lesion, stroke, or focal infection)
- New-onset seizure (within 1 week of presentation)
- Papilledema
- Abnormal level of consciousness
- Focal neurologic deficit

Patients with these clinical risk factors should have a CT scan to identify a possible mass lesion and other causes of increased intracranial pressure.

However, it has been suggested that a normal CT scan does not always mean that performance of an LP is safe and that certain clinical signs of impending herniation (i.e., deteriorating level of consciousness, particularly a Glasgow coma scale <11; brainstem signs including pupillary changes, posturing, or irregular respirations; or a very recent seizure) may be predictive of patients in whom an LP should be delayed [42].

Those who underwent immediate LP without CT received antibiotics 1.6 hours earlier than those who underwent CT prior to LP. Treatment delay resulted in a significantly increased risk of fatal outcome, with a relative increase in mortality of 13 percent per hour of delay [43].

A study of 815 adults with bacterial meningitis in Sweden demonstrated a decrease in mortality if there was adherence to the Swedish guidelines in contrast with the IDSA or European guidelines [43]. However, this finding may be because, in clinical practice, patients who have a CT before LP are often not started on antibiotics before neuroimaging, despite recommendations to the contrary.

If LP is delayed or deferred, blood cultures should be obtained, and antimicrobial therapy should be administered empirically before the imaging study, followed as soon as possible by the LP. In addition, dexamethasone (0.15 mg/kg intravenously [IV] every 6 hours) should be given shortly before or at the same time as the antimicrobial agents if the clinical and laboratory evidence suggests bacterial meningitis with a plan to stop therapy if indicated when the evaluation is complete. Adjunctive dexamethasone should not be given to patients who have already received antimicrobial therapy because it is unlikely to improve patient outcome [8].

Prior administration of antimicrobials tends to have minimal effects on the chemistry and cytology findings [44] but can reduce the yield of Gram stain and culture [25–27]. However, a pathogen can still be cultured from the CSF in most patients up to several hours after the administration of antimicrobial agents [41], with the possible exception of the meningococcus. This issue was addressed in a review of 128 children with bacterial meningitis in whom LP was first performed after initiation of therapy and serial LPs were obtained [41]. Among patients with meningococcal infection, CSF culture was negative in three of nine samples obtained within 1 hour. In contrast, 4–10 hours was required before CSF cultures were sterile in patients with pneumococcal meningitis.

Relative contraindications Although there are no absolute contraindications to performing an LP, caution should be used in patients with evidence of raised intracranial pressure (e.g., mass effect on CNS imaging or clinical signs of impending herniation), thrombocytopenia or another bleeding diathesis, or spinal epidural abscess.

Opening pressure The opening pressure is typically elevated in patients with bacterial meningitis. In the series of 301 adults cited above, the mean opening pressure was approximately 350 mm H2O (normal up to 200 mm H2O) [35]. However, there is a wide range of values as illustrated in a report of 296 episodes of community-acquired bacterial meningitis: 39% had values ≥300 mm H2O, while 9% had values below 140 mm H2O [7].

The opening pressure with the patient lying in the lateral decubitus position should be measured and documented.

CSF Analysis

Overview When clinical findings strongly suggest meningitis, CSF analysis including Gram stain and culture will help differentiate between bacterial and viral infection if the Gram stain and culture is positive. Normal CSF values are less than 50 mg/dL of protein, a CSF-to-serum glucose ratio greater than 0.6, less than 5 white blood cells/microL, and a lactate concentration less than 3.5 mEq/L.

There are some CSF findings that, in the appropriate clinical setting (e.g., unexplained fever and headache), are highly suggestive of bacterial meningitis. The usual CSF findings in patients with bacterial meningitis are a white blood cell count of 1000–5000/microL (range of <100 to >10,000) with a percentage of neutrophils usually greater than 80%, protein >200 mg/dL, and glucose <40 mg/dL (with a CSF/serum glucose ratio of ≤0.4).

An observational study found that bacterial meningitis was highly probable (≥99% certainty) when CSF glucose concentration is below 34 mg/dL (1.9 mmol/L), CSF protein concentration above 220 mg/dL, and white blood cell count above 2000/microL, or a neutrophil count more than 1180/microL [47]. However, clinicians must recognize that many exceptions exist and that empiric antimicrobial therapy is warranted when bacterial meningitis is suspected clinically even if the CSF abnormalities are not diagnostic.

Determination of the CSF lactate concentration has been suggested as a useful test to differentiate bacterial from viral meningitis. Two meta-analyses that included 25 studies (1692 patients) and 31 studies (1885 patients) concluded that the diagnostic accuracy of CSF lactate was superior to that of CSF white blood cell count, glucose, and protein concentration in differentiating bacterial from aseptic meningitis [48, 49], although sensitivity was lower in patients who received antimicrobial treatment prior to lumbar puncture [49], and CSF lactate may be elevated in patients with other CNS diseases.

Pleocytosis It is important to note that a false-positive elevation of the CSF white blood cell (WBC) count can be found after traumatic lumbar puncture or in patients with intracerebral or subarachnoid hemorrhage in which both red blood cells and white blood cells are introduced into the subarachnoid space. If a traumatic lumbar puncture is suspected and the peripheral WBC count is not abnormally low or high, a good rule of thumb for estimating the adjusted WBC count is to subtract 1 WBC for every 500–1500 red blood cells (RBCs) measured in the CSF.

Generalized seizures may also induce a mild transient CSF pleocytosis, although this has not been well studied [50, 51]. However, CSF pleocytosis should not be ascribed to seizure activity alone unless the fluid is clear and colorless, the opening pressure and CSF glucose are normal, the CSF Gram stain is negative, and the patient has no clinical evidence of bacterial meningitis.

Despite these typical CSF findings, the spectrum of CSF values in bacterial meningitis is so wide that the absence of one or more of the typical findings is of little value (Table 9.1) [35, 37, 45]. For example, in a review of 296 episodes of community-acquired bacterial meningitis, 50% had a CSF glucose above 40 mg/dL (2.2 mmol/L), 44% had a CSF protein below 200 mg/dL, and 13% had a CSF white blood cell count below 100/microL [41]. In another series of 696 episodes of community-acquired bacterial meningitis, 12% had none of the characteristic CSF findings of bacterial meningitis [36].

Table 9.1 Spinal fluid analysis for meningitis

Etiology	Opening pressure	WBC count	Protein	Glucose	CSF/serum glucose ratio
Normal	<180 mm H_2O*	≤5 cells/mm³	15–45 mg/dL	45–80 mg/dL	0.6–0.7
Bacterial	>180 mm H_2O	>100 cells/mm³	>45 mg/dL	<40 mg/dL	<0.4
		PMNs predominant			
Viral, *Borrelia burgdorferi, Treponema pallidum, Bartonella henselae*	<180 mm H_2O	25–500 cells/mm³	15–45 mg/dL	45–80 mg/dL	0.6–0.7
		Lymphocyte predominant			
Fungi, *Mycobacterium tuberculosis,* sarcoid, lymphoma, leptomeningeal metastases, partially treated bacterial meningitis	Normal or increased	25–500 cells/mm³	>45 mg/dL	<40 mg/dL	<0.6
		Lymphocyte predominant			

Gram stain A Gram stain should be obtained whenever there is suspicion of bacterial meningitis. It has the advantage of suggesting the bacterial etiology 1 day or more before culture results are available [38]. The following findings may be seen:

1. Gram-positive diplococci suggest pneumococcal infection.
2. Gram-negative diplococci suggest meningococcal infection.
3. Small pleomorphic gram-negative coccobacilli suggest *Haemophilus influenzae* infection.
4. Gram-positive rods and coccobacilli suggest *Listeria monocytogenes* infection.

The reported sensitivity of Gram stain for bacterial meningitis has varied from 60% to 90%; however, the specificity approaches 100% [45].

The Gram stain is positive in 10–15% of patients who have bacterial meningitis but negative CSF cultures [7]. As noted above, the yield of both Gram stain and culture may be reduced by prior antibiotic therapy [38, 41].

Rapid tests Several rapid diagnostic tests have been developed to aid in the diagnosis of bacterial meningitis. Latex agglutination tests detect the antigens of the common meningeal pathogens in the CSF, although these tests are no longer routinely recommended because results do not appear to modify the decision to administer antimicrobial therapy and false-positive results have been reported [8]. An immunochromatographic test for detection of *S. pneumoniae* in CSF was found to be 100% sensitive and specific for the diagnosis of pyogenic pneumococcal meningitis [46]. More studies are needed, however, before this test can be routinely recommended.

Polymerase chain reaction Nucleic acid amplification tests, such as the polymerase chain reaction (PCR), have been evaluated in patients with bacterial meningitis. One study evaluated a multiplex PCR assay for detection of *N. meningitidis*, *S. pneumoniae*, and *H. influenzae* type B and had an overall specificity and positive predictive value of 100%; the negative predictive value was >99% [52]. The sensitivity and specificity of CSF PCR for the diagnosis of pneumococcal meningitis is 92–100% and 100%, respectively [53].

Problems with false-positive results have been reported with PCR. However, further refinements in this technique may make it useful for the diagnosis of bacterial meningitis, especially when results of CSF Gram stain and culture are negative, especially in patients who have received prior antimicrobial therapy. Use of PCR for the two most common meningeal pathogens (*S. pneumoniae* and *N. meningitidis*) is routinely recommended in the UK guidelines for patients presenting with meningitis [11].

In the absence of a positive Gram stain, which has almost 100% specificity (i.e., very few false positives), studies in both adults and children have concluded that, in the setting of an elevated CSF white blood cell count, no single CSF biochemical variable can reliably exclude bacterial meningitis [45, 54].

Critical Care Management of Meningitis

The choice of antimicrobial therapy is based on the age of the patient, underlying risk factors for disease (e.g., immunocompromise, trauma, neurosurgery), and patterns of antimicrobial resistance in the community. According to the Infectious Diseases Society of America (IDSA) practice guidelines for the management of bacterial meningitis, poor outcomes are associated with advanced clinical severity of disease, and empiric antimicrobial therapy for suspected or proven bacterial meningitis should be initiated as soon as possible after the diagnosis of bacterial meningitis is suspected [29]. Results from CSF Gram stain, culture, and susceptibility testing will allow modifications and refinements in empiric antimicrobial therapy. Due to the emergence of penicillin-resistant *S. pneumoniae* infections, current empiric standard therapy for suspected adult bacterial meningitis includes vancomycin and a third-generation cephalosporin, such as ceftriaxone or cefotaxime [55]. In cases of suspected *Listeria* infection (e.g., age > 65, alcoholism, pregnancy, atypical CSF profile), empiric therapy should include ampicillin or penicillin G, as cephalosporins have limited activity against this organism (Fig. 9.2).

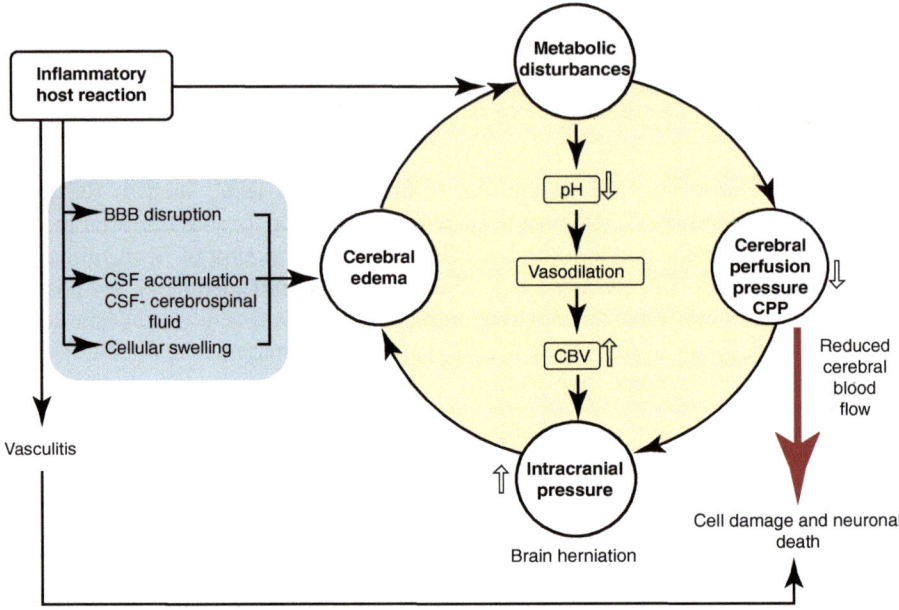

Fig. 9.2 Vicious cycle of pathophysiologic alterations leading to neuronal injury during bacterial meningitis. BBB blood-brain barrier, CBV cerebral blood volume, CSF cerebrospinal fluid

Adjunctive corticosteroid therapy for bacterial meningitis is started in patients to treat the underlying cerebral edema, inflammation, and increased intracranial pressure (ICP). Adjunctive corticosteroids improve outcomes in infants and children with *H. influenzae* type B and in adults with *S. pneumoniae* meningitis [56, 57]. A randomized, double-blind, placebo-controlled trial evaluating the efficacy of corticosteroid therapy found that the addition of corticosteroids reduced the risk of unfavorable outcome from 25% to 15% and reduced mortality from 15% to 7% [57]. The benefit was greatest in patients with intermediate severity of disease and *S. pneumoniae* infection. Practice guidelines published in 2004 from the IDSA state that consideration should be given to administer adjunctive dexamethasone in patients with suspected or proven bacterial meningitis and adjunctive dexamethasone should be initiated in all adult patients with suspected or proven pneumococcal meningitis [29]. Recent studies in the developing world suggest no clear benefit with adjunctive corticosteroid therapy in children and adults [58, 59], and these data were analyzed in a large meta-analysis, which questioned the mortality benefit for corticosteroid therapy in patients in the developing world [60, 61]. The underlying etiology of different responses to corticosteroid therapy in the developed world and the developing world is not clear. A recent observational study from the Netherlands found that mortality from bacterial meningitis had decreased from 30% to 20% after steroid therapy became widely used as a general standard of care [62]. Administration of corticosteroid therapy in cases of *S. pneumoniae* meningitis was also found to preferentially benefit patients >55 years of age in another study from a developed

Table 9.2 Recommendations for antimicrobial therapy in adult patients with presumptive pathogen identification by positive Gram stain

Microorganism	Recommended therapy	Alternative therapies
Streptococcus pneumoniae	Vancomycin plus a third-generation cephalosporin[a, b]	Meropenem, fluoroquinolene[c]
Neisseria meningitidis	Third-generation cephalosporin[a]	Penicillin G, ampicillin, chloramphenicol, fluoroquinolone, aztreonam
Listeria monocytogenes	Ampicillin[d] or penicillin G[d]	Trimethoprim-sulfamethoxazole, meropenem
Streptococcus agalactiae	Ampicillin[d] or penicillin G[d]	Third-generation cephalosporin[a]
Haemophilus influenzae	Third-generation cephalosporin[a]	Chloramphenicol, cefepime, meropenem, fluoroquinolone
Escherichia coli	Third-generation cephalosporin[a]	Cefepime, meropenem, aztreonam, fluoroquinolone, trimethoprim-sulfamethoxazole

Note: In children, ampicillin is added to the standard therapeutic regimen of cefotaxime or ceftriaxone plus vancomycin when *L. monocytogenes* is considered and to an aminoglycoside if a gram-negative enteric pathogen is of concern
[a]Ceftriaxone or cefotaxime
[b]Some experts would add rifampin if dexamethasone is also given
[c]Gatifloxacin or moxifloxacin
[d]Addition of an aminoglycoside should be considered

country [60, 62]. Based on the IDSA guidelines and recent data, patients with suspected or proven *S. pneumoniae* meningitis in the developed world should receive adjunctive dexamethasone therapy. Data to support initiation of adjunctive dexamethasone therapy in patients in the developing world with bacterial meningitis is less clear and must be left to the discretion of the treating physician (Tables 9.2 and 9.3).

Encephalitis

Encephalitis is an inflammation of brain tissue that leads to alterations in level of consciousness (LOC), cognition, and behavior. It can also cause fever, headache, seizures, cranial nerve disorders, and motor deficits, including paralysis. Encephalitis results from various identifiable etiologies.

Viral encephalitis. Many viruses are transmitted to humans by arthropods, such as mosquitoes and ticks, and are called arthropod-borne viruses or arboviruses. Arboviruses include Japanese encephalitis virus (JEV), West Nile virus (WNV), Eastern equine encephalitis virus (EEEV), St. Louis encephalitis virus (SLEV), chikungunya virus (CKNV), and others. Arbovirus infections such as WNV, EEEV, and SLEV are designated by the Council of State and Territorial Epidemiologists and the CDC as nationally notifiable infectious diseases [63].

Table 9.3 Recommendations for empirical antimicrobial therapy for purulent meningitis based on patient age and specific predisposing condition

Predisposing factor	Common bacterial pathogens	Antimicrobial therapy
Age		
< 1 month	*Streptococcus agalactiae, Escherichia coli, Listeria monocytogenes, Klebsiella* species	Ampicillin plus cefotaxime or ampicillin plus an aminoglycoside
1–23 months	*Streptococcus pneumoniae, Neisseria meningitidis, S. agalactiae, Haemophilus influenzae, E. coli*	Vancomycin plus a third-generation cephalosporin[a, b]
2–50 years	*N. meningitidis, S. pneumoniae*	Vancomycin plus a third-generation cephalosporin[a, b]
>50 years	*S. pneumoniae, N. meningitidis, L. monocytogenes*, aerobic gram-negative bacilli	Vancomycin plus ampicillin plus a third-generation cephalosporin[a, b]
Head trauma		
Basilar skull fracture	*S. pneumoniae, H. influenzae*, group A β-hemolytic streptococci	Vancomycin plus a third-generation cephalosporin[a]
Penetrating trauma	*Staphylococcus aureus*, coagulase-negative staphylococci (especially *Staphylococcus epidermidis*), aerobic gram-negative bacilli (including *Pseudomonas aeruginosa*)	Vancomycin plus cefepime, vancomycin plus ceftazidime, or vancomycin plus meropenem
Postneurosurgery	Aerobic gram-negative bacilli (including *P. aeruginosa*), *S. aureus*, coagulase-negative staphylococci (especially *S. epidermidis*)	Vancomycin plus cefepime, vancomycin plus ceftazidime, or vancomycin plus meropenem
CSF shunt	Coagulase-negative staphylococci (especially *S. epidermidis*), *S. aureus*, aerobic gram-negative bacilli (including *P. aeruginosa*), *Propionibacterium acnes*	Vancomycin plus cefepime,[c] vancomycin plus ceftazidime,[c] or vancomycin plus meropenem[c]

[a]Ceftriaxone or cefotaxime
[b]Some experts would add rifampin if dexamethasone is also given
[c]In infants and children, vancomycin alone is reasonable unless Gram stains reveal the presence of gram-negative bacilli

JEV is the leading cause of encephalitis, with an estimated 67,900 annual cases worldwide. The Advisory Committee on Immunization Practices (ACIP) recommends JEV vaccination for all travelers who plan to spend 1 month or more in JEV-endemic regions (Asia) during the transmission season (in temperate regions of China, Japan, the Korean Peninsula, and eastern parts of Russia, transmission occurs mainly during the summer and fall; it may take place year-round in Southeast Asia).15 ACIP also recommends vaccination for short-term travelers going to areas with known outbreaks and short-term travelers who are unsure of their itineraries [64].

WNV continues to pose a significant disease burden in human populations, with new emerging or reemerging strains. Between 1999 and 2013, more than 39,000 cases of clinical WNV were reported to the CDC. In 2012, the CDC reported the highest number of human WNV cases in the United States since 2003. The majority of individuals present with signs and symptoms such as fatigue, fever, and headache. They may also present with myalgia, muscle weakness, rash, difficulty concentrating, neck pain, arthralgia, gastrointestinal symptoms, photophobia, and maculopapular or morbilliform rash involving the neck, trunk, arms, or legs [65].

Approximately 75% of individuals infected with WNV remain asymptomatic. Those who progress to WNV encephalitis present for clinical care with a prolonged altered mental status greater than 24 hours, seizures, and focal neurologic abnormalities.

Of the 5674 cases of WNV reported to the CDC in 2012, 51% were determined to be West Nile neuroinvasive disease (WNND), amounting to the highest number of human neuroinvasive cases caused by a mosquito-borne or arbovirus in US history. Prior to 2012, WNND accounted for less than 1% of symptomatic cases per year. WNND is characterized by meningitis, encephalitis, and acute flaccid paralysis and occurs in 1 in 150 WNV-infected individuals. In 2012, 286 deaths occurred from WNV/WNND, the most WNV-associated fatalities on record in the United States. Among patients who meet clinical criteria for WNND, acute case fatality is 5–10% [65, 66].

Herpes simplex virus type 1 (HSV-1), varicella-zoster virus (VZV), and enterovirus are three of the most commonly identified etiologic agents associated with acute encephalitis. Herpes is the most common cause of sporadic encephalitis in Western countries, with an incidence of approximately two to four cases per million per year. Herpes simplex virus encephalitis (HSE) is the most common nonepidemic form of viral encephalitis in Western countries. Affecting the limbic structures of the brain, HSE causes fever, alterations in LOC, personality change, memory dysfunction, seizures, and focal neurologic deficits. The most common focal neurologic findings include aphasia, ataxia, involuntary movements including myoclonus, and cranial nerve dysfunction. However, HSV-1 can cause severe necrotizing encephalitis with high mortality approaching 70% without treatment. Clinical presentation, brain imaging such as magnetic resonance imaging (MRI), and cerebral spinal fluid (CSF) analysis are necessary for the diagnosis of HSE. Unilateral or bilateral temporal lobe involvement is the classic finding of HSE seen on MRI [67, 68].

Because HSV, VZV, and enterovirus are three of the most commonly identified etiologic agents in acute encephalitis, they should be routinely screened for in CSF analysis. If HSE is still suspected despite negative testing from the first CSF analysis, a second CSF analysis should be repeated within 3–7 days [67–69].

The prevalence of HSE is not increased in immunocompromised hosts, but the presentation may be subacute or atypical in these patients. HSE has a bimodal distribution by age, with the first peak occurring in patients under age 20 and a second peak occurring in patients over age 50. HSE in younger patients usually represents primary infection, whereas HSE in older patients typically reflects reactivation of latent infection. Untreated HSE is progressive and often fatal in 7–14 days. Even with treatment, permanent neurologic deficits are common, affecting more than 50% of survivors [74].

Bacterial Encephalitis

Rates of bacterial encephalitis in the United States have declined in the last decade due in large part to highly effective vaccination programs. Because of vaccination, the incidence of bacterial encephalitis fell from 0.44 cases per 100,000 between 1998 and 1999 to 0.19 cases between 2006 and 2007.

Diagnosis of Encephalitis

A thorough health and travel history can help identify potential causes of encephalitis and should include a review of all recent travel, infections, and vaccinations. The history should also include any report of a recent bite from a potentially rabid animal or exposure to mosquitoes, ticks, or rodents. In addition, the season in which illness occurs, and the disease currently prevalent in the community, may provide clues to the diagnosis [75].

Other relevant history that can provide clues to the diagnosis include drug and alcohol use, occupational or recreational exposure to rural or outdoor settings (farmers, hunters, campers, forest workers), and the immune status of the patient. Although pathologic examination and testing of brain tissue are considered to be the diagnostic gold standard for encephalitis, they are rarely done due to potential morbidity associated with an invasive neurosurgical procedure. In the absence of pathologic brain tissue confirmation, encephalitis is diagnosed based on selected clinical, lab, electroencephalography (EEG), and neuroimaging features [75]. In addition to brain imaging, CSF polymerase chain reaction (PCR) analysis is considered a standard diagnostic study for HSE. The benefit of PCR is that the replication of viral DNA can result in both a rapid and specific diagnosis that can facilitate targeted therapies early [75].

An LP is the most common approach to access CSF for pressure measurement and sample analysis. Before performing an LP, evidence of a space-occupying brain lesion causing suspected or known increased ICP should first be ruled out because removal of CSF could precipitate cerebral bleeding or brain herniation.

Because the spinal cord terminates at the L2 level, the spinal needle used for an LP enters or punctures the L4–L5 intervertebral space to avoid damage to the spinal cord. The subarachnoid space of the lumbar cistern is punctured and accessed. This location is used both to measure spinal fluid opening and closing pressure and to remove CSF for analysis [70, 71].

The spinal fluid usually is clear, and opening pressure is normally 10–20 cm H2O. Elevated opening pressure may contribute to the neurologic dysfunction in encephalitis and must be managed as part of the treatment plan [71].

Management Fever can increase cerebral metabolism, oxygen demand, and accumulation of leukocytes, which also increases with temperature. These changes in inflammatory processes could worsen the neurologic condition by disrupting the blood-brain barrier leading to brain tissue edema. Inflammation also increases the viscosity of CSF, which can interfere with absorption, leading to increased ICP, cerebral edema, and hydrocephalus [72]. Concerns for ICP elevation and cerebral mass effect due to brain tissue edema from inflammation should prompt rapid bedside assessment and direct neurologic imaging such as a non-contrast head computed tomography (CT) scan. Rapidly evolving hydrocephalus, seen on CT scan, typically requires the placement of a ventriculostomy for CSF drainage and ICP monitoring [72].

Altered LOC associated with unilateral or bilateral pupillary dilation and sluggish reaction or nonreactivity to light may indicate a neurologic emergency such as transtentorial brain tissue herniation from increased ICP [72].

A recent review addressed interventions designed to manage acute brain tissue herniation. Normal oxygenation (oxygen saturation greater than 90%) and hyperventilation to a PaCO2 of 30 ± 2 mm Hg (normal 35–45 mm Hg) and mean arterial pressure of at least 60 mm Hg are recommended. Hyperosmolar therapy with IV mannitol or hypertonic saline may also be indicated. When administering IV mannitol, it is important to anticipate and correct subsequent diuresis with 0.9% sodium chloride solution to avoid dehydration. Head-of-bed elevation to greater than or equal to 30 degrees can be effective in reducing or controlling increased ICP. Despite interventions, brain tissue edema, ICP elevation, and herniation may progress. Initiation of a pharmacologic-induced barbiturate coma with endotracheal intubation and mechanical ventilation, if not already done, or a surgical hemicraniectomy to relieve global ICP, may be necessary [75].

Encephalitis-associated seizure activity can worsen the patient's neurologic status and should be recognized and treated immediately. EEG monitoring is essential, and continuous EEG (cEEG) is recommended to improve diagnosis and to monitor the effect of antiepileptic drugs (AEDs) in real time [75].

For individuals with suspected or diagnosed seizures, first-line benzodiazepine agents such as lorazepam or midazolam are administered. Second-line AEDs, such as fosphenytoin, levetiracetam, or valproic acid, can be tailored to the specific clinical situation [75].

For patients who progress to medically refractory seizures, a third-line AED with anesthetic properties, such as barbiturates including pentobarbital or phenobarbital, or other agents such as propofol or ketamine, may be necessary. Depending on individual response to AEDs, it may be necessary to temporarily induce a pharmacologic burst suppression pattern on EEG using third-line agents as therapeutic serum levels of second-line AEDs are reached. Burst suppression, although not a specific treatment for long-term control of medically refractory seizures, can be beneficial to help recovery after brain injuries and to treat epilepsy that is refractory to conventional drug therapies. On cEEG, burst suppression is characterized by alternating patterns of generalized electrical silence, seen as a flat EEG pattern, which is interrupted by generalized bursts of chaotic electrical activity seen as spikes and waves. The goal of burst suppression on cEEG is from one to three bursts every 10 seconds [73, 75]. Aggressive seizure treatment and management requires ICU support due to potential complications from the seizure activity or the medications administered to control seizures such as hypotension, loss of protective airway reflexes, and impaired respiratory drive.

Treating Encephalitis

At time of presentation, it is important to consider empiric and broad-spectrum management for common etiologies of encephalitis. The foremost consideration is for HSV and the need to start IV antiviral medication (acyclovir) as early as possible. A delay in IV acyclovir treatment in individuals with suspected or known HSV-1 infection can result in an increased risk of severe permanent disability and death [76].

Any suspicion of bacterial infection may necessitate broader coverage with appropriate antibiotics and corticosteroids. In addition, results of the diagnostic evaluation may prompt administration of other appropriate antibacterial or antifungal agents [76].

Brain Abscess

Brain abscess is a focal area of necrosis with a surrounding membrane within the brain parenchyma, usually resulting from an infectious process or rarely from a traumatic process [77–79].

Etiology

Direct Local Spread

Brain abscess can originate from infections in head and neck sites: otitis media (5%) and mastoiditis (secondarily cause inferior temporal lobe and cerebellar brain abscesses), paranasal sinus infection (approximately 30–50% as the reported cause), infection from frontal or ethmoid sinuses that spreads to the frontal lobes, and dental infection that usually causes frontal lobar abscesses. Facial trauma, even from neurosurgical procedures, can result in necrotic tissue, and brain abscesses have been reported afterward. Metal fragments or other foreign bodies left in the brain parenchyma can also serve as a nidus for infection [80].

Generalized Septicemia and Hematogenous Spread

Various conditions can cause hematogenous seeding of the brain. The most common associated organ; pulmonary infections, such as lung abscess and empyema, often in hosts with bronchiectasis; or cystic fibrosis from an important encountered cause. Others include pneumonia, pulmonary arteriovenous malformation, and bronchopleural fistula. Other common reason is cyanotic congenital heart diseases in children which associated with more than 60% of cases. Bacterial endocarditis, ventricular aneurysms, and thrombosis are also among the causes. Skin, pelvic, and intraabdominal infections have been reported frequently as risk factors. Brain abscesses associated with bacteremia commonly cause multiple abscesses mostly in the distribution of the middle cerebral artery and usually at the gray-white matter junction.

The most common microbial pathogens isolated from brain abscess are *Staphylococcus* and *Streptococcus*. Among this class of bacteria, *Staphylococcus aureus* and viridans streptococci are the commonest.

Epidemiology

According to studies, the incidence of brain abscess is approximately 8% of intracranial masses in developing countries and 1–2% in the Western countries with almost four cases occurring per million. The prevalence of brain abscess in patients with AIDS is higher. Therefore, the prevalence rate has increased with the emanation of AIDS pandemic. Approximately 1500–2500 cases are diagnosed annually in the United States. The incidence of fungal brain abscess also has increased because of higher usage of broad-spectrum antibiotics and immunosuppressive agents like steroids. Prevalence is highest in adult men younger than 30 years, while pediatric disease occurs most frequently in children aged 4–7 years. Neonates are third in high-risk groups. Vaccination has reduced the prevalence of young children. Data suggests that brain abscesses are more predominant in males than in females with a male-to-female ratio varying between 2:1 and 3:1. Geographical and seasonal differences have no significant impact. In developing countries with poor living standards, brain abscess accounts for a disproportionate percentage of space-occupying intracranial lesions compared to developed nations [81, 82].

Pathophysiology

The histologic changes depend upon the stage of the infection. The early (first 1–2 weeks) lesion, often called focal cerebritis, is poorly demarcated and is evident by acute inflammatory changes like vascular congestion and localized edema. This early stage is commonly called cerebritis. After 2–3 weeks, necrosis and liquefaction occur, which is then covered by a distinct capsule consisting of an inner layer of granulation tissue, a middle collagenous layer, and an outer astroglial layer; surrounding brain parenchyma is often edematous.

History and Physical Exam

In about two-thirds of cases, symptoms are present for 2 weeks or less. The diagnosis is made at a mean of 8 days after the onset of symptoms. The course ranges from indolent to fulminant. Most manifestations of brain abscess tend to be nonspecific, resulting in a delay in establishing the diagnosis. Most symptoms are a direct result of the size and location of the space-occupying lesion or lesions. The triad of fever, headache, and the focal neurologic deficit is observed in less than half of patients. The frequency of common symptoms and signs is as follows:

- A headache (69–70%), the most common medical symptom.
- Mental status changes (65%): lethargy progressing to coma is indicative of severe cerebral edema and a poor prognostic sign.
- Focal neurologic deficits (50–65%) occur days to weeks after the onset of a headache.
- Pain is usually localized to the side of the abscess, and its onset can be gradual or sudden. The pain is most severe in intensity and not relieved by over-the-counter pain medications.
- Fever (45–53%).
- Seizures (25–35%) can be the first manifestation of brain abscess. Grand mal seizures are particularly frequent in frontal abscesses.
- Nausea and vomiting (40%) are mostly seen with raised intracranial pressure.
- Nuchal rigidity (15%) is most commonly associated with occipital lobe abscess or an abscess that has leaked into a lateral ventricle.
- Third and sixth cranial nerve deficits.
- Rupture of abscess usually presented with sudden worsening headache and followed by emerging signs of meningismus.

Evaluation

Routine Tests

CBC with differential and platelet count, ESR, serum C-reactive protein, serologic test, blood cultures (at least two; preferably before antibiotic therapy).

Lumbar Puncture

Rarely required and only should be performed with a prior CT and MRI scan after ruling out increased intracranial pressure because of the potential for cerebrospinal fluid (CSF) herniation and death. In circumstances of acute presentation of patients or suspicion of meningitis, blood cultures can be used for initiation of antibiotic therapy.

Stereotactic CT or Surgical Aspiration

Samples obtained can be employed for culture, Gram stain, serology, histopathology, and polymerase chain reaction.

Computed Tomography

Imaging findings depend on the stage of the lesion. Early cerebritis often appears as an irregular low-density area that does not enhance or may show infrequent patchy enhancement. As cerebritis evolves, a more conspicuous rim-enhancing lesion becomes visible. Enzmann et al. reported that CT findings of patchy enhancement in early cerebritis grow to a rim of enhancement in late cerebritis which later on forms the brain abscess. A key histopathologic difference is that rim enhancement of late cerebritis is not associated with collagen deposition as seen in an abscess where it surrounds a purulent cavity. Serial CT examinations in patients with late abscess show progressively decreasing edema and mass effect. Brain abscess wall is usually smooth and regular with 1 mm to 3 mm thickness with surrounding parenchymal edema. The ring of enhancement may not be uniform in thickness and can be relatively thin on the medial or ventricular surface in the deep white matter, where vascularity is less abundant. Edema and contrast enhancement are suppressed by administration of steroids. Multi-location with subjacent daughter abscesses or satellite lesions is frequently seen. Gas if present is suggestive of gas-forming organisms [82, 83].

Magnetic Resonance Imaging

MRI is the imaging modality of choice for diagnosis as well as follow-up of lesions. It is more sensitive for early cerebritis and satellite lesions particularly those present in the brainstem as well as estimating the necrosis and extent of the injury. It allows for higher contrast between cerebral edema and the brain and is also more sensitive for detecting the spread of inflammation into the ventricles and subarachnoid space [7, 8].

Conventional Spin Echo Imaging with Contrast

Classic MR imaging findings of an abscess include a contrast-enhanced rim surrounding a necrotic core. Rim is T1 isointense to hyperintense relative to white matter and T2 hypointense. On MRI characteristic smooth tri-laminar structure of the rim on T2W imaging proves helpful in differentiating from other ring-enhancing lesions. Central necrosis shows variable hyperintensity on T2 depending upon the degree of protein content and hypointense on T1.

Diffusion-Weighted Magnetic Resonance Imaging

DWI is capable of distinguishing brain abscess from other ring-enhancing brain lesions. Abscesses are typically hyperintense on DWI (indicating restricted diffusion), while neoplasms like glioma as lack restricted diffusion appearing hypointense or variable hyperintense much lower than an abscess [84].

Diffusion tensor imaging is based on three-dimensional diffusivity and commonly employed for evaluation of white matter tracts. Fractional anisotropy, a quantitative variable, is calculated by diffusion tensor imaging. This variable reflects the degree of tissue organization and quite higher in abscess supposedly due to organized leukocytes in the abscess cavity.

Proton MR spectroscopy probe tissue metabolism. Spectral analysis reveals elevated succinate, although not commonly seen is quite specific for an abscess. Other significant metabolites include high acetate, alanine, and lactate signals. Amino acids from neutrophil-driven protein breakdown suggest a pyogenic abscess. MR spectroscopy may be used to further differentiate anaerobic from aerobic metabolism by elevated succinate and acetate peaks which are only observed in anaerobic infections due to glycolysis and subsequent fermentation. Also, lactate peaks are lowest in strict anaerobes owing to metabolic lactate consumption [83].

Treatment/Management

A brain abscess can lead to elevated intracranial pressure and has significant morbidity and mortality. Management can be divided into medical and surgical approaches.

Medical management can be considered for deep-seated, small abscess (less than 2 cm), cases of co-existing meningitis, and few other selected cases. Usually, a combination of both medical and surgical approaches is considered [78].

CT and MRI brain offer clear guides in management by localizing the abscess and delineating details including dimensions and a number of abscesses. Usually, large abscesses (more than 2 cm) are considered for aspiration or excision based on surgical skills of the operator. While the approach for multiple abscesses includes long course (4–8 weeks) of high-dose antibiotics with or without aspirations, based on weekly CT scanning.

Selection of antibiotic regimen should be wisely made based on microorganisms isolated from blood or CSF. Certain antibiotics are unable to cross the blood-brain barrier and are not useful in treating brain abscess; these antibiotics include first-generation cephalosporins, aminoglycosides, and tetracyclines.

Specific antibiotic regimens according to microorganisms:

- Gram-positive bacteria including streptococci: third-generation cephalosporin (e.g., cefotaxime, ceftriaxone) or penicillin G is effective.
- *Staph. aureus* and *Staph. epidermis* are usually seen in association with penetrating brain trauma and/or neurosurgical procedure. These should be covered with vancomycin. It is also effective for *Clostridium* species. In cases of vancomycin resistance, linezolid, trimethoprim-sulfamethoxazole, or daptomycin can be considered.
- Fungal infections including *Candida* and *Cryptococcus* need to be treated with amphotericin B.
- *Aspergillus* and *Pseudallescheria boydii*: voriconazole can be considered.
- *Toxoplasma gondii* infection is treated with pyrimethamine and sulfadiazine, which can be combined with HAART in cases of HIV.

Steroids can be considered in select cases, especially to reduce the mass effect and improve antibiotic penetration and cerebral edema [85].

The surgical approach has a pivotal role in the management of brain abscess. The choice of the procedure depends on operator skills and preference. Strategies include ultrasound, or CT-guided needle aspirations via the stereotactic procedure, burr hole, and craniotomy for loculated multiple abscesses. Intravenous or intrathecal agents against specific microorganisms are considered with surgical therapy [86].

Prognosis

With the advent of antimicrobials and imaging studies as CT scanning and MRI, the mortality rate has reduced from 5% to 10%. Rupture of a brain abscess, however, is fatal. The long-term neurological sequelae after the infection are dependent on the early diagnosis and administration of antibiotics [87].

Cranial Subdural Empyema

Cranial subdural empyema (SDE) presents as a focal, loculated suppuration between the dura mater and the arachnoid [88]. Symptom onset is usually very rapid with initial complaints of fever and headache that follow recent craniofacial infection (otitis or sinusitis) or trauma [88]. Patients develop meningeal irritation, increased intracranial pressure, focal neurological signs or symptoms, altered consciousness, and seizures [89]. Causative organisms are dependent on the original site of infection. In cases of craniofacial infection, *S. anginosus* group with or without associated anaerobic organisms are common etiologic bacteria followed by *Staphylococcus* sp. and gram-negative organisms associated with otogenic sources [88]. Postsurgical SE is commonly associated with *S. aureus* infection in as many as 46% of cases [88]. Other hospital-acquired gram-negative rods, including *Pseudomonas* sp. and *Klebsiella pneumoniae*, contribute significantly as well to iatrogenic SE and should be considered when empiric therapy is initiated [90].

As with brain abscess, MRI is the preferred imaging modality to diagnose SE, and the CT scan is less sensitive, especially in cases of posterior fossa involvement. CSF examination is not recommended because the infection is localized and encapsulated, such that CSF examination often provides little useful diagnostic information and may increase the risk of cerebral herniation [91].

Treatment of SE is a medical emergency and requires a combined surgical and therapeutic approach. The optimum therapy for SE involves surgical drainage and antibiotic treatment based on Gram stain and cultures obtained at the time of the drainage procedure. Empiric antibiotic treatment should be initiated based on suspected organisms and the underlying risk factor for the development of SE. The goals of surgical therapy for cranial SE are to decompress the brain and evacuate the empyema. With appropriate management, mortality rates are 10% in patients with functional mental status at presentation, but mortality increases to 50% in patients that present later in infection with significant changes in mental status or semicomatose state [91, 92]. Thus, early and urgent intervention is vital to improving outcomes in patients with subdural empyema.

References

1. Schuchat A, Robinson K, Wenger JK, et al. Bacterial meningitis in the United States in 1995. Active Surveillance Team. N Engl J Med. 1997;337:970–6.
2. Uchihara T, Tsukagoshi H. Jolt accentuation of headache: the most sensitive sign of CSF pleocytosis. Headache. 1991;31:167.
3. Thomas KE, Hasbun R, Jekel J, Quagliarello VJ. The diagnostic accuracy of Kernig's sign, Brudzinski's sign, and nuchal rigidity in adults with suspected meningitis. Clin Infect Dis. 2002;35:46.
4. Nakao JH, Jafri FN, Shah K, Newman DH. Jolt accentuation of headache and other clinical signs: poor predictors of meningitis in adults. Am J Emerg Med. 2014;32:24.
5. Zoons E, Weisfelt M, de Gans J, et al. Seizures in adults with bacterial meningitis. Neurology. 2008;70:2109.
6. Kornelisse RF, Westerbeek CM, Spoor AB, et al. Pneumococcal meningitis in children: prognostic indicators and outcome. Clin Infect Dis. 1995;21:1390.
7. Durand ML, Calderwood SB, Weber DJ, et al. Acute bacterial meningitis in adults. A review of 493 episodes. N Engl J Med. 1993;328:21–8.
8. Tunkel AR, Hartman BJ, Kaplan SL, et al. Practice guidelines for the management of bacterial meningitis. Clin Infect Dis. 2004;39:1267–84. https://doi.org/10.1086/425368.
9. Brouwer MC, van de Beek D, Heckenberg SG, et al. Community-acquired Listeria monocytogenes meningitis in adults. Clin Infect Dis. 2006;43:1233.
10. Tunkel AR. Approach to the patient with central nervous system infection. In: Bennett JE, Dolin R, Blaser MJ, editors. Principles and practice of infectious diseases. 8th ed. Philadelphia: Elsevier Saunders; 2015. p. 1091.

11. McGill F, Heyderman RS, Michael BD, et al. The UK joint specialist societies guideline on the diagnosis and management of acute meningitis and meningococcal sepsis in immunocompetent adults. J Infect. 2016;72:405.
12. Beek D, Gans J, Spanjaard L, Weisfelt M, Reitsma JB, Vermeulen M. Clinical features and prognostic factors in adults with bacterial meningitis. N Engl J Med. 2004;351:1849–59.
13. Scheld WM, Koedel U, Nathan B, Pfister HW. Pathophysiology of bacterial meningitis: mechanism(s) of neuronal injury. J Infect Dis. 2002;186(Suppl 2):S225.
14. Arditi M, Mason EOJ, Bradley JS, et al. Three-year multicenter surveillance of pneumococcal meningitis in children: clinical characteristics, and outcome related to penicillin susceptibility and dexamethasone use. Pediatrics. 1998;102:1087–97.
15. Hortal M, Camou T, Palacio R, Dibarbourne H, Garcia A. Ten-year review of invasive pneumococcal diseases in children and adults from Uruguay: clinical spectrum, serotypes, and antimicrobial resistance. Int J Infect Dis. 2000;4:91–5.
16. Lopez R, Garcia E, Garcia P, Garcia JL. The pneumococcal cell wall degrading enzymes: a modular design to create new lysins. Microb Drug Resist. 1997;3:199–211.
17. Tuomanen E, Liu H, Hengstler B, Zak O, Tomasz A. The induction of meningeal inflammation by components of the pneumococcal cell wall. J Infect Dis. 1985;151:859–68.
18. Tuomanen E, Tomasz A, Hengstler B, Zak O. The relative role of bacterial cell wall and capsule in the induction of inflammation in pneumococcal meningitis. J Infect Dis. 1985;151: 535–40.
19. Yoshimura A, Lien E, Ingalls RR, Tuomanen E, Dziarski R. Cutting edge: recognition of gram-positive bacterial cell wall components by the innate immune system occurs via toll-like receptor 2. J Immunol. 1999;163:1–5.
20. Braun JS, Novak R, Gao G, Murray PJ, Shenep JL. Pneumolysin, a protein toxin of Streptococcus pneumoniae induces nitric oxide production from macrophages. Infect Immun. 1999;67:3750–6.
21. Friedland IR, Paris MM, Hickey S, et al. The limited role of pneumolysin in the pathogenesis of pneumococcal meningitis. J Infect Dis. 1995;172:805–9.
22. Medzhitov R. CpG DNA: security code for host defense. Nat Immunol. 2001;2:15–6.
23. Wagner H. Toll meets bacterial CpG-DNA. Immunity. 2001;14:499–502.
24. Deng GM, Liu ZQ, Tarkowski A. Intracisternally localized bacterial DNA containing CpG motifs induces meningitis. J Immunol. 2001;167:4616–26.
25. Chang L, Karin M. Mammalian MAP kinase signaling cascades. Nature. 2001;410:37–40.
26. Herlaar E, Brown Z. p38 MAPK signaling cascades in inflammatory disease. Mol Med Today. 1999;5:439–47.
27. Guha M, Mackman N. LPS induction of gene expression in human monocytes. Cell Signal. 2001;13:85–94.
28. Dziarski R, Jin YP, Gupta D. Differential activation of extra cellular signal-regulated kinase (ERK) 1, ERK2, p38, and c-Jun NH2-terminal kinase mitogen-activated protein kinases by bacterial peptidoglycan. J Infect Dis. 1996;174:777–85.
29. Shall S, de Murcia G. Poly (ADP-ribose) polymerase-1: what have we learned from the deficient mouse model. Mutat Res. 2000;460:1–15.
30. Hausmann EH, Berman NE, Wang YY, Meara JB, Wood GW. Selective chemokine mRNA expression following brain injury. Brain Res. 1998;788:49–59.
31. Kempski O. Cerebral edema. Semin Nephrol. 2001;21:303–7.
32. Scheld WM, Dacey RC, Winn HR, Welsh JE, Jane JA. Cerebrospinal fluid outflow resistance in rabbits with experimental meningitis. J Clin Invest. 1980;66:243–53.
33. Kaplan SL. Clinical presentations, diagnosis, and prognostic factors of bacterial meningitis. Infect Dis Clin N Am. 1999;13:579.
34. Brouwer MC, van de Beek D, Heckenberg SG, et al. Hyponatraemia in adults with community-acquired bacterial meningitis. QJM. 2007;100:37.
35. de Gans J, van de Beek D. European dexamethasone in adulthood bacterial meningitis study investigators. Dexamethasone in adults with bacterial meningitis. N Engl J Med. 2002; 347:1549.

36. van de Beek D, de Gans J, Spanjaard L, et al. Clinical features and prognostic factors in adults with bacterial meningitis. N Engl J Med. 2004;351:1849.
37. Aronin SI, Peduzzi P, Quagliarello VJ. Community-acquired bacterial meningitis: risk stratification for adverse clinical outcome and effect of antibiotic timing. Ann Intern Med. 1998;129:862.
38. Geiseler PJ, Nelson KE, Levin S, et al. Community-acquired purulent meningitis: a review of 1,316 cases during the antibiotic era, 1954-1976. Rev Infect Dis. 1980;2:725.
39. Brouwer MC, Thwaites GE, Tunkel AR, van de Beek D. Dilemmas in the diagnosis of acute community-acquired bacterial meningitis. Lancet. 2012;380:1684.
40. Hasbun R, Abrahams J, Jekel J, Quagliarello VJ. Computed tomography of the head before lumbar puncture in adults with suspected meningitis. N Engl J Med. 2001;345:1727.
41. Kanegaye JT, Soliemanzadeh P, Bradley JS. Lumbar puncture in pediatric bacterial meningitis: defining the time interval for recovery of cerebrospinal fluid pathogens after parenteral antibiotic pretreatment. Pediatrics. 2001;108:1169.
42. Joffe AR. Lumbar puncture and brain herniation in acute bacterial meningitis: a review. J Intensive Care Med. 2007;22:194.
43. Glimåker M, Sjölin J, Åkesson S, Naucler P. Lumbar puncture performed promptly or after neuroimaging in acute bacterial meningitis in adults: a prospective National Cohort Study Evaluating Different Guidelines. Clin Infect Dis. 2018;66:321.
44. Blazer S, Berant M, Alon U. Bacterial meningitis. Effect of antibiotic treatment on cerebrospinal fluid. Am J Clin Pathol. 1983;80:386.
45. Fitch MT, van de Beek D. Emergency diagnosis and treatment of adult meningitis. Lancet Infect Dis. 2007;7:191.
46. Saha SK, Darmstadt GL, Yamanaka N, et al. Rapid diagnosis of pneumococcal meningitis: implications for treatment and measuring disease burden. Pediatr Infect Dis J. 2005;24:1093.
47. Spanos A, Harrell FE Jr, Durack DT. Differential diagnosis of acute meningitis. An analysis of the predictive value of initial observations. JAMA. 1989;262:2700.
48. Huy NT, Thao NT, Diep DT, et al. Cerebrospinal fluid lactate concentration to distinguish bacterial from aseptic meningitis: a systemic review and meta-analysis. Crit Care. 2010;14:R240.
49. Sakushima K, Hayashino Y, Kawaguchi T, et al. Diagnostic accuracy of cerebrospinal fluid lactate for differentiating bacterial meningitis from aseptic meningitis: a meta-analysis. J Infect. 2011;62:255.
50. Schmidley JW, Simon RP. Postictal pleocytosis. Ann Neurol. 1981;9:81.
51. Tumani H, Jobs C, Brettschneider J, et al. Effect of epileptic seizures on the cerebrospinal fluid--a systematic retrospective analysis. Epilepsy Res. 2015;114:23.
52. Tzanakaki G, Tsopanomichalou M, Kesanopoulos K, et al. Simultaneous single-tube PCR assay for the detection of Neisseria meningitidis, Haemophilus influenzae type b and Streptococcus pneumoniae. Clin Microbiol Infect. 2005;11:386.
53. Werno AM, Murdoch DR. Medical microbiology: laboratory diagnosis of invasive pneumococcal disease. Clin Infect Dis. 2008;46:926.
54. Negrini B, Kelleher KJ, Wald ER. Cerebrospinal fluid findings in aseptic versus bacterial meningitis. Pediatrics. 2000;105:316.
55. Beek D, Gans J, Tunkel AR, Wijdicks EF. Community-acquired bacterial meningitis in adults. N Engl J Med. 2006;354:44–53.
56. McIntyre PB, Berkey CS, King SM, et al. Dexamethasone as adjunctive therapy in bacterial meningitis. A meta-analysis of randomized clinical trials since 1988. JAMA. 1997;278:925–31.
57. Gans J, Beek D. Dexamethasone in adults with bacterial meningitis. N Engl J Med. 2002;347:1549–56.
58. Nguyen TH, Tran TH, Thwaites G, et al. Dexamethasone in Vietnamese adolescents and adults with bacterial meningitis. N Engl J Med. 2007;357:2431–40.
59. Scarborough M, Gordon SB, Whitty CJ, et al. Corticosteroids for bacterial meningitis in adults in sub-Saharan Africa. N Engl J Med. 2007;357:2441–50.
60. Beek D, Farrar JJ, Gans J, et al. Adjunctive dexamethasone in bacterial meningitis: a meta-analysis of individual patient data. Lancet Neurol. 2010;9:254–63.

61. Brouwer MC, McIntyre P, de Gans J, Prasad K, van de Beek D. Corticosteroids for acute bacterial meningitis. Cochrane Database Syst Rev. 2010;(9):CD004405.
62. Brouwer MC, Heckenberg SG, Gans J, Spanjaard L, Reitsma JB, Beek D. Nationwide implementation of adjunctive dexamethasone therapy for pneumococcal meningitis. Neurology. 2010;75:1533–9.
63. Tenembaum S, Chitnis T, Ness J, Hahn JS. Acute disseminated encephalomyelitis. Neurology. 2007;68(16 Suppl 2):S23–36.
64. Chaudhuri A, Kennedy PG. Diagnosis and treatment of viral encephalitis. Postgrad Med J. 2002;78:575–83.
65. Petropoulou KA, Gordon SM, Prayson RA, Ruggierri PM. West Nile virus meningoencephalitis: MR imaging findings. AJNR Am J Neuroradiol. 2005;26:1986–95.
66. Ali M, Safriel Y, Sohi J, Llave A, Weathers S. West Nile virus infection: MR imaging findings in the nervous system. AJNR Am J Neuroradiol. 2005;26:289–97.
67. Gilden DH, Mahalingam R, Cohrs RJ, Tyler KL. Herpesvirus infections of the nervous system. Nat Clin Pract Neurol. 2007;3:82–94.
68. Domingues RB, Tsanaclis AM, Pannuti CS, Mayo MS, Lakeman FD. Evaluation of the range of clinical presentations of herpes simplex encephalitis by using polymerase chain reaction assay of cerebrospinal fluid samples. Clin Infect Dis. 1997;25:86–91.
69. Domingues RB, Fink MC, Tsanaclis AM, et al. Diagnosis of herpes simplex encephalitis by magnetic resonance imaging and polymerase chain reaction assay of cerebrospinal fluid. J Neurol Sci. 1998;157:148–53.
70. O'Sullivan CE, Aksamit AJ, Harrington JR, Harmsen WS, Mitchell PS, Patel R. Clinical spectrum and laboratory characteristics associated with detection of herpes simplex virus DNA in cerebrospinal fluid. Mayo Clin Proc. 2003;78:1347–52. https://doi.org/10.4065/78.11.1347.
71. Simko JP, Caliendo AM, Hogle K, Versalovic J. Differences in laboratory findings for cerebrospinal fluid specimens obtained from patients with meningitis or encephalitis due to herpes simplex virus (HSV) documented by detection of HSV DNA. Clin Infect Dis. 2002;35:414–9.
72. Whitley RJ, Soong SJ, Linneman C Jr, Liu C, Pazin G, Alford CA. Herpes simplex encephalitis. Clinical Assessment. JAMA. 1982;247:317–20.
73. Weil AA, Glaser CA, Amad Z, Forghani B. Patients with suspected herpes simplex encephalitis: rethinking an initial negative polymerase chain reaction result. Clin Infect Dis. 2002;34:1154–7.
74. Solomon T, Hart IJ, Beeching NJ. Viral encephalitis: a clinician's guide. Pract Neurol. 2007; 7:288–305.
75. Tunkel AR. Brain abscess. In: Mandell GL, Bennett JE, Dolin R, editors. Principles and practice of infectious diseases. 7th ed. Philidelphia: Churchill-Livingstone; 2010. p. 1265–78.
76. Kamei S, Sekizawa T, Shiota H, et al. Evaluation of combination therapy using aciclovir and corticosteroid in adult patients with herpes simplex virus encephalitis. J Neurol Neurosurg Psychiatry. 2005;76:1544–9.
77. Lange N, Berndt M, Jörger AK, Wagner A, Wantia N, Lummel N, Ryang YM, Meyer B, Gempt J. Clinical characteristics and course of primary brain abscess. Acta Neurochir. 2018;160(10):2055–62.
78. Widdrington JD, Bond H, Schwab U, Price DA, Schmid ML, McCarron B, Chadwick DR, Narayanan M, Williams J, Ong E. Pyogenic brain abscess and subdural empyema: presentation, management, and factors predicting outcome. Infection. 2018;46(6):785–92.
79. Chen M, Low DCY, Low SYY, Muzumdar D, Seow WT. Management of brain abscesses: where are we now? Childs Nerv Syst. 2018;34(10):1871–80.
80. Udayakumaran S, Onyia CU, Kumar RK. Forgotten? not yet. Cardiogenic brain abscess in children: a case series-based review. World Neurosurg. 2017;107:124–9.
81. Gorji GRS, Rassouli M, Staji H. Prevalence of cerebral toxoplasmosis among slaughtered sheep in Semnan, Iran. Ann Parasitol. 2018;64(1):37–42.
82. Maher G, Beniwal M, Bahubali V, Biswas S, Bevinahalli N, Srinivas D, Siddaiah N. Streptococcus pluranimalium: emerging animal streptococcal species as causative agent of human brain abscess. World Neurosurg. 2018;115:208–12.

83. Longo D, Narese D, Fariello G. Diagnosis of brain abscess: a challenge that magnetic resonance can help us win! Epidemiol Infect. 2018;146(12):1608–10.
84. Berndt M, Lange N, Ryang YM, Meyer B, Zimmer C, Hapfelmeier A, Wantia N, Gempt J, Lummel N. Value of diffusion-weighted imaging in the diagnosis of postoperative intracranial infections. World Neurosurg. 2018;118:e245–53.
85. Simjian T, Muskens IS, Lamba N, Yunusa I, Wong K, Veronneau R, Kronenburg A, Brouwers HB, Smith TR, Mekary RA, Broekman MLD. Dexamethasone administration and mortality in patients with brain abscess: a systematic review and meta-analysis. World Neurosurg. 2018;115:257–63.
86. Vieira E, Guimarães TC, Faquini IV, Silva JL, Saboia T, Andrade RVCL, Gemir TL, Neri VC, Almeida NS, Azevedo-Filho HRC. Randomized controlled study comparing 2 surgical techniques for decompressive craniectomy: with watertight duraplasty and without watertight duraplasty. J Neurosurg. 2018;129(4):1017–23.
87. Tunthanathip T, Kanjanapradit K, Sae-Heng S, Oearsakul T, Sakarunchai I. Predictive factors of the outcome and intraventricular rupture of brain abscess. J Med Assoc Thail. 2015;98(2):170–80.
88. Bonis P, Anile C, Pompucci A, Labonia M, Lucantoni C, Mangiola A. Cranial and spinal subdural empyema. Br J Neurosurg. 2009;23:335–40.
89. Nathoo N, Nadvi SS, Dellen JR. Cranial extradural empyema in the era of computed tomography: a review of 82 cases. Neurosurgery. 1999;44:748–53.
90. Mat Nayan SA, Mohd Haspani MS, Abd Latiff AZ, Abdullah JM, Abdullah S. Two surgical methods used in 90 patients with intracranial subdural empyema. J Clin Neurosci. 2009;16:1567–71.
91. Nathoo N, Nadvi SS, Dellen JR, Gouws E. Intracranial subdural empyemas in the era of computed tomography: a review of 699 cases. Neurosurgery. 1999;44:529–35.
92. Bockova J, Rigamonti D. Intracranial empyema. Pediatr Infect Dis J. 2000;19:735–7.

Chapter 10
Intracranial Pressure Monitoring and Management in Bacterial Meningitis

Ignacio J. Previgliano

Scope of the Problem

A controversial issue in bacterial meningitis' management is intracranial pressure (ICP) monitoring usefulness to manage raised ICP or diminished cerebral perfusion pressure (CPP).

Most of ICP monitoring recommendations are based on traumatic brain injury (TBI) research as is stated by Helbok et al. [1] "although the influence of ICP based care on outcome in non-TBI conditions appears less robust than in TBI, monitoring ICP and CPP can play a role in guiding therapy in select patients."

Reviewing the literature, ICP monitoring in meningitis is limited to case reports and descriptive series, most of them retrospective. Different Sweden groups have shown that there is no relationship between images and ICP [2], as well as that ICP target therapy [3, 4] diminishes mortality and improves outcome.

Kumar et al. [5] in a large prospective study compared ICP target therapy (maintaining intracranial pressure <20 mmHg using osmotherapy while ensuring normal blood pressure) and cerebral CPP target therapy (maintaining cerebral perfusion pressure ≥60 mmHg, using normal saline bolus and vasoactive therapy—dopamine and if needed noradrenaline) in children with acute central nervous system (CNS) infections having raised intracranial pressure and a modified Glasgow Coma Scale (GCS) score less than or equal to 8. They conclude that CPP management significantly reduced mortality, ICU and hospital length of stay, and functional outcome.

Coma, diagnosed as GCS ≤ 8, is one of the most important prognostic indicators for bad outcome [6] mainly due to the association with raised ICP.

I. J. Previgliano (✉)
Hospital General de Agudos J. A. Fernández, Buenos Aires, Argentina

Universidad Maimonides, Buenos Aires, Argentina

© Springer Nature Switzerland AG 2020   175
J. Hidalgo, L. Woc-Colburn (eds.), *Highly Infectious Diseases in Critical Care*,
https://doi.org/10.1007/978-3-030-33803-9_10

Taking into account this background, there are some pathophysiological events that give support to ICP monitoring in consciousness impairment bacterial meningitis patients.

One of them is the neurovascular unit's damage reflected by permeability alteration, thrombosis, and ischemia secondary to vasculitis, direct neuronal injury with damage cascade's initiation generating NMDA and free radicals, and anoikis [7, 8].

The other is Rosner's vasodilation (Vd)/vasoconstriction (Vc) cascade theory to explain autoregulation patency and cerebral blood flow (CBF) ensuring [9].

According to his first observations [10], there is a close relationship between CPP diminishing and ICP raising that is explained in Fig. 10.1.

The mechanism by which the cerebral vasculature maintains CBF almost constant across a wide range of pressure gradients is through vasoconstriction and vasodilatation. CPP is the stimulus to cerebral autoregulation. In normal conditions of low ICP, CPP is approximated by the mean arterial pressure. Modest increments in ICP (10–20 mmHg) united to similar decrements in MAP (70–80 mmHg) may result in a CPP of 50 mmHg, which denotes the lower limit of normal cerebral autoregulation. Vasoconstriction and vasodilation are mainly caused by changes in the cerebral arteries, especially in the arterioles.

The variable diameter effectively changes the cerebral vascular resistance, and, therefore, as the perfusion pressure is reduced, the cerebral vascular resistance is reduced in a way that approximately compensates for the reduction in the pressure gradient, and the blood flow can be maintained. At CPP levels between 110 and 120 mmHg, cerebral vascular resistance is nearly maximal; between 80 and 100 mmHg, vasodilation begins; and on the order of 10–15%, maximum vasodilation occurs with CPP between 50 and 60 mmHg, as is shown in Fig. 10.2. As seen there, radius change rate is logarithmic and not linear within the autoregulatory range, so as CPP drops below the lower limit of autoregulation, vessels collapse, and blood flow declines rapidly.

Taking into account this theory, a drop in CPP, which could be primary or secondary as explained in Fig. 10.3, generates a vasodilatory response in order to maintain a constant CBF, the ultimate goal of autoregulation. This response, sustained in

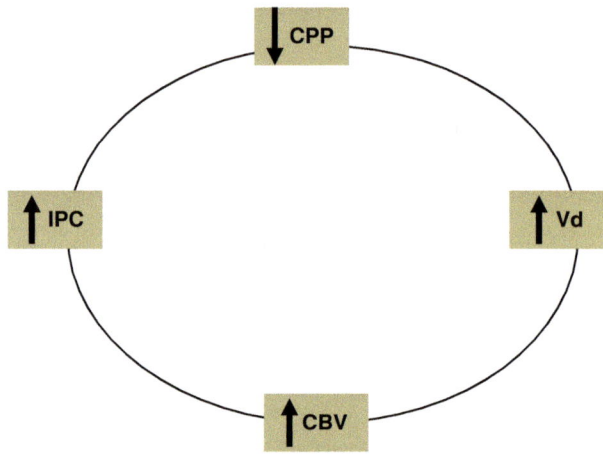

Fig. 10.1 Vasodilation cascade. A drop in CPP causes Vd in order to ensure CBF. Vd response increases cerebral blood volume (CBV) up to the point that exceeds cerebral compliance and generates ICP raising

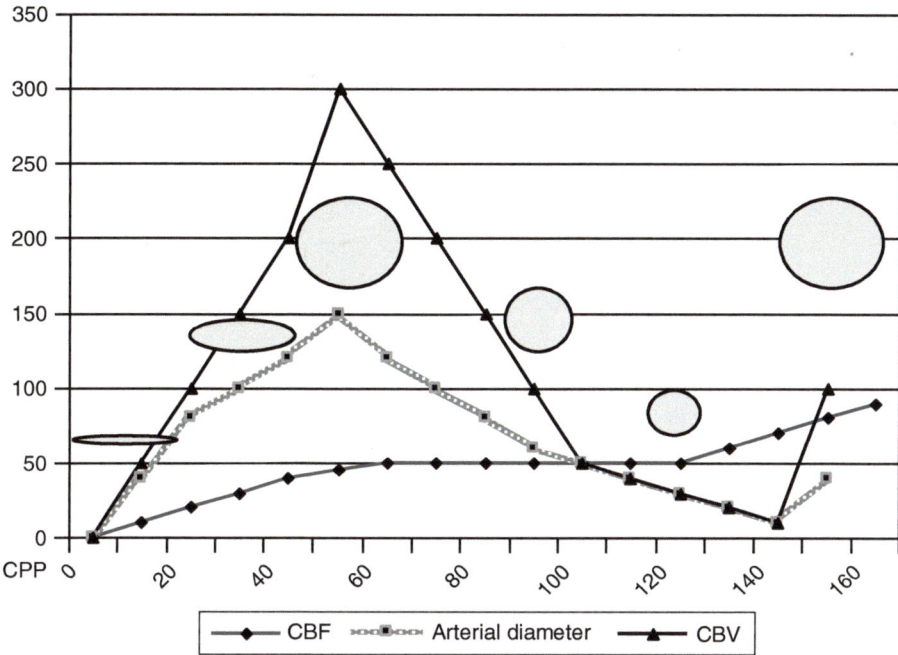

Fig. 10.2 Relative changes in CBV and arterial diameter, and absolute changes in CBF according to changes in CPP. See text for details

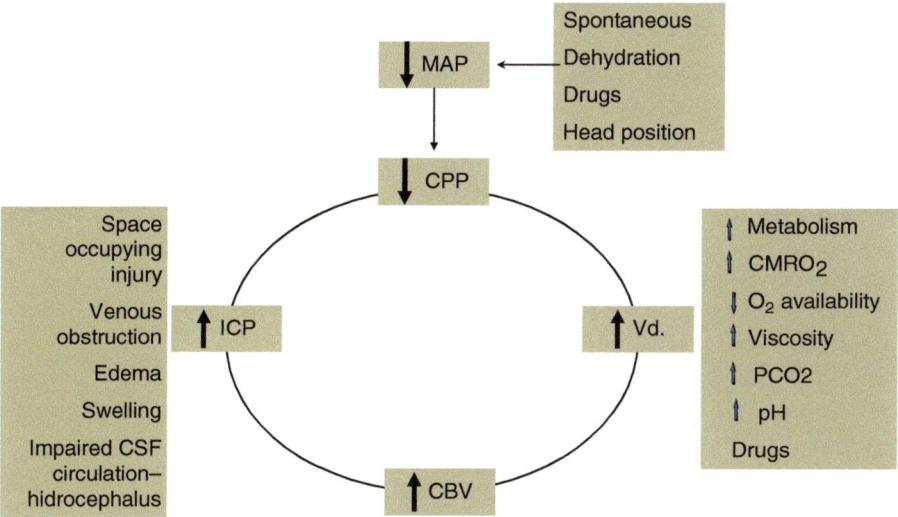

Fig. 10.3 Complex vasodilation cascade. Different pathophysiological conditions may trigger the vasodilatory cascade. They can appear isolated on in conjunction or as a chain of events

Fig. 10.4 The cascade of continuous ischemia. While these conditions are maintained, a vicious circle is established whose end result is permanent and persistent ischemia of brain tissue

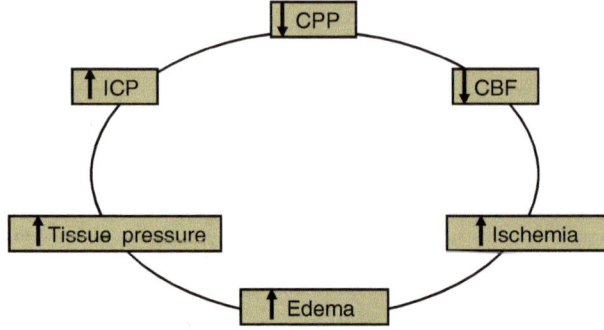

time, leads to an increment in cerebral blood volume (CBV) that in turns generates a raise in ICP due to diminished cerebral compliance in accordance with Monro-Kelly's law. This generates a vicious circle as seen in Fig. 10.4.

Bacterial meningitis associated with intracranial hypertension could be explained by means of Fig. 10.3. Systemic response to sepsis leads to hypotension, fever, changes in oxygen delivery, and acidosis and could evolve to septic shock that, in turn, will worsen the response developing multiorgan failure. In such condition, lactic acidosis and renal and respiratory failure will contribute to potentiate brain injury.

This theoretical construction is in accordance with the clinical picture that death is usually caused by brain tissue infarction secondary to herniation and brainstem compression, septic shock, and coagulation disturbances [11].

Indications for ICP Monitoring

Based on TBI lessons [1] and on poor outcome risk scores in bacterial meningitis [12, 13], possible candidates for intracranial pressure monitoring could be selected on the following bases:

(a) Age > 50 years old
(b) Glasgow Coma Scale <9, consider ≤10 points with more than two risk factors
(c) Space-occupying lesions (subdural empyema, brain abscess, hemorrhage)
(d) Compress or absent basal cisterns in CT scan
(e) CSF leucocyte count <1000 cell/mm³
(f) Gram + germs in CSF Gram's stain
(g) Ultrasound signs of raised ICP

Ultrasound Evaluation of Intracranial Pressure

Point-of-care ultrasound (POCUS) refers to the use, by a non-radiology specialist, of portable ultrasound at patient's bedside for diagnostic or therapeutic problems. The exam is for a well-defined purpose related to the improvement of patient outcomes [14] and focused and aimed at a goal: clinical question, procedure, or evolution control.

Exam findings are easily recognizable.

The exam is easy to learn, is carried out quickly at the patient's bedside, but generally is performed in suboptimal position and time conditions. Most importantly, the exam does not replace the specialized ecographist.

POCUS' concept is of particular interest in critical care as had been established by one of the pioneers, Dr. Lichtenstein [15]. Several focused examinations (FAST [16], RUSH [17], BLUE [18], FALLS [18]) have contributed to a better understanding of different pathological conditions in critical care.

Regarding neurocritical care, several formulas have been developed using transcranial Doppler flow velocities and pulsatility index. It can also been calculated using transcranial color-coded duplex (TCCD).

We have tested several of them [19] and finally decide to use Bellner's [20] formula for ICP and Belfort's [21] formula for CPP estimations.

Bellner's formula estimates ICP by means of PI as follows:

$$ICP = 10.93 \times PI - 1.28$$

Belfort's formula estimates CPP by means of TCD flow velocities and arterial pressure:

$$CPP = (MFV / (MFV - DFV) \times (MAP - DAP)$$

where MFV is mean flow velocity, DFV diastolic flow velocity, MAP mean arterial pressure, and DAP diastolic arterial pressure.

In our experience, by analyzing 290 patients with simultaneous invasive ICP and MAP monitoring, we found an r^2 of 0.84 for Bellner's formula and of 0.97 for Belfort's one.

Another way to estimate ICP is using optic nerve sheath diameter (ONSD) [22]. The optic nerve has the particularity that is wrapped by meninges as well as the CNS is, as is seen in Figs. 10.5 and 10.6. As ICP rises, CSF is displaced to the lower-pressure (or high-compliance) zones, one of them is ONS, which explains the diameter increment.

ONSD could be measured with a high-frequency linear transducer (7–10 MHz). The image is configured to see structures up to approximately 5 cm deep. Abundant ultrasound gel is applied to the closed eyelid.

By subtle movements, it is scanned from the top down (cranial to caudal) by slowly tilting the probe superiorly or inferiorly to visualize the optic nerve. It is identified as the hypoechoic structure with a regular path after the eyeball. After identifying the optic globe/optic nerve junction, a 3 mm transversal line is drawn; perpendicular to it, another 3 mm longitudinal is drawn. That is the point in which ONSD must be measured.

Three measurements are taken in parasagittal and transversal planes (Figs. 10.7 and 10.8). Although there are different ways to choose the right measurement, what we do in our practice is to elect the one that is coincident in both planes.

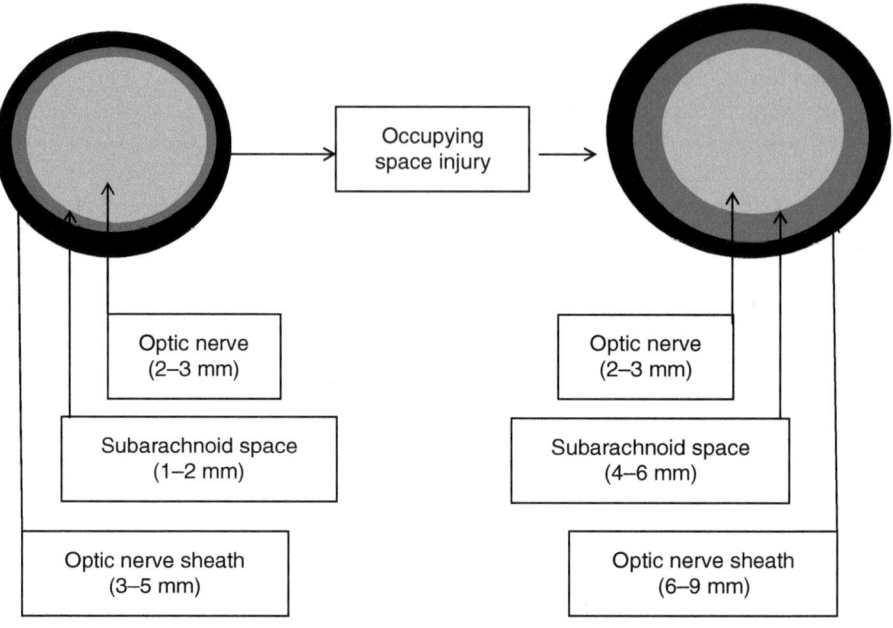

Fig. 10.5 Changes in ONSD. Optic nerve sheath (ONS) is composed of meningeal coverage (pia-mater, arachnoid, and duramater). According to Monro Kelly's law, CSF is displaced due to an increase in one of the intracranial compartments, ONSD increases (right)

Fig. 10.6 Optic nerve sheath. Nuclear magnetic resonance imaging clearly shows the continuity of the intracranial subarachnoid space with the subarachnoid space around the optic nerve

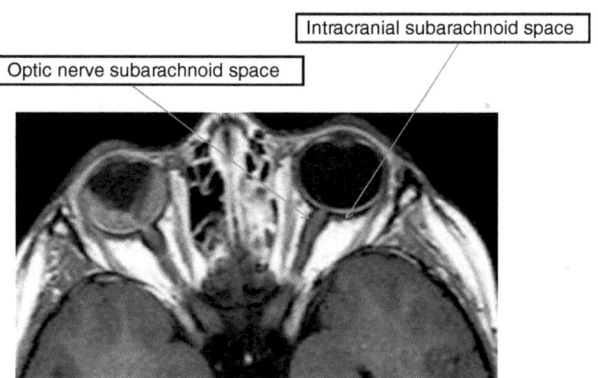

In their descriptive prospective study, Amin et al. [23] measured ONSD before lumbar puncture (LP) using ultrasonography in 50 non-traumatized patients who were candidates for LP due to varying diagnoses. Immediately after the sonography, the ICP of each patient was measured by LP. The ONSD of greater than 5.5 mm predicted an ICP of ≥ 20 cm H(2)O with sensitivity and specificity of 100% (95% CI, 100–100) ($P < 0.001$). These results were confirmed in Dubourg's systematic review and meta-analysis [24].

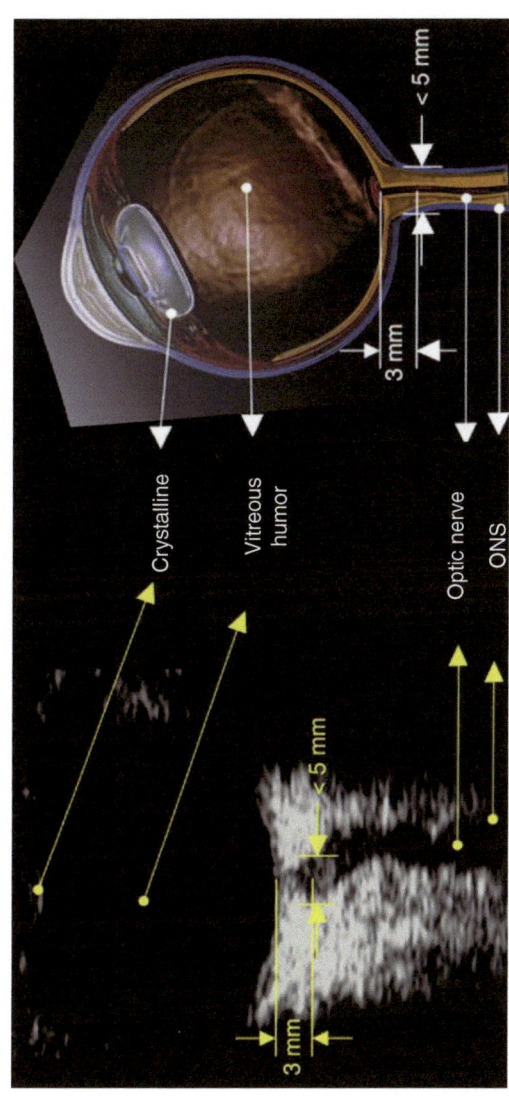

Fig. 10.7 Measurement of the optic nerve sheath in parasagittal plane. (Modified from Previgliano and Perez Ochoa [32])

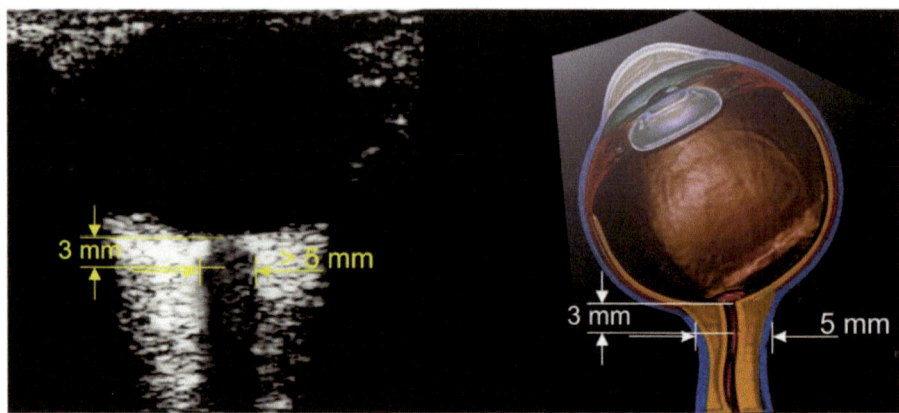

Fig. 10.8 Measurement of the optic nerve sheath in transversal plane. (Modified from Previgliano and Perez Ochoa [32])

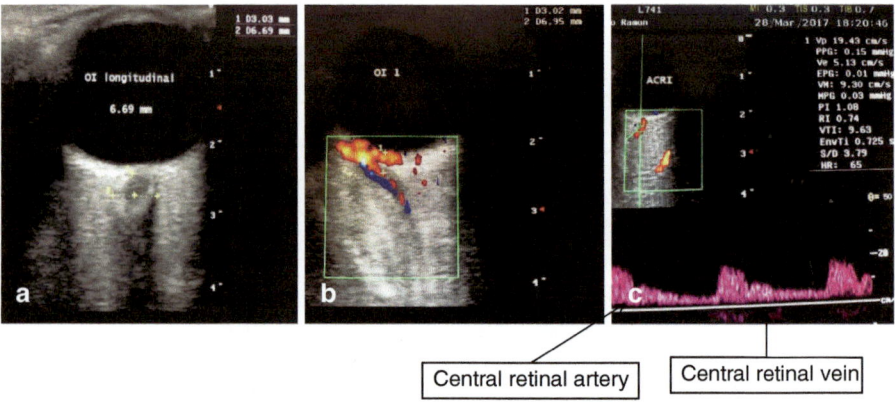

Central retinal artery   Central retinal vein

Fig. 10.9 Measurement of the optic nerve sheath in parasagittal (**a**) and transversal (**b**) planes. Both of them show pathological values. Doppler ultrasound of central retinal artery (**c**) with raised RI. Central retinal artery has the particularity that a venous ultrasound registry is below the arterial one

Another tool to confirm ONSD measurement is to use the central retinal artery resistance index (RI), which is raised due to the ONSD increment (Fig. 10.9).

Invasive ICP Monitoring

In Fig. 10.10, there is a scheme for ICP monitoring system placement.

Intraventricular catheters appear as the most valuable, taking into account that CSF production/reabsorption is one of the proposed pathophysiological mechanisms of raised ICP in meningitis. In Fig. 10.11, there is a scheme of its functioning.

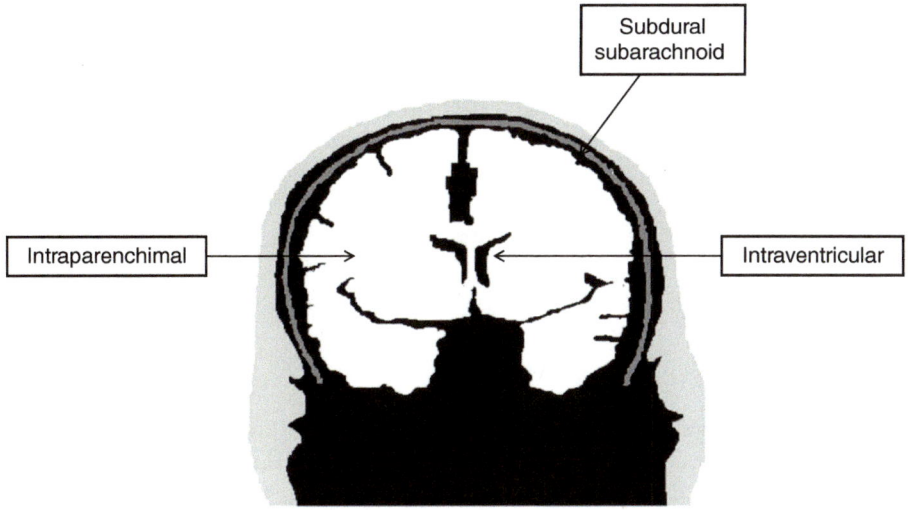

Fig. 10.10 Available spaces for ICP-monitoring devices

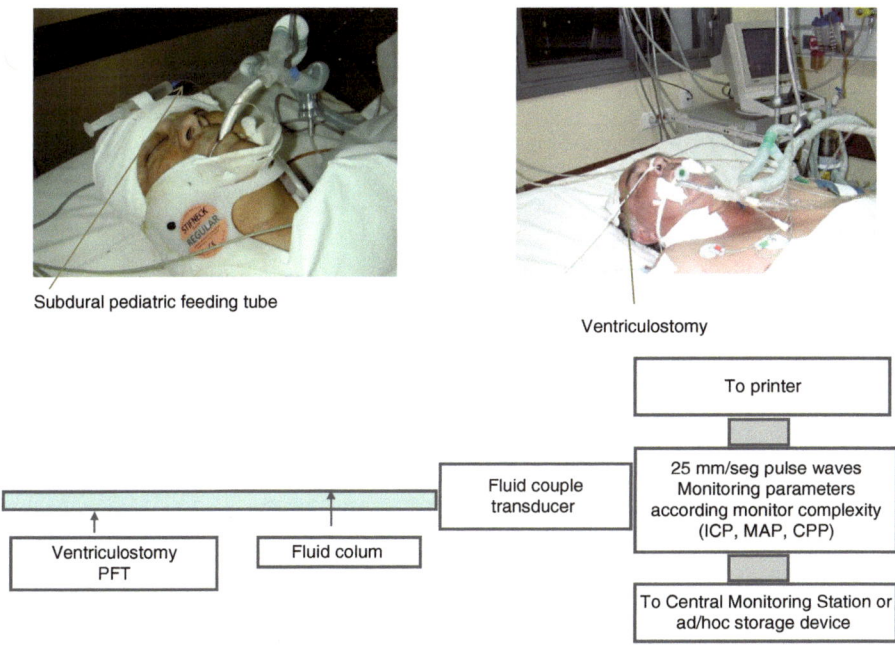

Fig. 10.11 Fluid couple external strain gauge devices principles of functioning

For low-income, low-resource environment, subdural or subarachnoid pediatric feeding tube connected to a pressure transducer (Fig. 10.11) is a good option. We tested it against fiber-optic device [25] in a 252 patient's cohort and found no differences in dysfunction, infection, and CDF fistula.

Other options are fiber-optic devices or microsensor tip devices that could be used intraparenchymal or intraventricular, which are more expensive. A scheme of functioning is drawn in Figs. 10.12 and 10.13.

Notwithstanding of the selected ICP monitoring device, all of them provide the same information:

1. Absolute ICP value
2. ICP waves
3. CPP calculation (MAP-ICP)

Absolute ICP values allow the identification of the threshold value to initiate intensive treatment. The Brain Trauma Foundation TBI guidelines recommend treating ICP above 22 mmHg.

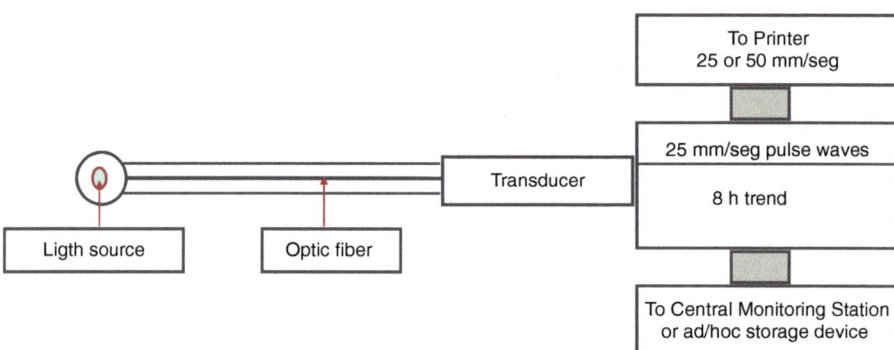

Fig. 10.12 Fiber-optic devices, principles of functioning

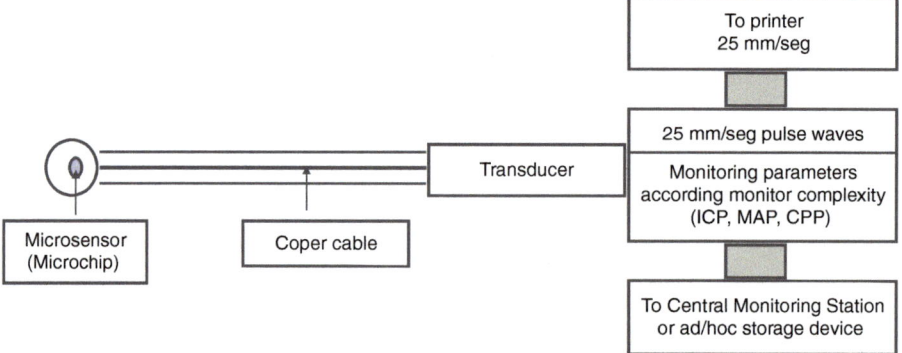

Fig. 10.13 Microsensor tip devices, principles of functioning

ICP waves include cerebral pulse waveform and pathological Lundberg's waves (Figs. 10.14 and 10.15). As shown in Fig. 10.14, P2 component of cerebral pulse waveform is related to cerebral compliance, so that the larger the wave size, the smaller the brain compliance.

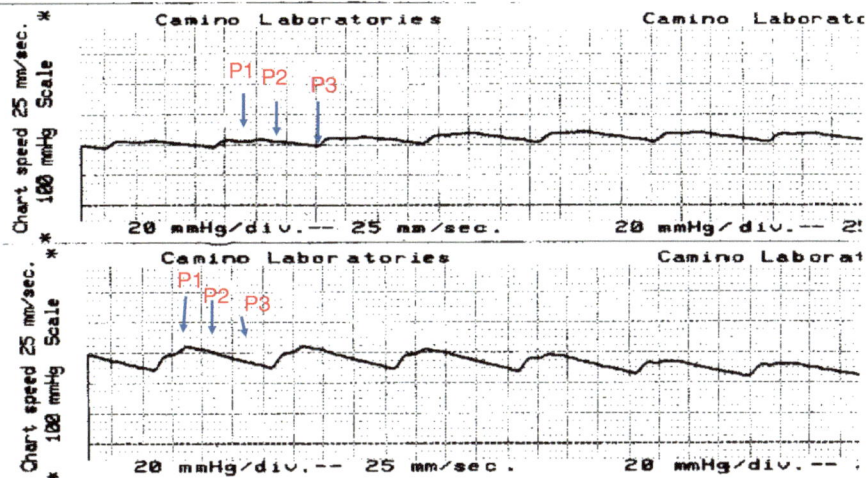

Fig. 10.14 The brain pulse wave is recorded at fast speeds and is the one seen on the monitor screen. It has three components: P1 (systolic impact), P2 (CSF movement, equivalent to cerebral compliance), and P3 (diastolic relaxation). In the inferior outline, there is an example of low cerebral compliance associated to an increase in ICP

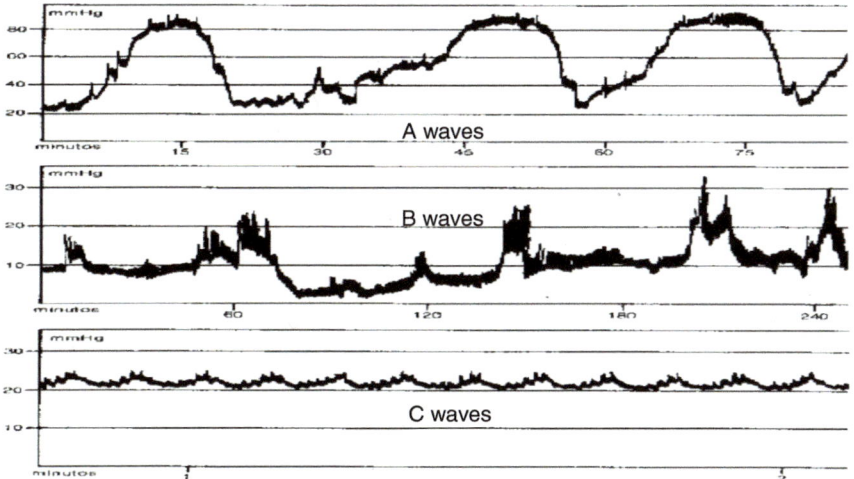

Fig. 10.15 Lundberg's waves. A waves: >40–50 mmHg for 15–20 min. Low cerebral compliance or inadequate CPP. B waves: variable amplitude, 0.5–2 min, pathological respiratory patterns. C waves: rhythmic and fast 6–8 min^{-1}, normal cardiorespiratory interaction

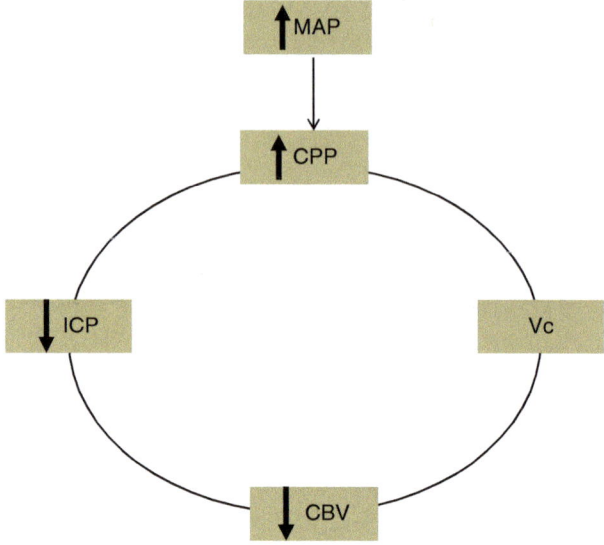

Fig. 10.16 Cushing's response explained by the vasoconstrictory cascade. See text for details

Lundberg's waves are named as A waves (or plateau waves), B waves, and C waves. In Fig. 10.15, there is a description of each of them. It is important to note Rosner's explanation of the origin and explanation of A waves, because it is part of his CPP management protocol basis. He described four phases that he has labeled the drift phase, plateau phase, ischemic response phase, and resolution phase. The drift phase is a premonitory stage in plateau wave development. Its characteristic is the gradual decline in CPP to levels of about 70 mmHg, mainly due to a slow fall in MAP. When CPP reaches 70 mmHg, there occurs a very rapid increase in ICP to "plateau" levels. If the MAP is able to stabilize the CPP above ischemic levels, the plateau wave continues. This is explained by the vasodilatory cascade. If the MAP continues to fall, the CPP reaches ischemic levels, and blood pressure will be elevated by a brainstem-mediated adrenergic discharge: a Cushing response (Fig. 10.16). This CPP restoration is a function of falling ICP even though MAP increase is responsible for this events' initiation, the resolution phase.

CPP calculation as MAP-ICP should be done with both transducers at the same level, preferably at the trago. The inverse relationship between CPP and ICP is a very important tool to guarantee an adequate CBF, maintaining CPP above 70 mmHg.

Treatment of Raised ICP

General Management

One of the fundamental concepts is to maintain adequate cerebral circulation. Any maneuver that can reduce arterial circulation or impair venous drainage should be avoided.

Patients should remain euvolemic (except in some special situations) and avoid episodes, albeit minimal, of arterial hypotension.

A central venous line will be placed to measure central venous pressure (PVC) that will ideally be maintained at around 8–12 cmH2O. In patients who require it, a Swan-Ganz catheter will be placed to assess pulmonary capillary pressure, minute volume, and other important data in the management of selected critical patients. If it is possible, avoid placing catheters in the jugular veins to avoid subsequent thrombosis and inadequate venous drainage.

The use of positive-end expiratory pressure (PEEP), in general, does not raise the ICP, although care should be taken when using high values, evaluating the behavior of ICP in the face of PEEP changes.

Many studies have shown that keeping the head elevated at no more than 25–30° above the horizontal decreases the ICP by favoring venous drainage and facilitating the passage of CSF to the spinal compartment.

Adequate oxygen availability should be maintained, which means a hematocrit equal to or greater than 30%, arterial oxygen saturation greater than 90%, and a normal or slightly increased cardiac output.

Agitated patients may receive sedation and analgesia if a source of pain is suspected. Morphine and fentanyl, in continuous intravenous infusion, are very good analgesic agents, and continuous infusion of midazolam or propofol can be used as sedation.

Neuromuscular blocking agents should be used with care, attempted only when ICP cannot be controlled with sedation and analgesia. The use of depolarizing agents will be avoided due to the possibility of an increase in ICP initially due to muscle contractions that temporarily reduce jugular venous return.

Metabolic disorders are extremely common in patients with acute brain injury. Fluid imbalances secondary to resuscitation, use of osmotherapy, diuretics, sodium metabolism disorders typical of these patients (diabetes insipidus, inadequate secretion of antidiuretic hormone, cerebral salt-wasting syndrome), and hyperglycemia give rise to their control and the need for their correction.

ICP Management

For didactical purposes, ICP management will be split in five different groups, based on the mechanisms of action of each of the therapeutic measures.

Evacuation of Space-Occupying Lesions

The most prevalent bacterial infections seen in the intensive care unit can be summarized as acute bacterial meningitis, subdural empyema, intracerebral abscess, and ventriculitis, which all commonly involve the brain parenchyma [26, 27]. The removal of a mass lesion almost always involves the surgical evacuation of it. There is no major controversy about the beneficial effects on ICP and the prognosis of mass removal that is believed to cause intracranial hypertension.

CSF Volume Reduction

CSF removal is usually performed when hydrocephalus is an important cause or contributing factor to the elevation of ICP, as seen in meningitis. CSF drainage can be a very effective method to reduce ICP.

Ventriculostomies can be placed in the intensive care unit, the operating room, or the emergency room. They allow the measurement of the ICP and the removal of CSF. It must be taken into account that to consider the ICP value reliable, the key that allows the CSF to exit must have been closed for at least 15 min.

When a ventriculostomy for CSF removal is placed, adequate circulation and resorption of the CSF must return to normal before it can be removed.

Intravascular Blood Volume Reduction

The most commonly used method to reduce intravascular blood volume is hyperventilation (HV). The usefulness of HV lays in the reactive vasoconstriction of intracranial arterioles in response to the decrease in carbon dioxide pressure (PCO_2). Kontos studies in the 1970s showed that changes in the pial arteries with variations in PCO_2 remained unchanged until brain death. Sometimes the reduction in ICP is accompanied by a significant decrease in jugular saturation of O2 (SjO_2) and tissue pressure of O2 (Pti O_2), which highlight the existence of ischemia or cerebral hypoflux.

The use of HV as a treatment in the neurological intensive care unit is controversial, since the decrease in ICP and the ischemia caused by vasoconstriction must be balanced. Our recommendation is to place a system that allows inferring cerebral oximetry to control HV. These devices could be a jugular bulb catheter placement or Pti O_2 catheter placement simultaneously with ventricular or intraventricular catheter settlement or near-infrared sensors.

Another physiological mechanism that affects CBV includes the notion of brain oxygen availability. When the hematocrit drops to around 30%, the reduction in blood viscosity has more effect on the cerebrovascular diameter than the reduction in oxygen content, and then the resulting effect is vasoconstriction and the reduction of CBV, with the consequent ICP reduction. When hematocrit drops below 30%, oxygen availability deteriorates significantly, causing vasodilation and increased CBF and ICP.

Mannitol and other osmotic agents also act producing vasoconstriction and reduction of VSC, data that will be expanded in the next topic.

Metabolic suppression caused by barbiturates, other anesthetics such as propofol, and possibly hypothermia results in ICP reduction.

Barbiturate coma therapy has generally been considered a second-order therapeutic alternative. The objective to achieve with this therapy is the electroencephalographic pattern of "burst suppression" (3–6 bursts/min). There is a good correlation between this pattern and maximum metabolic depression, and no more is gained by inducing electroencephalographic silence. Unfortunately, the adverse effects of high doses of barbiturates limit its usefulness. The most important are arterial hypotension and infections (due to suppression of leukocyte activity).

The most used barbiturates are pentobarbital and thiopental. The thiopental begins its action in seconds, and its effects are quickly dissipated by redistribution in fat and muscles. It also has an active metabolite that is pentobarbital.

The loading dose of thiopental is 5 mg/kg intravenously to pass in 10 min, and the maintenance dose is 3–5 mg/kg/h.

Although the low doses produce myosis, higher doses produce mydriasis and suppress the pupillary reflex to light, as well as prolong the duration of the ciliaspinal reflex, producing transient arreactive mydriasis that sometimes comes to be interpreted, erroneously, as a sign of herniation or brain death.

When the ICP control has been maintained for 24–48 h, therapy suspension should begin. Weaning of barbiturates should be slow, because serious raise in ICP may appear from rebound or seizures. The infusion will be reduced hourly to achieve a dose reduction of 50% per day.

Propofol, although structurally different, has clinical action and effects on brain electrical activity and intracranial dynamics similar to ultrashort-acting barbiturates such as thiopental. It produces a dose-dependent alteration of the sensory, from light sedation to general anesthesia, severe respiratory depression, and reduction of systemic vascular resistance.

Some data suggest that the hypotensive action of propofol may compromise CPP to the point of producing ischemia despite its beneficial effect on ICP. In contrast, sedative doses result in minimal hemodynamic alterations, without changes in the CPP.

The sedative doses are 0.1–0.3 mg/kg in intravenous bolus as a loading dose and maintenance of 0.6–6.0 mg/kg/h in intravenous infusion.

Its adverse effects include arterial hypotension, infection, propofol infusion syndrome, and pain at the injection site.

Hypothermia as a brain protection mechanism has been described for more than four decades.

The basis of this statement was based on the observation that patients drowned in frozen waters had a better recovery than those drowned in warm waters and spectacular "resuscitation" of patients with brain damage plus hypothermia.

Hypothermia is the treatment of choice for anoxic hypoxic encephalopathy, having demonstrated superiority over normothermia in several randomized controlled studies [28]. The purpose is to quickly induce hypothermia and slowly reheat the patient.

The range of hypothermia in which the best brain protection is obtained with the least hemodynamic changes in reperfusion is between 32 and 34 °C.

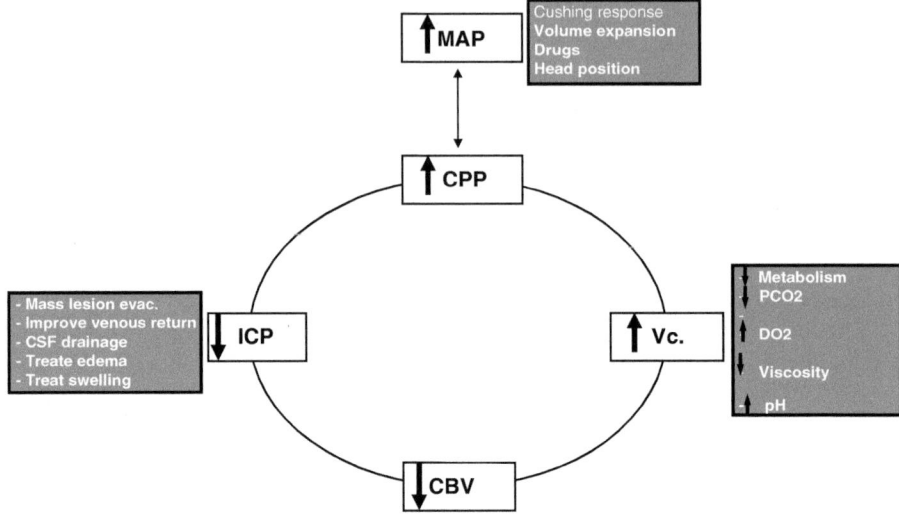

Fig. 10.17 Rosner's complex vasoconstriction cascade. See text for details

Complications of hypothermia include coagulation abnormalities, myocardial sensitivity to catecholamines, and increased ICP during reheating.

Following Rosner and Becker's elegant theoretical model, we can analyze the complex vasoconstrictor cascade shown in Fig. 10.17.

The increase in MAP as a function of increased CPP, as mentioned above, is the expression of the Cushing reflex.

Regarding vasoactive drugs, the first choice are norepinephrine and phenylephrine that have peripheral and cerebral vasoconstrictor activity. Dopamine should be avoided in doses greater than 15 ranges/kg/min, since the peripheral vasoconstrictor effect is associated with cerebral vasodilation.

However, despite emphasizing the importance of maintaining CPP at least 70 mmHg, an ICP of less than 20 mmHg should be attempted.

In patients receiving treatment with induced arterial hypertension for control of raised ICP, the risk of suffering from acute respiratory distress syndrome or renal failure is higher, as well as some patients could develop persistent intracranial hypertension probably due to hydrostatic edema induced by arterial hypertension in patients with blood-brain barrier rupture.

The effect of head position has been discussed, but it is easily proven in practice if one places the MAP transducer at the same height as that of the ICP and raises or lowers the head, while if one keeps the MAP transducer at heart level, this is not visualized.

Indomethacin produces a reduction in CBF, with a consequent decrease in the ICP, although its use is limited and controversial, since its risk-benefit ratio is not yet fully clarified. The dose of indomethacin is 50 mg in 100 ml of physiological solution to pass in 20 min as a loading dose and 500 mg in 500 ml of physiological solution to pass between 10 and 30 mg/h; the upper limit cannot be exceeded.

Reduction of Edema and Interstitial Fluid Volume

Edema and interstitial fluid volume reduction is the final strategy for intracranial volume and ICP lowering. This effect is the most commonly accepted mechanism for mannitol.

Mannitol also generates marked changes in blood rheology, decreasing viscosity (due to the fall of the hematocrit, and decrease in volume, and stiffness and cohesion of the red blood cell membranes, thus reducing the mechanical resistance to its passage through the microvasculature), producing alterations of vascular tone (vasoconstriction in areas with preserved self-regulation), and allowing to decrease the VSC and increase the minute heart volume. This also acts as a scrubber for free radicals of O2 and could exert a cytoprotective effect. It would also fulfill a role in the prevention of the "non-reflux" phenomenon and other aspects of reperfusion injury of global cerebral ischemia.

By reducing viscosity and therefore CBV, and increasing the CPP, ICP is reduced. If the CPP is low and autoregulation is present, ICP reduction in response to mannitol infusion is maximum. This type of response is fast and achieves ICP reductions in the first 30 min. The less rapid response of the ICP is believed to be due to osmotic dehydration of brain tissue.

Useful doses for this purpose range from 0.25 to 1.0 g/kg weight, usually given every 4 h in an intravenous infusion, according ICP thresholds.

The possibility of hypovolemia induced by osmotic diuresis and inappropriate correction of losses, hypernatremia (due to increased clearance of free water), and urinary losses of potassium, phosphate, and magnesium should be highlighted. Acute hyponatremia can be caused by plasma dilution immediately after the bolus of mannitol. An osmolality gap of less than 55 mmol/kg of water should be maintained to avoid renal failure and/or a plasma osmolality of less than 320 mmol/kg.

Hypertonic saline solutions are other treatments that act through this mechanism.

Another useful treatment to reduce interstitial edema includes the use of corticosteroids which are only indicated for edema associated with tumors and abscesses.

Increase of the Continent

In situations of intractable intracranial hypertension or in those where horizontal cerebral displacements announce the imminent herniation or vascular involvement of anterior and/or posterior cerebral arteries and where conventional ICH treatments have failed or are believed to increase displacement, an alternative remains. It consists of transforming the closed box (the skull) into a relatively open one, allowing the midline structures to return to normal, avoiding traditional herniations and transforming them into external herniations, not compromising arterial vascular structures and allowing significantly reducing ICP, improving cerebral perfusion, avoiding ischemia, and improving perfusion in the twilight area. We refer to decompressive craniectomies with dura plastic.

There are only anecdotal case reports of decompressive craniectomy for refractory ICP treatment in meningitis [3, 29–31].

Conclusion

ICP monitoring could be useful for bacterial meningitis patients with consciousness compromise.

Although experience is limited, several trials have demonstrated diminish in mortality and morbidity using ICP or CPP management as treatment options.

In Fig. 10.18, there is a summary of those different options that neurocritical and general intensivists should bear in mind.

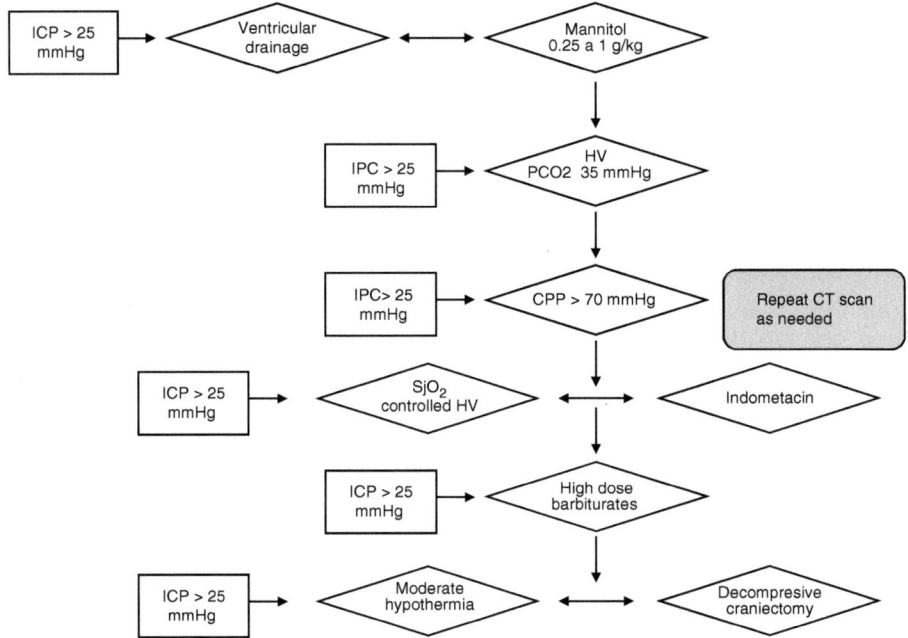

Fig. 10.18 Algorithm for intracranial hypertension treatment. See text for details

References

1. Helbok R, Olson DM, Le Roux PD, Vespa P. Participants in the international multidisciplinary consensus conference on multimodality monitoring. Intracranial pressure and cerebral perfusion pressure monitoring in non-TBI patients: special considerations. Neurocrit Care. 2014;21(Suppl 2):S85–94.
2. Larsen L, Poulsen FR, Nielsen TH, Nordström GH, Schulz MK, Andersen AB. Use of intracranial pressure monitoring in bacterial meningitis: a 10-year follow up on outcome and intracranial pressure versus head CT scan. Infect Dis. 2017;1:1–9.
3. Edberg M, Furebring M, Sjölin J, Enblad P. Neurointensive care of patients with severe community-acquired meningitis. Acta Anaesthesiol Scand. 2011;55:732–9.
4. Glimåker M, Johansson B, Halldorsdottir H, et al. Neuro-intensive treatment targeting intracranial hypertension improves outcome in severe bacterial meningitis: an intervention-control study. PLoS One. 2014;9(3):e91976.
5. Kumar R, Singhi S, Singhi P, Jayashree M, Bansal A, Bhatti A. Randomized controlled trial comparing cerebral perfusion pressure-targeted therapy versus intracranial pressure-targeted therapy for raised intracranial pressure due to acute CNS infections in children. Crit Care Med. 2014;42:1775–87.
6. Schutte C, van der Meyden C. A prospective study of Glasgow Coma Scale (GCS), age, CSF-neutrophil count, and CSF-protein and glucose levels as prognostic indicators in 100 adult patients with meningitis. J Infect. 1998;37:112–5.
7. Al-Obaidi MMJ, Desa MNM. Mechanisms of blood brain barrier disruption by different types of bacteria, and bacterial-host interactions facilitate the bacterial pathogen invading the brain. Cell Mol Neurobiol. 2018;38:1349–68.
8. Iadecola C. The neurovascular unit coming of age: a journey through neurovascular coupling in health and disease. Neuron. 2017;96(1):17–42.
9. Rosner MJ. Introduction to cerebral perfusion pressure management. Neurosurg Clin N Am. 1995;6(4):761–73.
10. Rosner MJ, Becker DP. Origin and evolution of plateau waves. Experimental observations and a theoretical model. J Neurosurg. 1984;60:312–24.
11. Täuber MG. Brain edema, intracranial pressure and cerebral blood flow in bacterial meningitis. Pediatr Infect Dis J. 1989;8:915–7.
12. Weisfelt M, van de Beek D, Spanjaard L, Reitsma JB, de Gans J. A risk score for unfavorable outcome in adults with bacterial meningitis. Ann Neurol. 2008;63:90–7.
13. Bijlsma MW, Brouwer MC, Bossuyt PM, Heymans MW, van der Ende A, Tanck MW, van de Beek D. Risk scores for outcome in bacterial meningitis: systematic review and external validation study. J Infect. 2016;73:393–401.
14. Moore CL, Copel JA. Point-of-care ultrasonography. N Engl J Med. 2011;364(8):749–57.
15. Neri L, Storti E, Lichtenstein D. Toward an ultrasound curriculum for critical care medicine. Crit Care Med. 2007;35:S290–304.
16. Rozycki GS, Ochsner MG, Schmidt JA, Frankel HL, Davis TP, Wang D, et al. A prospective study of surgeon-performed ultrasound as the primary adjuvant modality for injured patient assessment. J Trauma. 1995;39(3):492–8.
17. Lichtenstein DA. BLUE-protocol and FALLS-protocol: two applications of lung ultrasound in the critically ill. Chest. 2015;147:1659–70.
18. Perera P, Mailhot T, Riley D, Mandavia D. The RUSH exam: Rapid Ultrasound in SHock in the evaluation of the critically ill. Emerg Med Clin North Am. 2010;28:29–56.
19. Previgliano I, Corral MM, Vera D, Baccaro F, Valiño M, Groer C. Estimación de la Presión Intracraneana y de la Presión de Perfusión cerebral mediante el Doppler Transcraneano: ¿mito o realidad? Med Intensiva. 2008;25:0329.

20. Bellner J, Romner B, Reinstrup P, Kristiansson KA, Ryding E, Brandt L. Transcranial Doppler sonography pulsatility index (PI) reflects intracranial pressure (ICP). Surg Neurol. 2004;62:45–51.
21. Belfort MA, Tooke-Miller C, Varner M, et al. Evaluation of a noninvasive transcranial Doppler and blood pressure-based method for the assessment of cerebral perfusion pressure in pregnant women. Hypertens Pregnancy. 2000;19:331–40.
22. Helmke K, Hansen HC. Fundamentals of transorbital sonographic evaluation of optic nerve sheath expansion under intracranial hypertension II. Patient study. Pediatr Radiol. 1996;26:706–10.
23. Amini A, Kariman H, Arhami Dolatabadi A, et al. Use of the sonographic diameter of optic nerve sheath to estimate intracranial pressure. Am J Emerg Med. 2013;31:236–9.
24. Dubourg J, Javouhey E, Geeraerts T, Messerer M, Kassai B. Ultrasonography of optic nerve sheath diameter for detection of raised intracranial pressure: a systematic review and meta-analysis. Intensive Care Med. 2011;37:1059–68.
25. Gardella JL, Guevara M, Purves C, Moughty Cueto C. Intracranial pressure monitoring: infection and other complications with the subdural K-30 and the intraparenquimatous fiber optic. Rev Argent Neurocir. 2006;20:151–5.
26. Brouwer MC, van de Beek D. Management of bacterial central nervous system infections. Handb Clin Neurol. 2017;140:349–64.
27. Garvey G. Current concepts of bacterial infections of the central nervous system. Bacterial meningitis and bacterial brain abscess. J Neurosurg. 1983;59:735–44.
28. Schenone AL, Cohen A, Patarroyo G, et al. Therapeutic hypothermia after cardiac arrest: a systematic review/meta-analysis exploring the impact of expanded criteria and targeted temperature. Resuscitation. 2016;108:102–10.
29. Hoehne J, Friedrich M, Brawanski A, Melter M, Schebesch KM. Decompressive craniectomy and early cranioplasty in a 15-year-old boy with N. meningitidis meningitis. Surg Neurol Int. 2015;6:58.
30. Di Rienzo A, Iacoangeli M, Rychlicki F, Veccia S, Scerrati M. Decompressive craniectomy for medically refractory intracranial hypertension due to meningoencephalitis: report of three patients. Acta Neurochir. 2008;150:1057–65.
31. Baussart B, Cheisson G, Compain M, Leblanc PE, Tadie M, Benhamou D, Duranteau J. Multimodal cerebral monitoring and decompressive surgery for the treatment of severe bacterial meningitis with increased intracranial pressure. Acta Anaesthesiol Scand. 2006;50:762–5.
32. Previgliano I, Perez Ochoa L. Medición del diámetro de la vaina del nervio óptico y su correlación con hipertensión intracraneal. In: Tamagnone F, Previgliano I. POCUS Manual de ultrasonografía crítica. Rosario: Corpus; 2018.

Chapter 11
Rabies

Gerald Marín-García, Javier Pérez-Fernández, and Gloria Rodríguez-Vega

Epidemiology

Rabies remains a worldwide public health problem. Rabies cases have been reported in more than 150 countries with the highest incidence in Africa and Asia. The World Health Organization (WHO) estimates that rabies causes more than 58,000 deaths yearly [1]. In the USA, only one to three cases are reported annually [2]. This low incidence is attributed to canine vaccination programs as well as to the efficacy of modern prophylaxis. Rabies carries a significant financial burden in the world with an estimated 8.6 billion US dollars spent in 2015, a rise from over half a billion US dollars from 2005 [3].

Rabies is a neurological disorder that will lead to respiratory depression and coma. Given its low incidence in developed countries, clinicians must exercise a high clinical suspicion for its diagnosis and promptly start adequate treatment before neurological manifestations occur.

G. Marín-García
VA Caribbean Healthcare System, Pulmonary Critical Care Section, San Juan, PR, USA

J. Pérez-Fernández
Critical Care Section, Baptyist Hospital of Miami, Florida International University, Miami, FL, USA

G. Rodríguez-Vega (✉)
HIMA-San Pablo, Caguas, PR, USA

© Springer Nature Switzerland AG 2020
J. Hidalgo, L. Woc-Colburn (eds.), *Highly Infectious Diseases in Critical Care*,
https://doi.org/10.1007/978-3-030-33803-9_11

Etiology

Rabies is a bullet-shaped single-stranded ribonucleic acid (RNA) virus from the genus *Lyssavirus*. Like most of the *Lyssavirus*, it has a predilection for central nervous tissue. The virus has two functional units: internal nucleocapsid core and lipoprotein envelope. The virus is transmitted in the saliva, typically through a bite of an infected mammal. Canines are the most common worldwide animal vector, being involved in over 99% of all cases. Canine control and widespread mandatory vaccination campaigns have claimed elimination of dog-mediated rabies in Western Europe, Canada, the USA, Japan, and some Latin American countries [4]. In the USA, bats, racoons, foxes, and skunks are the main reservoirs of the virus. Bat rabies accounts for most human rabies cases in the Americas. Other less common mechanisms of infection have been reported such as organ donation or inhaled aerosolized virus while handling contaminated materials in research laboratories or in bat caves [5, 6].

Pathogenesis

Once a patient has been infected, the virus replicates in the muscle gaining access to the nervous system through the motor endplate and traveling via the peripheral nervous system to the spinal cord at a rate of 50–100 mm/day [7]. The retrograde migration accelerates from there, reaching the central nervous system (CNS). CNS spread occurs from cell to cell across the synaptic junction [7]. Once the CNS has been reached, systemic invasion can occur to highly innervated organs via anterograde axoplasmic flow. The most common involved organs include the salivary glands, heart, lungs, and intraabdominal organs. The incubation period will range from days to months and does not depend on the location of the bite. The prolonged incubation period is thought to be caused by the low titer of inoculum and by the existence of endogenous RNA silencing mechanisms that slow down viral replication but renders an incomplete immune response [8]. Isolated cases have been reported after several years of exposure [9]. The pathophysiology of rabies-caused damage remains unclear. In vitro studies have found that interaction between viral phosphoprotein P and neuronal mitochondria leads to an overproduction of reactive oxygen radicals and eventual neurotoxicity [10].

Clinical Manifestations

The clinical presentation of rabies can be heterogenous. In general, it has been reported in three different phases: prodromal, acute neurological, and coma.

Prodromal Phase

The prodromal phase occurs during the viral replication and the retrograde migration to the dorsal root ganglion. Neuropathic pain at the site of the bite with proximal radiation of the symptoms is described in half of the cases. During this phase, other nonspecific symptoms related to the acute inflammatory immune response may be present. These symptoms include general malaise, fever, chills, nausea, vomiting, pharyngitis, myalgias, and fatigue. This phase lasts from 2 to 10 days [11].

Neurological Phase

The acute neurological phase might present into two different forms: the furious (hyperactive) rabies and the paralytic rabies. The former is the most common form. Its presentation overlaps with the prodromal phase, and it is associated with symptoms such as anxiety, insomnia, and depression. Once this phase is reached, the classical hydrophobia and aerophobia can be observed, along with delirium. During this phase, we encounter the presence of muscle spasms in response to tactile, auditory, visual, or olfactory stimuli that, if severe enough, can lead to opisthotonos. Autonomic manifestations include tachycardia, salivation, lacrimation, and body temperature variability.

Approximately one third of the patients present with the paralytic form, making the diagnosis more difficult to entertain [8]. It usually starts at the site of inoculation and spreads symmetrically or asymmetrically in an ascending manner. As paralysis worsens, lower motor neuron findings such as fasciculations and decreased or loss deep tendon reflexes can be identified in the affected area. Fever and nuchal rigidity may also be encountered. This form will progress to respiratory failure.

Coma

Coma occurs as the natural progression of the disease, and in most cases, once the neurological phase is started, it will be unavoidable despite aggressive treatment. After coma has developed, most patients die within weeks due to intractable seizures caused by encephalitis, cardiac dysrhythmias, acute respiratory distress syndrome, or complications from prolonged mechanical ventilation.

Diagnosis

Rabies diagnosis is a medical challenge as it relies solely on clinical acumen. A detailed history to unveil possible exposures and a thorough physical examination are essential. Rabies should be part of the differential diagnosis in all patients who present with unexplained, acute, and progressive viral encephalitis. Even in areas where the disease is rare, clinicians need to remain suspicious as rabies may occur locally in wildlife or can be acquired during travel to enzootic areas. Imported cases of human and animal rabies continue to occur [5]. Due to its high mortality, any patient with compatible manifestations in whom a clinical suspicion is contemplated must receive treatment without delay.

Laboratory Testing

When a patient presents to the emergency department (ED) with an animal bite, appropriate consultation with local authorities must be performed. If the involved animal has a low probability of being rabid, such as a domesticated cat or dog, then quarantine for development of symptoms for 10 days can be undertaken. If there is a higher probability for rabies and the animal is captured, then euthanization followed by biopsies from cerebellum and brainstem is performed. A direct fluorescent antibody (DFA) tests is performed on a sample of the cerebral tissue from the animal. If the animal is not captured, then adequate post-exposure prophylaxis ensues [12].

Laboratories such as cell blood count and differential, complete metabolic panel or arterial blood gases are nonspecific for the diagnosis. Blood and cerebrospinal fluid cultures are only helpful to rule out other causes of encephalitis.

There is no gold standard laboratory test for the antemortem diagnosis of rabies. Rabies-specific antibodies for DFA test are of little value since they become positive late in the course of the disease. To date, the test with the highest antemortem diagnostic value in humans is a reverse-transcription, heminested polymerase chain reaction (RT-hnPCR). When this test is applied to three sequential samples of saliva, the sensitivity and specificity is 100%. If performed to skin biopsies from the back of the neck including hair follicles, sensitivity and specificity can be 98% and 100%, respectively [13]. These tests are limited by their widespread availability and the complexity of storing and handling the samples.

Imaging

As it is the case with laboratory tests, neuroimaging only helps in excluding other causes of neurologic symptoms. Head CT has no role in the diagnosis of rabies. Magnetic resonance imaging (MRI), however, has shown T2-weighted enhancement in nonspecific areas such as basal ganglia, brainstem, hippocampus, or hypothalamus. Enhancement along the brachial plexus of the bitten arm has been documented [14]. However, these findings have only been described in advanced phases of the disease of reported fatalities.

Treatment

The most effective treatment method is prevention. Anticipation of exposure in an endemic area warrants pre-exposure prophylaxis (PrEP). Once a patient has presumably been exposed, rabies immunoglobulin (RIG) and/or post-exposure prophylaxis (PEP) is recommended. Timely administration of such therapy is nearly 100% effective in preventing the disease. Once the disease has manifested, there are no other options except comprehensive supportive treatment in the ICU.

Pre-exposure Prophylaxis

Pre-exposure prophylaxis is indicated for people that have a high risk of exposure to rabies such as veterinarians, scientists that work directly with the virus, or people who are going to be in an endemic area without reliable access to health facilities if exposed. PrEP uses human diploid cells or embryonated egg vaccine, manufactured with attenuated virus [15].

Pre-exposure vaccination consists of a series of three intramuscular injections given on days 0, 7, and 21 or 28. Depending on the type of exposure risk, frequent antibody testing should be performed and booster administered as needed [16].

Post-exposure Prophylaxis

The post-exposure prophylaxis regimen will depend on the patient's prior vaccination status. If a patient has not been vaccinated, human rabies immunoglobulin (HRIG) must be administered as close to the inoculation site and as far away from the site of the vaccine administration as possible. The treatment must then be followed by rabies vaccines at days 0, 3, 7, and 14. Immunocompromised individuals must receive a fifth dose at day 28. HRIG should never be administered in the same syringe or in the same anatomical site as the first vaccine dose. However, subsequent doses of vaccine can be administered in the same anatomic location where the HRIG dose was administered. The recommended dose of HRIG is 20 IU/kg body weight for both adults and children [17]. If PrEP has been previously administered, immunoglobin is withheld, and booster vaccines are given at days 0 and 3 [16].

Symptomatic Rabies

Once a patient develops symptomatic rabies, supportive treatment needs to be carried out in the ICU. Invasive mechanical ventilation will be inevitable due to progression of muscle weakness leading to respiratory failure or cerebral edema.

Patients are at high risk for cardiac dysrhythmias and hypotension secondary to marked autonomic dysfunction. Disease-specific guidelines are non-existent. It has been reported in animal models that the rabies vaccine and RIG are associated with an accelerated progression of disease and mortality if administered once symptoms have started [18]. Death is almost unavoidable, and only a few cases of survival have been documented in the literature, most of them with adequate post-exposure pro-phylaxis prior the development of symptoms [19].

The controversial case of a 15-year-old girl that in 2004 survived rabies with good neurological outcome initiated the steps of an experimental approach now called the Milwaukee protocol. The protocol consists of the induction of coma to burst suppression pattern on EEG to protect from autonomic instability. The pro-tocol also recommends the use of N-methyl-D-aspartate (NMDA) antagonists such as ketamine and amantadine for neuroprotection from glutamine-induced toxicity. Amantadine was also used as a viral replication antagonist. The protocol emphasizes the prevention of cerebral vasospasm with medications such as nimodipine, vitamin C, and saproprotein and performing daily transcranial Dopplers for the first 2 weeks [20]. This protocol was applied in two other patients that survived rabies, but both patients had also received PEP. More than 30 cases have failed to survive despite the application of the Milwaukee protocol. For this reason and the absence of adequate clinical trials, most experts do not advocate for its application. Currently neither the CDC nor the WHO have specific recom-mendations on the treatment of symptomatic rabies other than supportive treat-ment [4, 16].

A palliative approach is acceptable if a patient is deemed to have a fatal outcome or has been documented that would not accept supportive measures such as mechan-ical ventilation. Once comfort measures are going to be pursued, the patient must be taken to a low-stimulation room. Agitation can be managed with antipsychotic drugs such as haloperidol or benzodiazepines. Dyspnea can be treated with opioids such as morphine. If hypersalivation is a feature, glycopyrrolate or scopolamine can be used [4].

Summary

Although a rare disease with approximately three cases per year in the USA, rabies continues to be a major health problem worldwide. The best treatment is prevention, either by animal vaccination and possible eradication of disease or the administra-tion of early prophylaxis upon recognizing patients at risk. Once symptoms have started, mortality is almost certain, and no guidelines exist regarding specific man-agement other than supportive care. Given its lethality and low incidence in some areas, clinicians must exercise a high index of suspicion and a very low threshold for initiating treatment in high-risk cases.

References

1. World Health Organization. Epidemiology and burden of disease [Internet]. 2019 [cited 4 Apr 2019]. Available from: https://www.who.int/rabies/epidemiology/en/World.
2. Centers for Disease Control and Prevention (CDC). Rabies surveillance in the U.S.: human rabies. Rabies [Internet]. cdc.gov. 2019 [cited 4 Apr 2019]. Available from: https://www.cdc.gov/rabies/location/usa/surveillance/human_rabies.html.
3. Hampson K, Coudeville L, Lembo T, Sambo M, Kieffer A, Attlan M, et al. Estimating the global burden of endemic canine rabies. PLoS Negl Trop Dis. 2015;9(4):e0003709.
4. World Health Organization. WHO expert consultation on rabies, third report, WHO technical report series, No. 1012. Geneva: World Health Organization; 2018.
5. Srinivasan A, Burton E, Kuehnert M, Rupprecht C, Sutker W, Ksiazek T, et al. Transmission of rabies virus from an organ donor to four transplant recipients. N Engl J Med. 2005;352(11):1103–11.
6. Davis AD, Rudd RJ, Bowen RA. Effects of aerosolized rabies virus exposure on bats and mice. J Infect Dis. 2007;195(8):1144–50.
7. Warrell M, Warrell D. Rabies and other lyssavirus diseases. Lancet. 2004;363(9424):1907.
8. Hemachudha T, Ugolini G, Wacharapluesadee S, Sungkarat W, Shuangshoti S, Laothamatas J. Human rabies: neuropathogenesis, diagnosis, and management. Lancet Neurol. 2013;12(5):498–513.
9. Boland TA, Mcguone D, Jindal J, Rocha M, Cumming M, Rupprecht CE, et al. Phylogenetic and epidemiologic evidence of multiyear incubation in human rabies. Ann Neurol. 2014;75(1):155–60.
10. Jackson AC. Diabolical effects of rabies encephalitis. J Neurovirol. 2015;22(1):8–13.
11. Hemachudha T, Laothamatas J, Rupprecht CE. Human rabies: a disease of complex neuro-pathogenetic mechanisms and diagnostic challenges. Lancet Neurol. 2002;1(2):101–9.
12. Centers for Disease Control and Prevention (CDC). Diagnosis in animals and humans. Rabies [Internet]. 2011 [cited 2 Apr 2019]. Available from: https://www.cdc.gov/rabies/diagnosis/animals-humans.html.
13. Dacheux L, Reynes JM, Buchy P, Sivuth O, Diop BM, Rousset D, et al. A reliable diagnosis of human rabies based on analysis of skin biopsy specimens. Clin Infect Dis. 2008;47(11):1410–7.
14. Laothamatas J, Hemachudha T, Mitrabhakdi E, Wannakrairot P, Tulayadaechanont S. MR imaging in human rabies. Am J Neuroradiol. 2003;24(6):1102–9.
15. Bernard KW, Roberts MA, Sumner J, Winkler WG, Mallonee J, Baer GM, Chaney R. Human diploid cell rabies vaccine. JAMA. 1982;247(8):1138–42.
16. Centers for Disease Control and Prevention (CDC). Travelers' health [Internet]. 2017 [cited 8 Apr 2019]. Available from: https://wwwnc.cdc.gov/travel/yellowbook/2018/infectious-diseases-related-to-travel/rabies#5245.
17. Manning SE, Rupprecht CE, Fishbein D, et al. Human rabies prevention--United States, 2008: recommendations of the Advisory Committee on Immunization Practices. MMWR Recomm Rep. 2008;57:1.
18. Willoughby RE. "Early death" and the contraindication of vaccine during treatment of rabies. Vaccine. 2009;27(51):7173–7.
19. Jackson AC. Rabies: scientific basis of the disease and its management. 3rd ed. Oxford: Elsevier Academic Press; 2013. p. 573–87.
20. Zeiler FA, Jackson AC. Critical appraisal of the milwaukee protocol for rabies: this failed approach should be abandoned. Can J Neurol Sci. 2015;43(01):44–51.

Chapter 12
Tetanus

Javier Pérez-Fernández, Gerald Marín-García, and Gloria Rodríguez-Vega

"Tetanus" was derived from a Greek word τέτανος (*tetanos*) with a meaning of "stretching or rigidity." It was already mentioned in the times of Hippocrates. Tetanus remains a worldwide burden of health. The World Health Organization (WHO) estimates that 16 countries have failed to eliminate maternal and neonatal tetanus with an excess of 30,000 reported annual cases [1]. Effective vaccination programs have led to the reduction of the disease [2]. The WHO has placed special emphasis on the reduction of neonatal and maternal tetanus.

Tetanus is seldom seen in the intensive care unit in most developed countries. In the USA, it has been a constant decline since the mid-1940s when national reporting began. Attributed factors to this decline have been the widespread use of the tetanus toxoid vaccines as well as improvements in the care of wounds and post-exposure use of tetanus immunoglobulin (TIG) [3]. The diagnosis of tetanus requires a high clinical suspicion index, and given the rarity of its occurrence, it might result in significant delays in both recognition and adequate management. Sporadic cases of tetanus occur in adults who did not get their vaccinations or those who do not stay up on their 10-year booster [4].

Tetanus is a disease characterized by muscle spasms leading to respiratory failure, cardiovascular dysfunction, and inherent problems of a prolonged ICU admission such as infections, anemia, thrombotic events, etc. The disease is fatal unless

J. Pérez-Fernández (✉)
Critical Care Section, Baptyist Hospital of Miami, Florida International University, Miami, FL, USA

G. Marín-García
VA Caribbean Healthcare System, Pulmonary Critical Care Section, San Juan, PR, USA
e-mail: gerald.marin@upr.edu

G. Rodríguez-Vega
HIMA-San Pablo, Caguas, PR, USA

© Springer Nature Switzerland AG 2020
J. Hidalgo, L. Woc-Colburn (eds.), *Highly Infectious Diseases in Critical Care*,
https://doi.org/10.1007/978-3-030-33803-9_12

prolonged and aggressive support is given to patients. The significant amount of resources necessary to support these patients becomes a challenge in some countries with healthcare limitations.

Etiology

Tetanus is caused by the spore-forming gram + anaerobic bacillus *Clostridium tetani*. *Clostridium tetani* spores are found on the soil and the gastrointestinal tract of many animals and humans. Spores can enter the organism by wounds. The incubation period is usually 7–10 days. Spores are resistant to boiling and antiseptics but can be eliminated by autoclave 121 °C for 15 min or 100 °C for 4 h [5]. Mechanisms of entry include puncture wounds, lacerations, or abrasions more commonly. With less frequency, it has been reported associated to tattoing, burns, frostbite, dental infections and in neonatal cases, umbilical cord manipulation with contaminated equipment. In both the USA and Europe, cases have been reported in intravenous drug users through the use of contaminated needles [6].

C. tetani secretes two exotoxins: tetanospasmin and tetanolysin. This last one produces tissue necrosis helping to recreate an anaerobic environment required by the bacilli to grow. Tetanospasmin, also known as tetanus toxin, is a neurotoxin that inhibits neurotransmitter release at the presynaptic membrane [7]. The effect of the neurotoxin can last several weeks *involving the nervous system* at different levels, central motor control, autonomic function, and neuromuscular junction.

Pathogenesis

After the entry of *C. tetani* spores into the organism, typically by a small wound, toxins are liberated. The neurotoxin adheres to proteins involved in neuro-exocytosis making them incapable of releasing transmitter. The toxin binds gangliosides on local nerve terminals. Via retrograde axonal transport, the toxin enters the neuron at the central nervous system. The involvement of the spinal neuron leads to some of the classical manifestations of tetanus. The most sensitive neurons are GABA and glycinergic cells. During the induction of palsy, both lines of cells are inhibited, and the motor system responds with intense, simultaneous, and sustained contractures (agonist and antagonist muscles) to afferent stimuli. These contractures are known as tetanic spasms.

Once toxin is fixed to the neurons, it cannot be neutralized. The process will reverse after new synapses are formed, a process that may take over 4–6 weeks to occur.

The involvement of the autonomic nervous system usually occurs at the second week producing an autonomic dysfunction syndrome with a myriad of signs including labile blood pressure, tachyarrhythmias, peripheral vasoconstriction, diaphoresis, and eventually bradycardia and hypotension.

The severity of tetanus depends on the involvement of certain muscle groups. Cases have been reported with only localized involvement versus others affecting the entire skeletal musculature [8].

Clinical Manifestations

With an incubation period oscillating between 3 and 21 days, it has been described that manifestations could present earlier in cases in which wounds are closer to the central nervous system. There is an association between severity and the incubation period, with more severe disease and increased lethality associated with shorter incubation terms.

Although the majority of cases follow some type of wound, no evidence of portal has been reported in up 25% of the cases [8]. Different entry wounds have been described accounting for minor skin-breaking traumas, ulcers, uterine lacerations after abortions, intravenous drug usage, postoperative wounds, or infected umbilical stumps [9].

For the purpose of clinical descriptions, there are four forms of clinical syndrome: generalized, focal, cephalic, and neonatal.

Generalized Tetanus

Characterized by diffuse muscle rigidity affecting any voluntary muscles. It represents 80% of the cases seen. The most common initial sign is spasm of the muscles of the jaw or "lockjaw." This is mostly induced by masseter trismus and results in difficulty opening the mouth. Neck rigidity, stiffness, and dysphagia can also be present. At a latter phase, muscle rigidity in the facial and vertebral muscles will produced risus sardonicus (sardonic smile) and opisthotonos and depending on the severity and treatment can lead into vertebral fractures [10].

As other group of muscles get involved, differential diagnosis might include peritonitis (abdominal muscles) or meningitis (nuchal rigidity). Special attention is required for laryngeal spasm that by itself can lead to asphyxia. Airway compromise can occur at any time during the course of the disease.

In about two thirds of the patients, reflex spams can occur, sometimes triggered by minimal stimulus. Such spasms are tonic-clonic and painful. In some instances and given the high frequency of the spasms, clinicians might suspect the presence of status epilepticus. Bone fractures, dislocations, and even renal failure motivated by rhabdomyolysis are all consequences of the uncontrolled and random muscle activity [11].

Spasms continue on the course of disease for weeks, producing paradoxical paralysis due to presynaptic inhibition of acetylcholine release at the neuromuscular junction. Apnea periods, urinary retention, and miscarriages (uterine musculature involvement) have been some of the effects described.

Generalized tetanus is in general associated with autonomic nervous dysfunction. Tachycardia, labile hypertension and hypotension, vasoconstriction, and diaphoresis are commonly present. Hyperthermia deserves special attention, which by itself represents autonomic dysfunction but is also possibly secondary to generalized muscle contractions and that might obscure the presence of secondary infections. In occasions, parasympathetic stimulation is associated with bronchial hypersecretion, bradycardia, and sinus arrest [12].

Localized Tetanus

Less common presentation. Rigidity of a group of muscles in the proximity of site of injury. The presence of circulating antitoxin without enough amount to eradicate the toxin is believed to be the cause for this "partial" development. Sometimes the clinicians might misdiagnose these with muscle spasms. Rare descriptions of generalizations from localized tetanus have been reported although in general associated with better prognosis [13].

Cephalic Tetanus

Rare manifestation and complications of traumatic scalp lesions, other head and neck trauma, dental extractions, or otitis media. It tends to have a shorter incubation period, between 1 and 14 days [14]. It manifests as trismus and cranial nerve paralysis. Any cranial nerve can be affected although the most commonly described is the facial nerve (VII) which is associated with lockjaw, facial palsy, or ptosis [14]. Trismus might develop later. Progression to generalized tetanus is associated with onerous prognosis [15].

Neonatal Tetanus

A form of generalized tetanus that occurs in newborns, especially in mothers that have not been vaccinated. It is important to mention that tetanus toxin does not cross the placenta and thus infections acquired by infants that did not carry over the immunity from the mother are usually associated with the manipulation of the umbilical stump with non-sterile instruments. The WHO has engaged in a massive worldwide campaign that has been able to reduce the death toll associated with neonatal tetanus in more than 90% [16].

Diagnosis and Laboratory Tests

The diagnosis of tetanus remains a clinical one, with little help from laboratory tests. In developed countries, it continues being a challenge that can delay significantly the management. The isolation of the bacilli from the wound area only occurs in less than one third of the cases.

The "spatula test" involves touching the posterior pharyngeal wall with a soft-tipped instrument. A positive test involves the involuntary contraction of the jaw ("biting down the spatula") with absence of a gag reflex. Available reports suggest that the specificity of this test could be as high as 100% with a sensitivity of 94% [17].

It is essential to always consider differential diagnosis such as malignant hyperthermia, atropine or strychnine poisoning, or hypercalcemia.

Blood cultures are of no value except for diagnosis of secondary infections. Laboratories in general offer little help on the diagnosis. Non-specific findings as leukocytosis or elevation of the creatinine as a result of the muscle degradation could be present. Elevation of the transaminases, increased catecholamine levels, and decreased serum cholinesterase as well as an increase of the creatinine phosphokinase (CPK) once spasms develop are commonly seen but do not direct the clinician to any conclusion. A report suggests that the elevation of cerebrospinal fluid (CSF) protein might be associated with disease severity [18].

Treatment

Treatment of tetanus is utmost related to intensive care units where patients are admitted for a prolonged period of time. Supportive management is essential in the survival of those patients [19].

Treatment goals must be aimed to the reduction of complications but source control and eradication of the etiologic agent are necessary steps.

The sequence of treatment steps should be summarized as limiting the production of the toxin (by eliminating the source, *B. tetani*) with antibiotics, limiting the reach of the tetanospasmin by management of the wound and administration of antitoxin, minimizing muscle contractures and spasms, and stabilizing the circulatory and autonomic systems. All these steps require admission to intensive care units and management by trained and skilled personnel. Even patients with mild forms, and considering the possibility of generalization of the disease, must be observed at the critical care unit for at least 1 or 2 weeks prior to transferring then to a lower acuity unit [20].

Several grading methods for severity have been postulated in order to determine some prognosis and/or allocation of resources. Some of those methods are based on clinical data and are modified by the course of the disease over time, describing whether patients are improving or not [21]. Some of these classifications are based on grades or clinical forms (mild to very severe) [22]. All these classifications add little to the management of patients as mild patients portend less risk of dying but still require significant monitoring and treatment. There is a linear correlation between the time of injury, the first appearance of the symptoms, and the severity of the course of the disease.

Aggressive supportive care should be exercised. Over 90% of the patients will typically require prolonged mechanical ventilation, and about two thirds will also need muscle paralysis to overcome significant spasms. Even in more severe cases, support therapies elevate survival rates to well over 80% at 1 year [23]. Advanced age has been associated with increased mortality [24].

Wound Care

Aggressive surgical treatment of the wound area is recommended, and it needs to occur as soon as the wound is discovered. It is believed that the removal of the spores is associated with improved survival. If foreign bodies are present, those need to be removed and wounds debrided and left open [10]. As *C. tetani* is anaerobic and spores are very resistant, the wound excision should always expose healthy tissue. In occasions, it might be required to amputate limbs if gangrene is present. In cases of neonatal or maternal tetanus, the indication for hysterectomy will depend on the presence of an infected wound. Regular wound care should be the rule for any skin breakage or surgical debris. There is not enough data to support the administration of local antibiotics or direct immunoglobulin instillation in the wound area.

Toxin Neutralization

Administration of human antitetanus immunoglobulin (HTIg) or equine antitetanus serum is standard therapy for tetanus. Once tetanospasmin has adhered to the nervous system, it cannot be neutralized. The aim for therapy should then be the neutralization of circulating tetanus toxin. Hence, antitoxin should be administered as soon as possible [25].

Administration of HTIg is intramuscular, in a dose range of 500–3000 units. If human immunoglobulin is not available, equine antitoxin (antitetanus serum) can be administered at doses of 1500–3000 units intramuscularly. Since no studies are available comparing head to head the efficacy of both therapies, the choice of one versus another depends more on hypersensitivity reactions associated with

ATS. Studies have failed to stablish the actual doses, and the doses listed are based on consensus [26].

Controversy persists on the route of administration. Intrathecal administration has been reported with variable outcomes [27, 28]. Cochrane reviews have found not enough evidence to support the recommendation [29], but a most recent meta-analysis favors its use [30]. If option is given to the intrathecal route, clinicians must be aware of the rare but reported adverse event of reversible paraplegia.

All patients should receive active immunization with three doses of tetanus toxoid, spaced at least 2 weeks apart, upon recovery of the acute infection with boosters given every 10 years throughout the life.

Antibiotics

Source control as part of the inhibition of further toxin production is a goal of the treatment. Metronidazole 500 mg intravenously every 6 h for 10 days is the treatment of choice [31]. Choices available include penicillin G, tetracycline, erythromycin, clindamycin, and chloramphenicol [32]. The GABA antagonist effect of penicillin has limited its use [33]. In addition, anaerobic environment associated with wounds nesting C. tetani is a nurturing media for polymicrobial flora with abundant beta-lactamase production.

Muscular Relaxants

Benzodiazepines are widely used as muscle relaxant agents. Their GABA agonist effect has been advantageous in the treatment of muscle spasms [12]. While diazepam has been favored historically, there is not enough data to suggest that other benzodiazepines such are midazolam or lorazepam are not equally effective [34].

Intravenous magnesium sulfate, a widely accepted therapy for eclampsia, is a physiological antagonist of calcium at the cellular level, and its effects are related to the prevention of catecholamine release and presynaptic neuromuscular blockade [35]. Several case reports demonstrated successful control of the tetanic spasms [36]. From the available evidence, magnesium sulfate does have a therapeutic benefit in controlling muscle spasms and reducing autonomic instability. The magnesium serum concentration recommended is that of 2–4 mmol/l [36]. No demonstrated benefit in mortality or ventilator dates has been established [37].

Baclofen, a GABA-B receptor agonist, has a poor blood-brain barrier penetration. Intrathecal administration is shown to limit spasms. Given the fact that the intrathecal route requires significant resources, such as tunneled intrathecal catheter and reservoir, might not be readily available in all circumstances [38]. With much less evidence than that for magnesium sulfate, baclofen infused 500–2000 µg seems to be effective to ameliorate muscle spasms although it is not favored by most [39].

Neuromuscular blockade can be necessary if sedatives fail to control spasms. Nondepolarizing agents are favored. Rapidly metabolized agents such as cisatracurium is preferred [13]. Patients must be fully sedated, and medications should be stopped daily to assess the need for continuation.

Propofol and dexmedetomidine have been reported to prevent muscular spasms [40]. Dantrolene can be effective in reducing hyperthermia induced by spasms and has been described in the treatment of tetanus [41].

Vaccination

Numerous formulations of vaccines are available. Vaccination consists on a three-dose administration within a period of 1 year. Acute tetanus infection does not create immunity. Patients affected must receive the vaccine with a 2-week interval from the recovery. Boosters are administered every 10 years.

It is also recommended the use of a booster and immunoglobulin in wound management of those wounds to be suspected as contaminated.

Summary

Albeit a rare disease with less than 100 cases per year in the USA and Europe, tetanus continues being a major health problem worldwide. Mortality has declined with extraordinary support measures available in most developed countries. However, given its rarity, high clinical suspicion must be exercise for its diagnosis. Early recognition and treatment are associated with better outcomes. Prolonged ICU stay is expected for those patients affected, and a great variety of supportive measures will be employed to guarantee the best outcomes.

Bibliography

1. WHO. Immunization, vaccines and biologicals: vaccines and diseases—maternal and neonatal tetanus elimination (MNTE). Geneva: WHO [updated 5 Apr 2017].
2. WHO. Expanded programme on immunization. Global Advisory Group—Part II. Wkly Epidemiol Rec. 1994;69(5):29–31, 34–5.
3. Wassilak SGF, Roper MH, Kretsinger K, Orenstein WA. Tetanus toxoid. In: Plotkin SA, Orenstein WA, Offit PA, editors. Vaccines. 5th ed. Philadelphia: Saunders; 2012. p. 746–72.
4. Faulkner AE, Tiwari TS. Chapter 16: Tetanus. In: VPD surveillance manual. www.cdc.gov/vaccines/pubs/surv-manual/chpt16-tetanus.html.
5. Hodowanec A, Bleck TP. In: Mandell GL, Douglas RG, Bennett JE, Dolin R, Blaser MJ, editors. Mandell, Douglas and Bennett's principles and practices of infectious diseases. 8th ed. Philadelphia: Elsevier. Tetanus Ch. 246. 2015;2757–63.

6. CDC. Tetanus among injecting-drug users—California, 1997. MMWR Morb Mortal Wkly Rep. 1998;47(8):149–51.
7. Mellanby J, Green J. How does tetanus toxin act? Neurscience. 1981;6:281–300.
8. Edmondson RS, Flowers MW. Intensive care in tetanus: management, complications and mortality in 100 cases. BMJ. 1979;1:1401–4.
9. Alfery DD, Rauscher LA. Tetanus: a review. Crit Care Med. 1979;7(4):176–81.
10. Brook I. Current concepts in the management of Clostridium tetani infection. Expert Rev Anti Infect Ther. 2008;6(3):327–36.
11. Weiss MF, Badalamenti J, Fish E. Tetanus as a cause of rhabdomyolysis and acute renal failure. Clin Nephrol. 2010;73:64–7.
12. Cook TM, Protheroe RT, Handel JM. Tetanus: a review of the literature. Br J Anaesth. 2001;87(3):477–87.
13. Edlich RF, Hill LG, Mahler CA, et al. Management and prevention of tetanus. J Long Term Eff Med Implants. 2003;13(3):139–54.
14. Seo DH, Cho DK, Kwon HC, Kim TU. A case of cephalic tetanus with unilateral ptosis and facial palsy. Ann Rehabil Med. 2012;36(1):167–70.
15. Doshi A, Warrell C, Dahdaleh D, Kullmann D. Just a graze? Cephalic tetanus presenting as a stroke mimic. Pract Neurol. 2014;14(1):39–41.
16. UNICEF. Elimination of maternal and neonatal tetanus.Archived from the original on 21 Feb 2014. Retrieved 17 Feb 2014.
17. Apte NM, Karnad DR. Short report: the spatula test: a simple bedside test to diagnose tetanus. Am J Trop Med Hyg. 1995;53(4):386–7.
18. Idoko JA, Amiobonomo AE, Anjorin FI, Oyeyinka GO, Elechi C. Cerebrospinal fluid changes in tetanus: raised proteins and immunoglobulins in patients with severe disease. Trans R Soc Trop Med Hyg. 1990;84(4):593–4.
19. Trujillo MH, Castillo A, Espana J, Manzo A, Zerpa R. Impact of intensive care management on the prognosis of tetanus. Analysis of 641 cases. Chest. 1987;92(1):63–5.
20. Udwadia FE, Lall A, Udwadia ZF, Sekhar M, Vora A. Tetanus and its complications: intensive care and management experience in 150 indian patients. Epidemiol Infect. 1987;99(3): 675–84.
21. Miranda-Filho DB, Ximenes RA, Barone AA, Vaz VL, Vieira AG, Albuquerque VM. Clinical classification of tetanus patients. Braz J Med Biol Res. 2006;39(10):1329–37.
22. Thwaites CL, Yen LM, Glover C, Tuan PQ, Nga NT, Parry J, et al. Predicting the clinical outcome of tetanus: the tetanus severity score. Tropical Med Int Health. 2006;11(3):279–87.
23. Mahieu R, Reydel T, Maamar A, Tadie JM, et al. Admission of tetanus patients to the ICU: a retrospective multicenter study. Ann Intensive Care. 2017;7:112–8.
24. Filia A, Bella A, von-Hunolstein C, Pinto A, et al. Tetanus in Italy 2001-2010: a continuing threat in older adults. Vaccine. 2014;32:639–44.
25. Ataro P, Mushatt D, Ahsan S. Tetanus: a review. South Med J. 2011;104(8):613:7.
26. Blake PA, Feldman RA, Buchanan TM, Brooks GE, et al. Serology therapy of tetanus in the United States 1965–1971. JAMA. 1976;235(1):42–4.
27. Miranda-Filho DB, Ximenes RA, Barone AA, Vaz VL, Vieira AG, Albuquerque VM. Randomised controlled trial of tetanus treatment with antitetanus immunoglobulin by the intrathecal or the intramuscular route. BMJ. 2004;328:615.
28. Geeta MG, Khrisnakumar P, Matthews L. Intrathecal tetanus immunoglobulin in the management of tetanus. Indian J Pediatr. 2007;74:43–5.
29. Abrutyn E, Berlin JA. Intrathecal therapy in tetanus, a meta-analysis. JAMA. 1991;266:2262–7.
30. Kabura L, Illibagiza D, Menten J, Van der Ende J. Intrathecal vs. intramuscular administration of human antitetanus immunoglobulin or equine tetanus antitoxin in the treatment of tetanus: a meta-analysis. Tropical Med Int Health. 2006;11:1075–81.
31. Ganesh K, Kotach: VM, Krishnan A, Karnad DR. Benzathine penicillin, metronidazole and benzyl penicillin in the treatment of tetanus: a randomized, controlled trial. Ann Trop Med Parasitol. 2004;98(1):59–63.

32. Campbell JL, Lam TM, Huynh TL, To SD, et al. Microbiologic characterization and antimicrobial susceptibility of Clostridium tetani isolated from wounds of patients with clinically diagnosed tetanus. Am J Trop Med Hyg. 2009;80(5):827–31.
33. Ahmadsyah I, Salim A. Treatment of tetanus: an open study to compare the efficacy of procaine penicillin and metronidazole. Br Med J Clin Res Ed. 1985;291:648–50.
34. Okoromah CN, Lesi FE. Diazepam for treating tetanus. Cochrane Database Syst Rev. 2004;(1):CD003954.
35. Karanikolas M, Velissaris D, Marangos M, Karamouzos V, Fligou F, et al. Prolonged high-dose intravenous magnesium therapy for severe tetanus in the intensive care unit: a case series. J Med Case Rep. 2010;4:100.
36. Attygalle D, Rodrigo N. Magnesium as first line therapy in the management of tetanus: a prospective study of 40 patients. Anaesthesia. 2002;57:811–7.
37. Thwaites CL, Yen LM, Loan HT, Thuy TT, Thwaites GE, Stepniewska K, Soni N, et al. Magnesium sulphate for treatment of severe tetanus: a randomised controlled trial. Lancet. 2006;368:1436–43.
38. Muller H, Borner U, Zierski J, Hempelmann G. Intrathecal baclofen for treatment of tetanus-induced spasticity. Anesthesiology. 1987;66:76–9.
39. Santos ML, Mota-Miranda A, Alves-Pereira A, Gomes A, Correia J, Marcal N. Intrathecal baclofen for the treatment of tetanus. Clin Infect Dis. 2004;38:321–8.
40. Girgin NK, Iscimen R, Gurbet A, Kahveci F, Kutlay O. Dexmedetomidine sedation for the treatment of tetanus in the intensive care unit. Br J Anaesth. 2007;99:599–600.
41. Sternlo JE, Andersen LW. Early treatment of mild tetanus with dantrolene. Intensive Care Med. 1990;16:345–6.

Chapter 13
Malaria

Jorge Hidalgo, Pedro Arriaga, and Bruno Alvarez Concejo

Introduction

Plasmodium spp. are a protozoan parasite that causes malaria. It has been a companion to the human species since our inception, before we started our long journey out of Africa 60.000 years ago, and has shaped our population, genetics, and behaviors like no other organism [1, 2]. Malaria presentation ranges from a mild febrile illness to a life-threatening disease with multisystem organ failure. Severe malaria belongs in the intensive care unit due to the multitude of potential complications, remaining a major cause of mortality worldwide. In the context of a globalized community and changing climate, borders' relevance is ever decreasing. Critical care providers familiar with this disease will be equipped to deliver timely and appropriate care in the face of this changing epidemiology.

Epidemiology

Malaria is intrinsically linked to the *Anopheles* mosquito, and only a minority of its species are appropriate vectors [3]. Disease incidence is influenced by interactions between environmental factors affecting vector survival and certain characteristics

J. Hidalgo
Division of Critical Care, Karl Heusner Memorial Hospital, Belize City, Belize

P. Arriaga
St Michaels Hospital, Toronto, ON, Canada

B. A. Concejo (✉)
University of Texas Southwestern, Dallas, TX, USA
e-mail: Bruno.alvarezconcejo@phhs.org

© Springer Nature Switzerland AG 2020

J. Hidalgo, L. Woc-Colburn (eds.), *Highly Infectious Diseases in Critical Care*,
https://doi.org/10.1007/978-3-030-33803-9_13

of the vector itself, like resilience, population density, efficiency, and biting habits [3, 4]. As such, in conditions of natural disasters, war, and poverty, most of the potential anopheline vector species will triumph, but only a few of them could be responsible for ongoing endemic infections in certain regions, e.g., *Anopheles gambiae* complex in Africa.

Humans have attempted, and partially succeeded, at altering that balance. Although once prevalent throughout much of the inhabited world, after World War II, malaria was eradicated from the United States, Canada, Europe, and Russia. Nonetheless, it persisted in the tropics. During the ensuing decades, improvement in malaria control was few, and morbidity worsened in many areas due to resistance of mosquitoes to insecticides and resistance of the parasite itself to antimalarials [3, 4].

Only recently, a new large effort to control and eventually eradicate malaria has been initiated including renewed ways of delivering insecticides (e.g., impregnating nets or indoor residual spraying), prompt treatment, and prophylactic treatment of high-risk groups [5]. This has led to documented decrease in levels of morbidity and mortality in parts of Africa, Asia, and Oceania with relatively low levels of transmission intensity [6]. Despite these efforts, epidemiologic changes in the coming years are hard to predict given the unproven impact of the above measures on highly endemic regions and the potential implications of climate change [7].

Malaria in Endemic Countries

In 2017, 219 million cases and 435.000 deaths attributed to malaria were identified, remaining endemic in 91 countries [8]. This disease remains a disproportionate burden in tropical and subtropical regions of Africa, Asia, and Central and South America (Fig. 13.1). Children and pregnant women constitute the main high-risk groups. The first one accumulates most of the deaths, and the second one is susceptible to significant morbidity in their offspring when infected by *P. falciparum*, including many deaths secondary to low birth weight.

Malaria mortality is influenced by the complex interaction between immunity and specific *Plasmodium* spp. virulence. Wherever there is year-round transmission, *P. falciparum* is usually primarily involved, and, although adults are usually immune, children remain vulnerable and accumulate most of the mortality. This is the case in sub-Saharan Africa, where the World Health Organization reports 90% of malaria deaths occur [8]. In other regions of Asia and Central and South America, transmission is intense but concentrated over a few months out of the year. As such, people remain susceptible into their adulthood, but since both *P. falciparum* and *P. vivax* have similar incidence, mortality is lessened. These later regions are the most influenced by changing economic, social, or environmental landscapes [4].

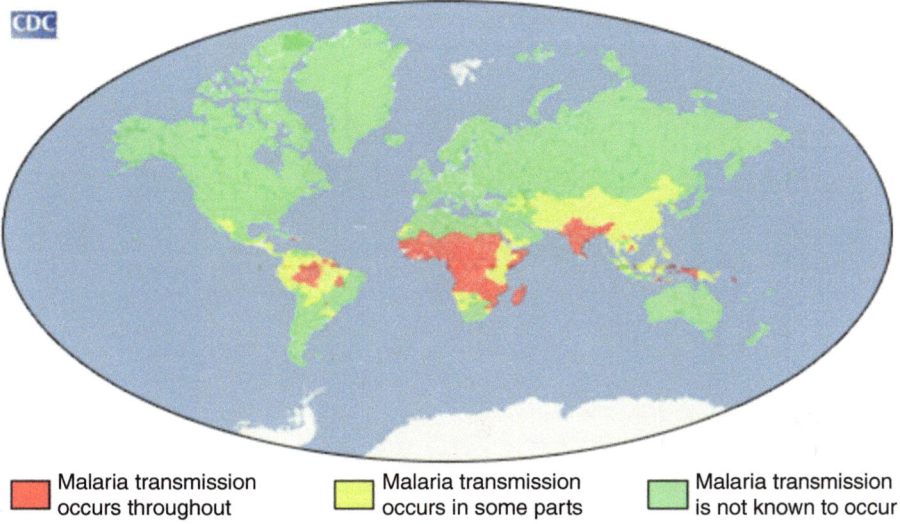

Malaria transmission occurs throughout

Malaria transmission occurs in some parts

Malaria transmission is not known to occur

Fig. 13.1 Malaria distribution worldwide. (Source CDC)

In highly endemic countries, the effects of malaria are far-reaching. Beyond mortality, it exerts a major toll on child development and significant school and work absenteeism. In this way, millions of dollars are lost among the poorest citizens of the poorest countries of the world [8, 9]. Interestingly, a direct correlation has been made between malaria elimination and income growth, with recognized factors including increase in productivity, foreign investment, and economic networks within the country [9].

Malaria in Travelers

In recent decades, there has been a progressive increase in international travels, both for business and tourism. Consequently, there has been a progressive increase in tropical disease diagnosed in returning travelers [10, 11]. Among them, malaria is the most common documented cause of febrile illness in travelers returning from the tropics to developed countries, representing 5–29% of patients presenting to a specialist and 26–75% of the patients admitted to the hospital [10, 12–15].

In the United States, almost all the cases occur in patients that have recently traveled to regions with ongoing transmission. Nonetheless, malaria is also rarely transmitted when imported parasites are transmitted by local anopheline mosquitoes, by blood products or through congenital spread of infection [16]. As of 2015, the CDC reports an upgoing trend in cases of malaria reported in the United States, with the reduction seen between 2014 and 2015 attributable to changing traveling patterns in the face of the Ebola outbreak in West Africa (Fig. 13.2) [16].

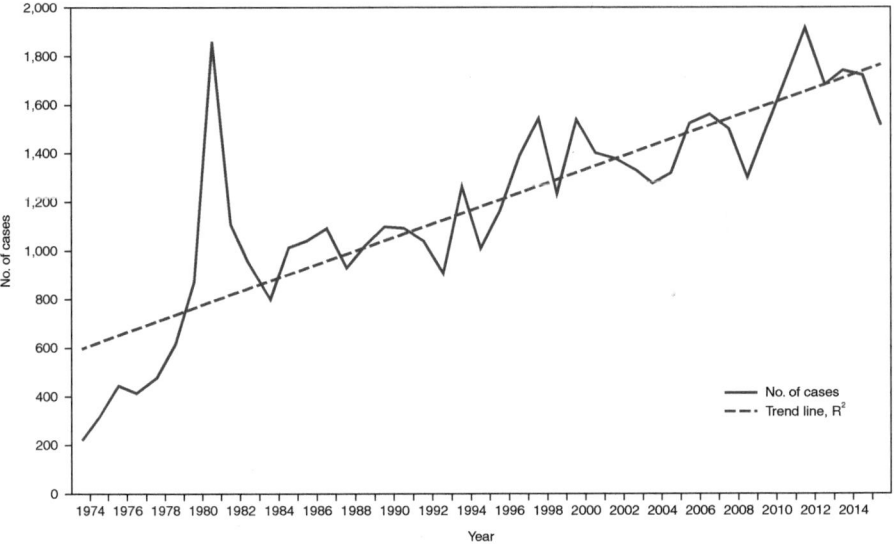

Fig. 13.2 Malaria cases in the United States. (Source CDC)

Plasmodium: A Closer Look

The genus *Plasmodium* encompasses over 200 species, of which only 5 are considered infectious to human beings. *P. falciparum* produces the highest levels of blood parasitemia and sequesters in key tissues, and it is the main cause of severe malaria. *P. vivax* usually produces milder disease, but it is increasingly recognized as a cause of severe malaria as well, especially in Asia and South America [3]. Two sympatric subspecies of *P. ovale* exist, *P.o. curtisi* and *P.o. wallikeri*, and tend to produce milder disease, as does *P. malariae* [17]. All these species are transmitted by the female *Anopheles* mosquito. *P. knowlesi* is believed to be mainly a zoonotic infection transmitted from macaques, and its importance is increasingly recognized, especially in Malaysia [18, 19]. Co-infections with different species can be seen in up to 10–30% of cases [20].

Parasite Life Cycle

Female mosquitoes carry sporozoites in their salivary glands, which may determine specific feeding habits including increased attraction for humans and more frequent and smaller feeds [21, 22]. These motile sporozoites are inoculated, circulate to the liver, and actively infect hepatocytes, causing asymptomatic liver infection (Fig. 13.3). Once they invade hepatocytes, they will mature over 7–10 days to produce schizonts. These schizonts rupture, releasing thousands of merozoites into the

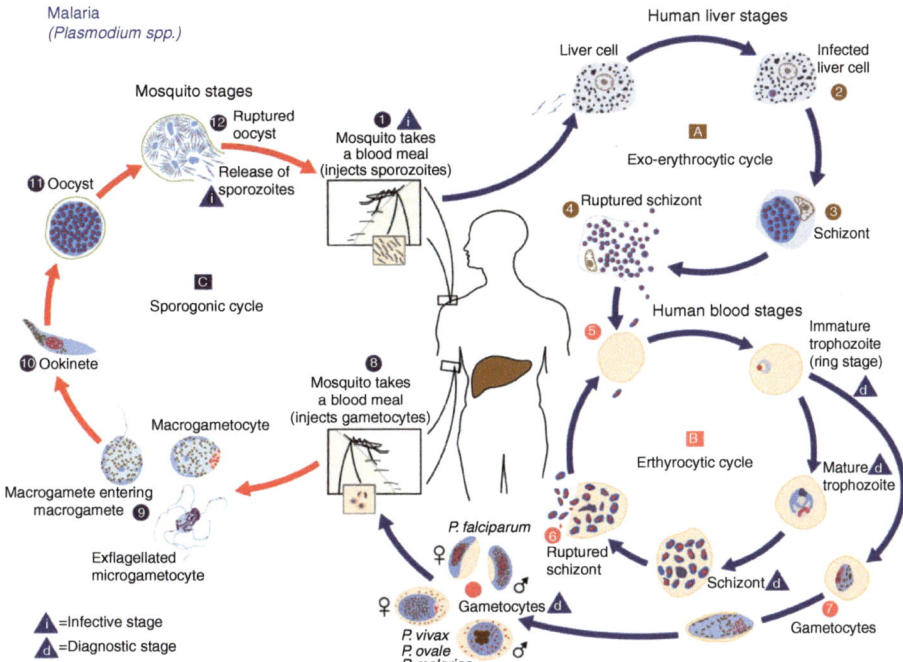

Fig. 13.3   Malaria life cycle. (Source CDC)

bloodstream that quickly invade erythrocytes, beginning the asexual erythrocyte stage (Fig. 13.3). Merozoites develop into trophozoites that will become schizonts over a period of 48 h in the cases of *P. falciparum*, *P. vivax*, and *P. ovale*, 72 h in the cases of *P. malariae*, and 24 h in the case of *P. knowlesi*. Schizonts will then rupture, causing hemolysis and releasing many merozoites with every cycle causing clinical illness. Some erythrocytic parasites will develop into sexual gametocytes. When taken up by the mosquito, a female and a male gametocyte have the capability of fusing to produce a zygote. After multiple steps, sporozoites are generated in the anopheline salivary glands, completing the cycle. *P. vivax* and *P. ovale* generate hypnozoites in the liver that can lead to recurrent disease months or years after the initial infection (Fig. 13.3).

Pathogenicity

A key pathogenic characteristic of *P. falciparum* is its ability to mediate adherence of infected erythrocytes to endothelial cells. Erythrocytes that are infected with more mature stages of this parasite remain within small tissue vessels, including the brain. This process is termed cytoadherence, and it is thought to be caused by the expression of *Plasmodium falciparum* erythrocyte membrane protein 1 (Pfemp1) in the erythrocyte membrane. Parasites avoid passing through the spleen where abnormal erythrocytes would be cleared while also being more likely to cause local tissue damage. This protein is member of the var family and continuously changes among more than 60 subtypes, impairing antigen recognition and host response [23, 24]. Moreover, subtypes of Pfemp1 may confer tissue specificity, as is the case with the affinity to endothelial protein C receptor and cerebral malaria [25]. The severity of disease is associated with both the increased parasitemia and a higher biomass of sequestered parasites [26].

Reinforcing a previously made point, *P. falciparum*'s life cycle requires a year-around transmission to survive, only possible in regions of the world with a high endemic rate. Given their capability to develop into hypnozoites, *P. vivax* and *P. ovale* can inhabit subtropical areas with marked seasonal patterns, remaining dormant until optimal conditions are met.

Immunity

Human immunity against malaria is still incompletely understood. Nonspecific host defense mechanisms control the infection initially [27]. After that, both humoral and cellular immunities are thought to contribute to protection.

In endemic countries where *P. falciparum* is prevalent, disease occurs primarily in children. The first few months of life are normally spared, likely due to protection conferred by maternal antibodies. Young children are infected frequently, experiencing repeated febrile malaria illness and being at high risk of severe disease. With repeated exposure, children develop partial immunity. Gradually, they gain protection against severe malaria and then increasingly to symptomatic illness and eventually strong protection against infection. Nonetheless, antimalarial immunity is incomplete, and malaria can occur in individuals of any age, and asymptomatic parasitemia is common in adults and older children living in areas with high transmission rates.

It is important to underline this only occurs in regions where there is constant exposure, year-round, but it is absent in areas where exposure is more seasonal or episodic. A corollary is adults that return to a highly endemic area after extended stay in a non-endemic area are at increased risk.

Genetics

No other disease has shaped human genetics as much as malaria [28]. Erythrocytes are the main host cell for *Plasmodium* species in our bodies, and certain changes may render them more or less susceptible to infection. Specific changes in hemoglobin generate environments that are more hostile to the parasite, e.g., decrease parasite growth at low oxygen tension or reduce cytoadherence [29].

Over the millennia, these changes have accumulated in certain regions, corresponding to the distribution of malaria prior to modern interventions [28]. Simultaneously, these changes have shaped the epidemiology of *Plasmodium*, probably the best example being *P. vivax*. As mentioned above, it is dependent on the presence of Duffy antigen in the erythrocyte membranes. As the population in Africa accumulated mutations rendering their erythrocytes Duffy-negative, *P. vivax* has all but disappeared from Africa, and it is now located in Asia and Central and South America [30, 31].

Clinical Presentation

Uncomplicated Malaria

Most cases of malaria, including when caused by *P. falciparum* malaria, present as a mild febrile illness. The incubation period is typically 12–14 days with *P. falciparum* and a little longer for the non-falciparum species. The incubation period may be longer in patients that have received certain antibiotics (tetracyclines, trimethoprim-sulfamethoxazole, quinolones, or macrolides) or inhabitants of endemic areas. Non-falciparum malaria is more likely to present with highly synchronous infections, leading if untreated to regular cycles of fever every 48 (*P. vivax* and *P. ovale*) or 72 (*P. malariae*) hours, often with minimal symptoms between episodes. Nonspecific symptoms are common like headache, malaise, myalgias, arthralgias, rigors, confusion, nausea, vomiting, diarrhea, abdominal pain, etc. Physical exam findings maybe include signs of anemia, jaundice, splenomegaly, and mild hepatomegaly, but may well be absent. Rash and lymphadenopathy are not typical in malaria and should trigger suspicion for alternative possibilities. Laboratory studies commonly show anemia, thrombocytopenia, and liver and renal function abnormalities.

Severe Falciparum Malaria .

Severe malaria has a specific definition by the World Health Organization, applicable to both endemic and non-endemic cases (Table 13.1) [32]. It is mostly caused by *P. falciparum*, although *P. vivax* is increasingly recognized as a cause in certain regions.

Severe malaria is normally a rapidly progressing disease. One series of imported malaria reported a median of 9.5 days (IQR 3-14) between return from a malaria-endemic area and hospital admission [33]. Progression to severe disease is highly variable, but the best available evidence reported a mean duration of symptoms of 5.5 days before ICU admission [34].

Table 13.1 Criteria for severe malaria

Impaired consciousness: A Glasgow coma score <11 in adults or a Blantyre coma score <3 in children

Prostration: Generalized weakness so that the person is unable to sit, stand, or walk without assistance

Multiple convulsions: More than two episodes within 24 h

Acidosis: A base deficit of >8 mEq/L or, if not available, a plasma bicarbonate level of <15 mmol/L or venous plasma lactate ≥5 mmol/L. Severe acidosis manifests clinically as respiratory distress (rapid, deep, labored breathing)

Hypoglycemia: Blood or plasma glucose <2.2 mmol/L (<40 mg/dL)

Severe malarial anemia: Hemoglobin concentration ≤5 g/dL or a hematocrit of ≤15% in children <12 years of age (<7 g/dL and <20%, respectively, in adults) with a parasite count >10,000/μL

Renal impairment: Plasma or serum creatinine >265 μmol/L (3 mg/dL) or blood urea >20 mmol/L

Jaundice: Plasma or serum bilirubin >50 μmol/L (3 mg/dL) with a parasite count 100,000/μL

Pulmonary edema: Radiologically confirmed or oxygen saturation <92% on room air with a respiratory rate >30/min, often with chest indrawing and crepitations on auscultation

Significant bleeding: Including recurrent or prolonged bleeding from the nose, gums, or venepuncture sites; hematemesis or melena

Shock: Compensated shock is defined as capillary refill ≥3 s or temperature gradient on leg (mid to proximal limb), but no hypotension. Decompensated shock is defined as systolic blood pressure <70 mmHg in children or <80 mmHg in adults, with evidence of impaired perfusion (cool peripheries or prolonged capillary refill)

Hyperparasitemia: *P. falciparum* parasitemia >10%

Adapted from World Health Organization, Global Malaria Programme [32]

Diagnosis

Fever in a Returning Traveler: A Framework

Tropical disease accounts for up to 20–30% of critical care admissions in certain countries of Asia, Africa, and South America [35]. Critical care physicians in these areas of the world are familiar with the different presentations of different infectious agents, and their index of suspicion is high at baseline. People are traveling more than ever before and are being exposed to these pathogens, often presenting upon returning from traveling [11]. Modifying the base rate of disease based on certain epidemiological factors is one the hardest things we are required to do as diagnosticians [36]. Having a framework may reduce the change of experiencing biases. A thorough review is out of the scope of this chapter, but the astute clinician will be aware of the importance of understanding malaria's place within a diagnostic schema. We refer the interested reader to specific reviews on the topic, great examples being the recent articles by Fink et al. or Thwaites et al. or the critical care-focused by Karnad et al. [35, 37, 38].

In brief, the differential diagnosis of severe malaria is broad and varies depending on specific travel history. Consider both local and foreign causes of infectious disease, as well as non-infectious causes of fever. Prioritize highly contagious diseases, like hemorrhagic fevers, measles, Middle Eastern respiratory syndrome-coronavirus virus (MERS-CoV), and others explored in this book. Obtain a detailed travel history with special emphasis on all the locations the patient might have visited (including layovers), activities that he/she engaged in, as well as exposures (e.g., mosquito bites, fresh water, or sexual commerce). The incubation period is crucially important in this presentation, as is the physical examination (e.g., conjunctival suffusion, skin rash, jaundice, or hepatosplenomegaly). Probably most relevant for critical care physicians, the pattern of organ involvement might also suggest specific etiologies [35].

Diagnosing Malaria

High index of suspicion is essential for diagnosing malaria, and any individual with a febrile illness and risk factors should be investigated. As mentioned above, it is the most common identifiable cause of fever in the returning traveler and in many areas of the world. Keeping an open mind to other possibilities will be key while attempting to perform a formal diagnosis and trying to identify the specific *Plasmodium* species (Fig. 13.4).

Thick and thin blood smears continue to be standard of care. In this procedure, one drop of blood is allowed to dry on a slide, erythrocytes are lysed, and parasites are then stained with Giemsa. Parasites are easily identified by trained personnel, and parasite density can be estimated on the basis of counts relative to those of leukocytes. However, thick blood smears do not allow identification of erythrocyte morphology, helpful in species diagnosis, and are difficult for those with limited training. Giemsa-stained thin blood smear offers an improved means of characterizing parasite morphology, but the process is much less efficient than for thick smears. As such, thick smear is standard of care in areas of high endemic burden, while thin are reserved for areas in which there is more trained personnel, with more time available to them. Finally, it is paramount to understand that a negative blood film does not exclude malaria and might very well be positive 8–12 h later [32, 39].

Antigen detection is a new way of diagnosing malaria. Multiple simple tests are now available that use calorimetric detection of one or two antigens in an assay that requires limited training and only a few minutes. The most used assays in Africa use histidine-rich protein-2, only able to detect *P. falciparum* [32]. Other assays are able to detect all human malarial species, as they detect lactate dehydrogenase and aldolase. Combination tests, that aim to detect both *P. falciparum* and *Plasmodium* spp., are now available. Issues are arising with standardization given the heterogeneity of manufacturers and tests available.

Other diagnostic techniques available include serology and polymerase chain reaction (PCR). Serology utility is limited since the antibody response is slow and tends to persist for a long period of time. PCR is likely the most sensitive test available to date and useful for research purposes. Nonetheless, it is not scalable as it is time and resource intensive. Furthermore, patients might have a not clinically significant parasitemia that would still be detected.

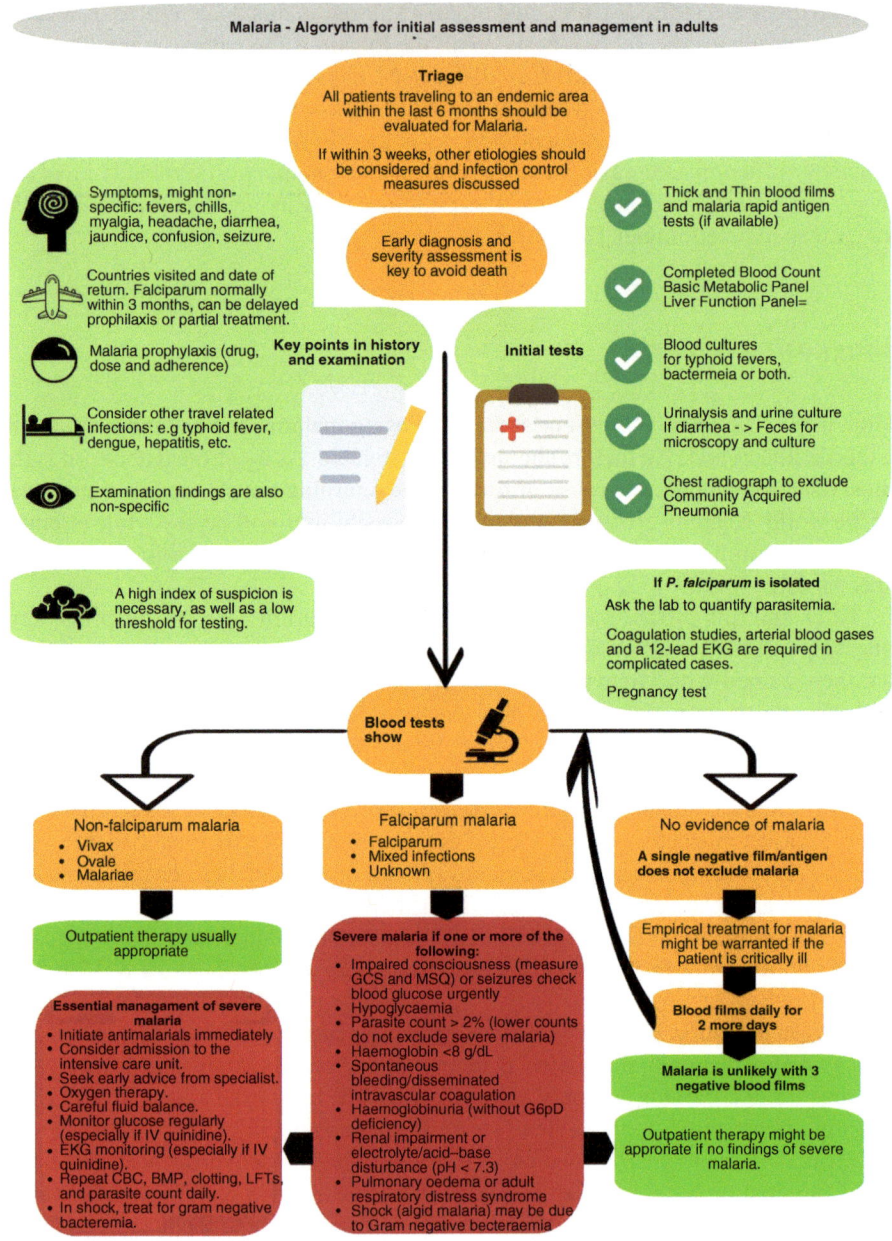

Fig. 13.4 Algorithm for initial diagnosis and management of suspected Malaria in the returning traveler. (Source http://www.hpa.org.uk/webc/HPAwebFile/HPAweb_C/1240212774627)

Treatment

Antimalarials: Overview and Resistance Emergence

Early in the twentieth century, there was a pressure to find a substitute for quinine as a treatment for malaria. This led to the discovery of primaquine and quinacrine and finally chloroquine in 1934 [40]. The United States later generalized its use, making it the drug of choice by the end of World War II [41]. Chloroquine quickly became one of the most important drugs ever developed against an infectious agent [40]. It is key to understand this in the context of the discovery of DDT and other vector control measures. Optimism was such that WHO launched an eradication campaign in 1955. Although we fell short and it had to be cancelled on 1969, the extraordinary impact that chloroquine had in vulnerable areas like the sub-Saharan Africa is undeniable [40, 41].

Its widespread use was not without consequence. *P. falciparum* initially found to develop resistance in the 1950s–1960s in foci in Colombia and Southeast Asia [42]. Resistance steadily spread during the 1960s, finally getting to Africa in the 1980s [42]. *P. vivax* was found to develop resistance to chloroquine first in Papua New Guinea in 1989 but is now found in Asia and South America [40].

Quinine, in the 1970s, would take back its place as the drug of choice [4, 39, 40]. The most common dose dependent is cinchonism (nausea, vomiting, blurred vision, reversible hearing loss, and headache). Despite this and other side effects like hypoglycemia, it would remain the treatment of choice until 2005, when the first trials comparing it with artemisinin(s) derivatives were published.

Artemisins, derived from the Chinese herb *qinghausu* or wormwood, have been used by Chinese traditional healers for millennia but have been adopted in the Western world only recent years. One of its derivatives, artesunate, was recently found in two large randomized control trials to be superior to quinine. SEAQUAMAT randomized patients in South and Southeast Asia, almost all adults, and found a reduction in mortality in patients treated with artesunate compared with quinine (15% vs. 22%) [43]. The subsequent AQUAMAT focused on children in 11 countries in sub-Saharan Africa and demonstrated a similar reduction in mortality (8.5% vs. 10.9%) [44].

In the acute setting, while treating severe malaria, intravenous quinine therapy requires close monitoring of QTc interval as well as capillary blood glucose, while artesunate is safe in both of those regards. Nonetheless, the latter cannot be used as a single agent due to its short biological half-life, as it leads to prompt recrudescence. Availability of artesunate is limited to specialized centers, and access to it might prove challenging. It is important to recognize that treatment with quinine should not be delayed while attempting to obtain artesunate.

For outpatient or consolidation treatment, artemisin combination treatments (ACTs) are now the standard of care for *P. falciparum* and recommended by the WHO in 3-day regimens [32]. This treatment combines artesunate with other active antimalarial agents, some of them are once daily (e.g., artesunate-mefloquine), while others require twice-daily dosing (e.g., artemether-lumefantrine). These therapies should be used in every patient confirmed to have *P. falciparum*, or in which the species involved is in doubt, after an initial administration of parenteral artesunate.

Chloroquine remains the treatment of choice for non-falciparum malaria and the few areas that have not registered any resistance (primarily Central America and the Caribbean). For *P. vivax* and *P. ovale*, it should always be given to eradicate hepatic hypnozoites. Also, chloroquine-related compounds are found on ACTs active against *P. falciparum*.

The development of resistance to quinine has been relatively slow [45]. It had been in use for over two centuries by the time the first resistance was first described. As a comparison, for chloroquine and proguanil, it only took 12 and 1 year, respectively [46]. Quinine resistance has been extensively documented in Asia and South America, but it seems relatively uncommon in Africa [47–51]. Quinine normally retains some efficacy, although its activity might be delayed or diminished. A recent meta-analysis of multiple randomized clinical trials demonstrates that the recrudescence rates after quinine treatment have been relatively stable for over 30 years [52]. With all the side effects and drawbacks pointed before, quinine seems to remain a viable treatment option.

Artesunate resistance was first reported in western Cambodia, and it was further confirmed by randomized control trials [53]. This was characterized by decreased clearance of parasites in vivo but hardly any sign on susceptibilities in vitro. Of note, the rapid parasite elimination is one of the main advantages of artemisin therapies and accounts for a significant part of its rapidity of therapeutic response and could drastically affect outcomes. Sadly, this has continued to be reported in other areas of the Southeast Asian subcontinent [49, 53, 54]. Worrisome laboratory data points the possibility of extreme artemisin resistance and, under the appropriate in vitro conditions, was accompanied with more complex patterns of multiple drug resistance [55]. As of now, contentment of resistant strains and judicious use of current available therapies and multiple agent regimens in the face of clinical failures are the only measures available.

Treatment of Severe Malaria

As any septic patient, treatment should immediately follow or be concurrent with treatment. Stabilizing the patient and isolating and treating the causative agent, here with parenteral antimalarials, is imperative. Although both *P. vivax* and *P. knowlesi* are increasingly recognized as causes of severe malaria, *P. falciparum* should be assumed to be the causative agent until proven otherwise.

Initial Stabilization

Aggressive fluid resuscitation is considered an intrinsic part of initial sepsis management, but evidence is mounting it might be detrimental in patients with malaria due to difference in pathogenesis and increased vascular permeability [56, 57].

In adults with malaria, the base deficit is the strongest predictor of mortality, and the degree of acute kidney injury (AKI) is an additional risk factor [58, 59]. Hypovolemia is present in severe malaria and can exacerbate both conditions [60, 61]. Nonetheless, the microvascular pathology of malaria is unique since impaired tissue perfusion is mostly caused by sequestration of infected erythrocytes [56]. The degree of acidosis and AKI is intrinsically related to sequestration, especially in the kidney and liver [56, 62, 63]. We have increasing evidence that fluid resuscitation cannot reverse this pathological process.

The recent FEAST trial suggested that among sub-Saharan African children with a particular definition of shock, saline and albumin bolus resuscitation appeared to increase mortality when compared to no-bolus strategy. Malaria was the reason for the admission in 57% in these children [64]. It is hard to translate these results directly to resource-rich countries, as it might be safe to assume the time of presentation to the hospital might be prolonged, as well the potential effect of the absence of tools like mechanical ventilators. Moreover, children with severe malaria rarely develop AKI, as opposed to 45% of adult patients.

More evidence is mounting fluid resuscitation might be detrimental, even with close monitoring. In a completely different study, they evaluated liberal vs. conservative fluid strategy while monitoring extracellular water with a well-validated tool, PiCCO™ [65]. Even though only hypovolemic patients were recruited, the acid-base status deteriorated after a reasonable amount of fluids (mean 5450 mL over the first 24 h). Pulmonary edema—secondary to increased pulmonary vascular permeability—was common, unpredictable, and exacerbated by fluid loading. Lactate, the strongest mortality predictor, was correlated with the degree of visualized microvascular sequestration of parasitized erythrocytes (i.e., decreased flow velocity by orthogonal polarized spectroscopy) and not impacted by fluid resuscitation [66]. In fact, 70% of patients' acid-base status deteriorated after fluid resuscitation [65].

Multiple studies have associated fluid resuscitation with worse outcomes in malaria [64, 65, 67]. Beyond early initiation of antimalarials, we recommend against overzealous liberal fluid resuscitation and for a rapid escalation to vasopressor therapy for hemodynamic management. Clinicians should be vigilant of the various complications associated with increased vascular permeability seen in this disease.

Antimalarials

Standard therapy for severe malaria is parenteral quinine, under continuous cardiac monitoring. As mentioned above, evidence is mounting that artesunate is superior, in terms of efficacy and safety profile, but availability is still a major issue. In the United States, IV quinine is not available in all hospitals, and IV artesunate should be requested on a name patient basis to the Center for Disease Control. As such, treatment should be started with whatever agent may be administered first (Table 13.2). After the three initial doses, patients that tolerate the oral route should receive oral medications, including the regimen mentioned above [32].

Table 13.2 Complicated falciparum malaria or unable to tolerate oral medications

IV artesunate	2.4 mg/kg every 12 h on day 1 and then daily for 2 additional days
Or	
IV quinidine gluconate	10 mg/kg over 1–2 h and then 0.02 mg/kg/min or 15 mg/kg over 4 h and then 7.5 mg/kg over 4 h every 8 h
Or	
IV quinidine dihydrochloride	20 mg/kg over 4 h and then 10 mg/kg every 8 h
Or	
IM artemether	3.2 mg/kg IM and then 1.6 mg/kg/day

Adjunctive Measures

Adjunctive measures as exchange transfusion have been proposed in the treatment of severe falciparum malaria. Although it seems to address the issue at its core, the evidence to support its use is still lacking. There are several case reports documenting successful use, but the only retrospective review available showed no improve in parasite clearance or outcomes [68–70].

Complications

Cerebral Malaria

Cerebral malaria is more common in children from Africa. Patients may present with stupor, coma, seizures, decerebrated posturing, and raised intracranial pressure. More strictly, cerebral malaria is defined by coma (GCS < 9) in a patient with malaria in which all other causes have been ruled out. More broadly, any patient with altered mental status should be presumed to have cerebral malaria after ruling out common causes like hypoglycemia. Cerebral malaria is associated with worse outcomes [71].

Patients with cerebral malaria have subclinical seizures [72]. Although prophylactic anticonvulsants reduce seizure incidence, a meta-analysis showed they may in fact worsen outcomes [73]. The main criticism is that the trials reported thus far were mainly done with phenobarbital, so the increase in mortality was attributed to respiratory depression. Whether the use of other antiepileptics is of any use remains to be determined. Regardless, current evidence discourages routine electroencephalogram monitoring and use of prophylactic phenobarbital. Clinical seizures should be treated appropriately.

Cerebral edema is a well-recognized complication of severe malaria. Multiple interventions have been tested in randomized clinical trials without success, including steroids and mannitol [74–76]. As such, no adjunctive therapies are currently recommended for cerebral malaria at the moment.

Severe Anemia and Coagulopathy

Anemia in patients with malaria is more than just a hemolytic process. It also involves dyserythropoiesis and removal of infected erythrocytes from the circulation by the spleen. Uninfected erythrocytes can be indirectly affected by antigens, antibody activation, and minor alterations in red cell membranes. WHO defines severe anemia as a Hgb of <5 mg/dL [32]. However, this degree of anemia is mainly seen in endemic areas and is likely to be multifactorial [77, 78]. It is exceptionally rare on imported cases [33, 34, 66]. Transfusion thresholds are currently the same as with any other critically ill patient.

Coagulopathy is seen in 5% to >20% of patients with severe malaria [33, 34]. Severe thrombocytopenia is common in severe and non-severe malaria secondary to increased platelet destruction, sequestration within the spleen, or both. Disseminated intravascular coagulation occurs in 5–10% of patients and should be treated with supportive transfusions [33, 34, 66].

Metabolic Changes

Lactic acidosis is a marker of poor prognosis [4, 58, 65]. It has been attributed mainly to microvascular obstruction secondary to parasite cytoadherence and leading to hypoperfusion. Other factors contributing are thought to be direct production of lactate by the parasite and decreased clearance in the setting of liver dysfunction [58]. As we have pointed out before, this differs from other Type A lactic acidosis, and treating it as we would any other might result in deleterious effects [65, 79].

Hypoglycemia defined by a blood sugar <40 mg/dL (<2.2 mmol/L) is common in severe malaria, and it is associated with worse outcomes specially in children [32, 80, 81]. This seems to be applicable to imported cases of malaria, where although the prevalence is smaller, it is correlated with worse outcomes [33, 66]. The pathogenesis is incompletely understood but likely involves direct glucose consumption by the parasite as well as impaired gluconeogenesis in the liver, paired with hyperinsulinemia [82]. It has also been shown to be more frequent when patients are treated with quinine as compared to artesunate (combined HR < 0.55) [83].

Clinical features include decreased level of consciousness and seizures. Blood glucose should be regularly assessed specially in patient treated with quinine. Early enteral feeding is recommended for any critically ill patient but could be particularly beneficial in patients with malaria [84, 85].

Pulmonary Complications

The WHO includes as pulmonary manifestations for malaria deep breathing, respiratory distress, and pulmonary edema [32]. Tachypnea might be caused by fever, anemia, and metabolic acidosis but also primary lung pathology like pulmonary edema and acute respiratory distress syndrome (ARDS). The reported incidence of

ARDS varies, in part due to the use of different definitions, but ranges from 3% to 30% [33, 34, 66, 86]. It is more common in adults as compared to children [57, 86]. It portends a worse prognosis [34, 87, 88].

Pulmonary complications of malaria are attributed to direct toxicity by the cytoadherence of *P. falciparum* paired with a hyperactive host response [86, 89]. Concurrent bacteria pneumonia and pulmonary edema are other important causes of respiratory distress in this population.

Acute Kidney Injury

Acute kidney injury (AKI) is mainly associated with *P. falciparum* although it has been described with other species [90]. The WHO uses a different criterion (>265 mmol/L or ≥ 3 mg/dL) to qualify severe malaria than what is currently used in any other disease [32]. Interestingly, acute kidney injury is more frequent in patients with primoinfection [90–92]. As such, AKI is much more frequent in patients with imported malaria (ranging from 23% to >50%) as compared to endemic cases (1–5%) [33, 34, 66, 91].

The pathophysiology is likely multifactorial with cytoadherence in glomerular and tubular vasculature likely playing a major role, but with contribution from hypovolemia, hemolysis, immune-complex deposition, and cytokine release [62, 90].

All patients should be screened for AKI, which may be absent initially [90]. Once discovered, the treatment is mainly supportive with avoidance of further nephrotoxic agents, maintenance fluids, and controlling electrolytes and acid-base disturbances, including renal replacement therapy when indicated. Improving perfusion with dopamine and epinephrine has been tested and failed to improve renal outcomes [93]. The prognosis is usually good, with complete resolution in most cases upon infection control [33].

Jaundice

Hyperbilirubinemia can be multifactorial. It may occur in the setting of hemolysis, cholestasis, and hepatocyte dysfunction. Bilirubin can be significantly elevated, but transaminases are normally less affected. In a cohort of critically ill patients, Krishnan et al. found that hyperbilirubinemia to more than 6 mg/dL was seen in 26% of patients and a transaminase level more than three times the upper limit of normal was seen in less than half. The patients with elevated transaminases had a higher incidence of hypoglycemia and worse mortality [94].

Interactions with Other Infections

In endemic areas, concurrent gram-negative infection, especially non-typhoidal *Salmonella* has been shown in up 10% of children [93, 95, 96]. Some community studies point to up to two thirds of community bacteremia to be related to co-infection with malaria. When this happens, it is associated with a worse prognosis [95, 96].

Rates of community-acquired bacterial infection have been reported to be between 5% and 10% in patients admitted to intensive care units with imported cases of malaria [33, 34]. Community-acquired pneumonia is the commonest.

The use of prophylactic antibiotics remains controversial. Bacterial co-infection should be suspected in patients with significant neutrophilia or focal signs of infection. In these cases, blood cultures should be drawn and therapy de-escalated or tailored based on culture results. As with any other critically ill patient, physicians should remain vigilant for nosocomial infections, including ventilator-associated pneumonia or catheter-related sepsis, with common stewardship practices (i.e., monitor for extubating readiness or limiting use of urinary catheters) applying in a similar manner.

Prognosis

Patients with *P. falciparum* malaria tend to respond well if treatment is started promptly. The mortality rate in those with uncomplicated *P. falciparum* is about 0.1%. Nonetheless in the critical care population, high-level parasitemia or clinical features might determine worse outcomes. However, with aggressive support, even individuals with severe disease can often experience complete recoveries. As an example, Marks et al. report a mortality of only 4% and Antinori et al. a mortality of 0% [33, 97]. Moreover, *non-falciparum* malaria usually responds well to treatment and makes an uneventful recovery.

Resistance emergence and changing epidemiology might be the greatest challenge we will face in the future. A judicious use of existing therapies, careful monitoring, and attention to other co-occurring complications will help us navigate the changing landscape of the treatment of malaria in our critical care units.

References

1. Tanabe K, Mita T, Jombart T, Eriksson A, Horibe S, Palacpac N, et al. Plasmodium falciparum accompanied the human expansion out of Africa. Curr Biol. 2010;20(14):1283–9.
2. Bruce-Chwatt LJ. Paleogenesis and paleo-epidemiology of primate malaria. Bull World Health Organ. 1965;32:363–87.
3. Ashley EA, Pyae Phyo A, Woodrow CJ. Malaria. Lancet. 2018;391(10130):1608–21.
4. White NJ, Pukrittayakamee S, Hien TT, Faiz MA, Mokuolu OA, Dondorp AM. Malaria. Lancet. 2014;383(9918):723–35.
5. Cotter C, Sturrock HJ, Hsiang MS, Liu J, Phillips AA, Hwang J, et al. The changing epidemiology of malaria elimination: new strategies for new challenges. Lancet. 2013;382(9895): 900–11.
6. Noor AM, Kinyoki DK, Mundia CW, Kabaria CW, Mutua JW, Alegana VA, et al. The changing risk of Plasmodium falciparum malaria infection in Africa: 2000-10: a spatial and temporal analysis of transmission intensity. Lancet. 2014;383(9930):1739–47.

7. Caminade C, Kovats S, Rocklov J, Tompkins AM, Morse AP, Colon-Gonzalez FJ, et al. Impact of climate change on global malaria distribution. Proc Natl Acad Sci U S A. 2014;111(9):3286–91.
8. World Health Organization. World malaria report 2017. Geneva: WHO; 2017.
9. Gallup JL, Sachs JD. The economic burden of malaria. Am J Trop Med Hyg. 2001;64(1–2 Suppl):85–96.
10. Leder K, Torresi J, Libman MD, Cramer JP, Castelli F, Schlagenhauf P, et al. GeoSentinel surveillance of illness in returned travelers, 2007-2011. Ann Intern Med. 2013;158(6):456–68.
11. Harvey K, Esposito DH, Han P, Kozarsky P, Freedman DO, Plier DA, et al. Surveillance for travel-related disease--GeoSentinel Surveillance System, United States, 1997-2011. MMWR Surveill Summ. 2013;62:1–23.
12. Gautret P, Schlagenhauf P, Gaudart J, Castelli F, Brouqui P, von Sonnenburg F, et al. Multicenter EuroTravNet/GeoSentinel study of travel-related infectious diseases in Europe. Emerg Infect Dis. 2009;15(11):1783–90.
13. Mizuno Y, Kudo K. Travel-related health problems in Japanese travelers. Travel Med Infect Dis. 2009;7(5):296–300.
14. Parola P, Soula G, Gazin P, Foucault C, Delmont J, Brouqui P. Fever in travelers returning from tropical areas: prospective observational study of 613 cases hospitalised in Marseilles, France, 1999–2003. Travel Med Infect Dis. 2006;4(2):61–70.
15. Stienlauf S, Segal G, Sidi Y, Schwartz E. Epidemiology of travel-related hospitalization. J Travel Med. 2005;12(3):136–41.
16. Mace KE, Arguin PM, Tan KR. Malaria surveillance—United States, 2015. MMWR Surveill Summ. 2018;67(7):1–28.
17. Phillips MA, Burrows JN, Manyando C, van Huijsduijnen RH, Van Voorhis WC, Wells TNC. Malaria. Nat Rev Dis Primers. 2017;3:17050.
18. Brock PM, Fornace KM, Parmiter M, Cox J, Drakeley CJ, Ferguson HM, et al. Plasmodium knowlesi transmission: integrating quantitative approaches from epidemiology and ecology to understand malaria as a zoonosis. Parasitology. 2016;143(4):389–400.
19. Davidson G, Chua TH, Cook A, Speldewinde P, Weinstein P. The role of ecological linkage mechanisms in Plasmodium knowlesi transmission and spread. EcoHealth. 2019; https://doi.org/10.1007/s10393-019-01395-6.
20. Ginouves M, Veron V, Musset L, Legrand E, Stefani A, Prevot G, et al. Frequency and distribution of mixed Plasmodium falciparum-vivax infections in French Guiana between 2000 and 2008. Malar J. 2015;14:446.
21. Das S, Muleba M, Stevenson JC, Pringle JC, Norris DE. Beyond the entomological inoculation rate: characterizing multiple blood feeding behavior and Plasmodium falciparum multiplicity of infection in Anopheles mosquitoes in northern Zambia. Parasit Vectors. 2017;10(1):45.
22. Busula AO, Verhulst NO, Bousema T, Takken W, de Boer JG. Mechanisms of Plasmodium-enhanced attraction of mosquito vectors. Trends Parasitol. 2017;33(12):961–73.
23. Flick K, Chen Q. Var genes, PfEMP1 and the human host. Mol Biochem Parasitol. 2004;134(1):3–9.
24. Marks M, Gupta-Wright A, Doherty JF, Singer M, Walker D. Managing malaria in the intensive care unit. Br J Anaesth. 2014;113(6):910–21.
25. Turner L, Lavstsen T, Berger SS, Wang CW, Petersen JE, Avril M, et al. Severe malaria is associated with parasite binding to endothelial protein C receptor. Nature. 2013;498(7455):502–5.
26. Dondorp AM, Desakorn V, Pongtavornpinyo W, Sahassananda D, Silamut K, Chotivanich K, et al. Estimation of the total parasite biomass in acute falciparum malaria from plasma PfHRP2. PLoS Med. 2005;2(8):e204.
27. Buffet PA, Safeukui I, Deplaine G, Brousse V, Prendki V, Thellier M, et al. The pathogenesis of Plasmodium falciparum malaria in humans: insights from splenic physiology. Blood. 2011;117(2):381–92.
28. Wellems TE, Hayton K, Fairhurst RM. The impact of malaria parasitism: from corpuscles to communities. J Clin Invest. 2009;119(9):2496–505.

29. Bunn HF. The triumph of good over evil: protection by the sickle gene against malaria. Blood. 2013;121(1):20–5.
30. Gething PW, Elyazar IR, Moyes CL, Smith DL, Battle KE, Guerra CA, et al. A long neglected world malaria map: Plasmodium vivax endemicity in 2010. PLoS Negl Trop Dis. 2012;6(9):e1814.
31. Howes RE, Battle KE, Mendis KN, Smith DL, Cibulskis RE, Baird JK, et al. Global epidemiology of Plasmodium vivax. Am J Trop Med Hyg. 2016;95(6 Suppl):15–34.
32. World Health Organization, Global Malaria Programme. WHO guidelines approved by the Guidelines Review Committee. In: Guidelines for the treatment of malaria. 3rd ed. Geneva: World Health Organization; 2015.
33. Marks ME, Armstrong M, Suvari MM, Batson S, Whitty CJ, Chiodini PL, et al. Severe imported falciparum malaria among adults requiring intensive care: a retrospective study at the hospital for tropical diseases, London. BMC Infect Dis. 2013;13:118.
34. Bruneel F, Tubach F, Corne P, Megarbane B, Mira JP, Peytel E, et al. Severe imported falciparum malaria: a cohort study in 400 critically ill adults. PLoS One. 2010;5(10):e13236.
35. Karnad DR, Richards GA, Silva GS, Amin P. Tropical diseases in the ICU: a syndromic approach to diagnosis and treatment. J Crit Care. 2018;46:119–26.
36. Tversky A, Kahneman D. Judgment under uncertainty: heuristics and biases. Science (New York, NY). 1974;185(4157):1124–31.
37. Fink D, Wani RS, Johnston V. Fever in the returning traveller. BMJ. 2018;360:j5773.
38. Thwaites GE, Day NP. Approach to fever in the returning traveler. N Engl J Med. 2017;376(6):548–60.
39. Karnad DR, Nor MBM, Richards GA, Baker T, Amin P. Intensive care in severe malaria: report from the task force on tropical diseases by the World Federation of Societies of Intensive and Critical Care Medicine. J Crit Care. 2018;43:356–60.
40. Wellems TE, Plowe CV. Chloroquine-resistant malaria. J Infect Dis. 2001;184(6):770–6.
41. Coatney GR. Pitfalls in a discovery: the chronicle of chloroquine. Am J Trop Med Hyg. 1963;12:121–8.
42. Payne D. Spread of chloroquine resistance in Plasmodium falciparum. Parasitol Today. 1987;3(8):241–6.
43. Dondorp A, Nosten F, Stepniewska K, Day N, White N. Artesunate versus quinine for treatment of severe falciparum malaria: a randomised trial. Lancet. 2005;366(9487):717–25.
44. Dondorp AM, Fanello CI, Hendriksen IC, Gomes E, Seni A, Chhaganlal KD, et al. Artesunate versus quinine in the treatment of severe falciparum malaria in African children (AQUAMAT): an open-label, randomised trial. Lancet. 2010;376(9753):1647–57.
45. Achan J, Talisuna AO, Erhart A, Yeka A, Tibenderana JK, Baliraine FN, et al. Quinine, an old anti-malarial drug in a modern world: role in the treatment of malaria. Malar J. 2011;10:144.
46. Peters W. Antimalarial drug resistance: an increasing problem. Br Med Bull. 1982;38(2):187–92.
47. Legrand E, Volney B, Meynard JB, Mercereau-Puijalon O, Esterre P. In vitro monitoring of Plasmodium falciparum drug resistance in French Guiana: a synopsis of continuous assessment from 1994 to 2005. Antimicrob Agents Chemother. 2008;52(1):288–98.
48. Mayxay M, Barends M, Brockman A, Jaidee A, Nair S, Sudimack D, et al. In vitro antimalarial drug susceptibility and pfcrt mutation among fresh Plasmodium falciparum isolates from the Lao PDR (Laos). Am J Trop Med Hyg. 2007;76(2):245–50.
49. Miotto O, Almagro-Garcia J, Manske M, Macinnis B, Campino S, Rockett KA, et al. Multiple populations of artemisinin-resistant Plasmodium falciparum in Cambodia. Nat Genet. 2013;45(6):648–55.
50. Tinto H, Rwagacondo C, Karema C, Mupfasoni D, Vandoren W, Rusanganwa E, et al. In-vitro susceptibility of Plasmodium falciparum to monodesethylamodiaquine, dihydroartemisinin and quinine in an area of high chloroquine resistance in Rwanda. Trans R Soc Trop Med Hyg. 2006;100(6):509–14.
51. Pradines B, Mabika Mamfoumbi M, Parzy D, Owono Medang M, Lebeau C, Mourou Mbina JR, et al. In vitro susceptibility of Gabonese wild isolates of Plasmodium falciparum

to artemether, and comparison with chloroquine, quinine, halofantrine and amodiaquine. Parasitology. 1998;117(Pt 6):541–5.

52. Myint HY, Tipmanee P, Nosten F, Day NP, Pukrittayakamee S, Looareesuwan S, et al. A systematic overview of published antimalarial drug trials. Trans R Soc Trop Med Hyg. 2004;98(2):73–81.

53. Dondorp AM, Nosten F, Yi P, Das D, Phyo AP, Tarning J, et al. Artemisinin resistance in Plasmodium falciparum malaria. N Engl J Med. 2009;361(5):455–67.

54. Akunuri S, Shraddha P, Palli V, MuraliSantosh B. Suspected Artesunate resistant malaria in South India. J Global Infect Dis. 2018;10(1):26–7.

55. Tyagi RK, Gleeson PJ, Arnold L, Tahar R, Prieur E, Decosterd L, et al. High-level artemisinin-resistance with quinine co-resistance emerges in P. falciparum malaria under in vivo artesunate pressure. BMC Med. 2018;16(1):181.

56. Dondorp AM, Ince C, Charunwatthana P, Hanson J, van Kuijen A, Faiz MA, et al. Direct in vivo assessment of microcirculatory dysfunction in severe falciparum malaria. J Infect Dis. 2008;197(1):79–84.

57. Charoenpan P, Indraprasit S, Kiatboonsri S, Suvachittanont O, Tanomsup S. Pulmonary edema in severe falciparum malaria. Hemodynamic study and clinicophysiologic correlation. Chest. 1990;97(5):1190–7.

58. Day NP, Phu NH, Mai NT, Chau TT, Loc PP, Chuong LV, et al. The pathophysiologic and prognostic significance of acidosis in severe adult malaria. Crit Care Med. 2000;28(6):1833–40.

59. Hanson J, Lee SJ, Mohanty S, Faiz MA, Anstey NM, Charunwatthana P, et al. A simple score to predict the outcome of severe malaria in adults. Clin Infect Dis. 2010;50(5):679–85.

60. Sitprija V, Napathorn S, Laorpatanaskul S, Suithichaiyakul T, Moollaor P, Suwangool P, et al. Renal and systemic hemodynamics, in falciparum malaria. Am J Nephrol. 1996;16(6):513–9.

61. Davis TM, Krishna S, Looareesuwan S, Supanaranond W, Pukrittayakamee S, Attatamsoonthorn K, et al. Erythrocyte sequestration and anemia in severe falciparum malaria. Analysis of acute changes in venous hematocrit using a simple mathematical model. J Clin Invest. 1990;86(3):793–800.

62. Nguansangiam S, Day NP, Hien TT, Mai NT, Chaisri U, Riganti M, et al. A quantitative ultrastructural study of renal pathology in fatal Plasmodium falciparum malaria. Trop Med Int Health. 2007;12(9):1037–50.

63. Prommano O, Chaisri U, Turner GD, Wilairatana P, Ferguson DJ, Viriyavejakul P, et al. A quantitative ultrastructural study of the liver and the spleen in fatal falciparum malaria. Southeast Asian J Trop Med Public Health. 2005;36(6):1359–70.

64. Maitland K, Kiguli S, Opoka RO, Engoru C, Olupot-Olupot P, Akech SO, et al. Mortality after fluid bolus in African children with severe infection. N Engl J Med. 2011;364(26):2483–95.

65. Hanson JP, Lam SW, Mohanty S, Alam S, Pattnaik R, Mahanta KC, et al. Fluid resuscitation of adults with severe falciparum malaria: effects on acid-base status, renal function, and extravascular lung water. Crit Care Med. 2013;41(4):972–81.

66. Santos LC, Abreu CF, Xerinda SM, Tavares M, Lucas R, Sarmento AC. Severe imported malaria in an intensive care unit: a review of 59 cases. Malar J. 2012;11:96.

67. Nguyen HP, Hanson J, Bethell D, Nguyen TH, Tran TH, Ly VC, et al. A retrospective analysis of the haemodynamic and metabolic effects of fluid resuscitation in Vietnamese adults with severe falciparum malaria. PLoS One. 2011;6(10):e25523.

68. Zodda D, Procopio G, Hewitt K, Parrish A, Balani B, Feldman J. Severe malaria presenting to the ED: a collaborative approach utilizing exchange transfusion and artesunate. Am J Emerg Med. 2018;36(6):1126.e1–4.

69. Sagmak Tartar A, Akbulut A, Gokmen Sevindik O, Akbulut HH, Demirdag K. A case of severe Plasmodium falciparum malaria co-infected with HIV improved with exchange transfusion. Turkiye Parazitol Derg. 2017;41(4):219–22.

70. Lin J, Huang X, Qin G, Zhang S, Sun W, Wang Y, et al. Manual exchange transfusion for severe imported falciparum malaria: a retrospective study. Malar J. 2018;17(1):32.

71. Hunt NH, Golenser J, Chan-Ling T, Parekh S, Rae C, Potter S, et al. Immunopathogenesis of cerebral malaria. Int J Parasitol. 2006;36(5):569–82.
72. Crawley J, Smith S, Muthinji P, Marsh K, Kirkham F. Electroencephalographic and clinical features of cerebral malaria. Arch Dis Child. 2001;84(3):247–53.
73. Meremikwu M, Marson AG. Routine anticonvulsants for treating cerebral malaria. Cochrane Database Syst Rev. 2002;(2):CD002152.
74. Roberts I, Yates D, Sandercock P, Farrell B, Wasserberg J, Lomas G, et al. Effect of intravenous corticosteroids on death within 14 days in 10008 adults with clinically significant head injury (MRC CRASH trial): randomised placebo-controlled trial. Lancet. 2004;364(9442): 1321–8.
75. Mohanty S, Mishra SK, Patnaik R, Dutt AK, Pradhan S, Das B, et al. Brain swelling and mannitol therapy in adult cerebral malaria: a randomized trial. Clin Infect Dis. 2011;53(4):349–55.
76. Warrell DA, Looareesuwan S, Warrell MJ, Kasemsarn P, Intaraprasert R, Bunnag D, et al. Dexamethasone proves deleterious in cerebral malaria. A double-blind trial in 100 comatose patients. N Engl J Med. 1982;306(6):313–9.
77. White NJ. Anaemia and malaria. Malar J. 2018;17(1):371.
78. Haldar K, Mohandas N. Malaria, erythrocytic infection, and anemia. Hematology Am Soc Hematol Educ Program. 2009;2009:87–93.
79. Kraut JA, Madias NE. Lactic acidosis. N Engl J Med. 2014;371(24):2309–19.
80. Willcox ML, Forster M, Dicko MI, Graz B, Mayon-White R, Barennes H. Blood glucose and prognosis in children with presumed severe malaria: is there a threshold for "hypoglycaemia"? Trop Med Int Health. 2010;15(2):232–40.
81. Jallow M, Casals-Pascual C, Ackerman H, Walther B, Walther M, Pinder M, et al. Clinical features of severe malaria associated with death: a 13-year observational study in the Gambia. PLoS One. 2012;7(9):e45645.
82. Taylor TE, Molyneux ME, Wirima JJ, Fletcher KA, Morris K. Blood glucose levels in Malawian children before and during the administration of intravenous quinine for severe falciparum malaria. N Engl J Med. 1988;319(16):1040–7.
83. Sinclair D, Donegan S, Isba R, Lalloo DG. Artesunate versus quinine for treating severe malaria. Cochrane Database Syst Rev. 2012;(6):CD005967.
84. Mehta NM, Skillman HE, Irving SY, Coss-Bu JA, Vermilyea S, Farrington EA, et al. Guidelines for the provision and assessment of nutrition support therapy in the pediatric critically ill patient: Society of Critical Care Medicine and American Society for Parenteral and Enteral Nutrition. JPEN J Parenter Enteral Nutr. 2017;41(5):706–42.
85. Maude RJ, Hoque G, Hasan MU, Sayeed A, Akter S, Samad R, et al. Timing of enteral feeding in cerebral malaria in resource-poor settings: a randomized trial. PLoS One. 2011;6(11):e27273.
86. Taylor WRJ, Hanson J, Turner GDH, White NJ, Dondorp AM. Respiratory manifestations of malaria. Chest. 2012;142(2):492–505.
87. Robinson T, Mosha F, Grainge M, Madeley R. Indicators of mortality in African adults with malaria. Trans R Soc Trop Med Hyg. 2006;100(8):719–24.
88. Marsh K, Forster D, Waruiru C, Mwangi I, Winstanley M, Marsh V, et al. Indicators of life-threatening malaria in African children. N Engl J Med. 1995;332(21):1399–404.
89. Mohan A, Sharma SK, Bollineni S. Acute lung injury and acute respiratory distress syndrome in malaria. J Vector Borne Dis. 2008;45(3):179–93.
90. Das BS. Renal failure in malaria. J Vector Borne Dis. 2008;45(2):83–97.
91. Mishra SK, Das BS. Malaria and acute kidney injury. Semin Nephrol. 2008;28(4):395–408.
92. Eiam-Ong S. Malarial nephropathy. Semin Nephrol. 2003;23(1):21–33.
93. Nadjm B, Amos B, Mtove G, Ostermann J, Chonya S, Wangai H, et al. WHO guidelines for antimicrobial treatment in children admitted to hospital in an area of intense Plasmodium falciparum transmission: prospective study. BMJ. 2010;340:c1350.
94. Krishnan A, Karnad DR. Severe falciparum malaria: an important cause of multiple organ failure in Indian intensive care unit patients. Crit Care Med. 2003;31(9):2278–84.

95. Scott JA, Berkley JA, Mwangi I, Ochola L, Uyoga S, Macharia A, et al. Relation between falciparum malaria and bacteraemia in Kenyan children: a population-based, case-control study and a longitudinal study. Lancet. 2011;378(9799):1316–23.
96. Berkley J, Mwarumba S, Bramham K, Lowe B, Marsh K. Bacteraemia complicating severe malaria in children. Trans R Soc Trop Med Hyg. 1999;93(3):283–6.
97. Antinori S, Corona A, Castelli A, Rech R, Borghi B, Giannotti C, et al. Severe Plasmodium falciparum malaria in the intensive care unit: a 6-year experience in Milano, Italy. Travel Med Infect Dis. 2017;17:43–9.

Chapter 14
Tuberculosis Multidrug Resistance (MDR-TB)

Juan Ignacio Silesky-Jiménez

Overview

Tuberculosis (TB) is an infectious disease caused by *Mycobacterium tuberculosis* and is a pathology of the human being, that is, it is an obligately human disease, since there are no animal reservoirs that maintain and perpetuate it. Currently, it is among the ten causes of death by an infectious agent worldwide [1].

Its existence has been known since antiquity, even from the Paleolithic period in the Stone Age, about 3.3 million years ago [2].

However, it is very important to note that it was not until Robert Koch presented two ideas at the Berlin Physiological Society in March 1882, where he postulated that the cause of this disease was due to an infectious agent and the other that said etiological agent is what we know as *Mycobacterium tuberculosis* [3]. However, it was not until 1944 where the effectiveness of streptomycin in the organism in vitro is described, by Schatx and Waksman, who initiate the development of the treatment antibiotic against this bacteria [4].

Since then he has taken special interest during the history of medicine, the development of drugs against this disease called antiphimic antibiotics, and even the development of surgical techniques in the field of thoracic surgery, for the treatment of people with this disease; the latter has been resumed in the twenty-first century for the treatment of patients with multidrug-resistant tuberculosis (MDR-TB).

During the history of mankind, tuberculosis has caused epidemic periods, during the eighteenth and nineteenth century, in Europe and the United States.

Already by the twentieth century, there has been an overall decline in this disease, especially in developing countries or in developed countries, persisting a high

J. I. Silesky-Jiménez (✉)
University of Costa Rica, San José, Costa Rica

© Springer Nature Switzerland AG 2020   235
J. Hidalgo, L. Woc-Colburn (eds.), *Highly Infectious Diseases in Critical Care*,
https://doi.org/10.1007/978-3-030-33803-9_14

incidence in countries with low or middle income and with emerging economies. The problem for human health has been aggravated by the appearance of strains of mycobacteria resistant to existing drugs and the association of people infected with the human immunodeficiency virus (HIV) [3, 5–11].

For example, according to the WHO Global Tuberculosis Report 2018 [1], the annual global incidence in 2017 was 10.0 million people (5.8 million were men, 3.2 million women, and one million children), with an annual mortality of 1.3 million (range between 1.2 and 1.4 million), without HIV and also in 300, 000 people with HIV. The majority of cases, in their two thirds, were in eight countries: India (27%), China (9%), Indonesia (8%), the Philippines (6%), Pakistan (5%), Nigeria (4%), Bangladesh (4%), and South Africa (3%); all of the above plus 22 countries (Angola, Brazil, Korea, DR Congo, Ethiopia, Kenya, Mozambique, Myanmar, Russian Federation, Thailand, UR Tanzania, Cambodia, Central African Republic, Congo, Lesotho, Liberia, Namibia, Papua New Guinea, Sierra Leone, Viet Nam, Zambia, Zimbabwe) are considered to be the 30 countries with the highest burden of tuberculosis by the WHO, which account for 87% of the cases worldwide. Some regions have a lower incidence such as Europe (3%) and America (3%), for example, it is observed in the United States in 2016, of 9287 new cases [12].

In the same Global TB Report 2018 of the WHO [1], it is reported that, in 2017, about 558, 000 (range between 483, 000 and 639, 000) people presented drug-resistant tuberculosis, with 82% having multidrug-resistant tuberculosis (multidrug-resistant TB (MDR-TB)), in which 3 countries in the world concentrate about half of the cases, such as India (24%), China (13%), and the Russian Federation (10%).

In this way, the World Health Organization (WHO), since 1993, has declared tuberculosis as an emerging global disease, and by May 2014, the World Health Assembly declared and proposed the strategy and new international objectives to stop tuberculosis, which are summarized in the following table (Fig. 14.1) [13]:

MDR-TB Definition and Causes

The *Mycobacterium tuberculosis* is an obligated aerobic bacteria [14], which has developed resistance thru various mechanisms, which have produced according to the WHO [15] by several types of drug-resistant TB which are:

1. Monoresistance: Resistance to one first-line anti-TB drug only.
2. Polydrug resistance: Resistance to more than one first-line anti-TB drug, other than both isoniazid and rifampicin.
3. Multidrug resistance (MDR): Resistance to at least both isoniazid and rifampicin.
4. Rifampicin resistance (RR): Resistance to rifampicin detected using phenotypic or genotypic methods, with or without resistance to other anti-TB drugs. It includes any resistance to rifampicin, whether monoresistance, multidrug resistance, polydrug resistance, or extensive drug resistance.

Vision	A world free of tuberculosis – zero deaths, disease and suffering due to tuberculosis
Goal	End the global tuberculosis epidemic
Milestones for 2025	75% reduction in tuberculosis deaths (compared with 2015) 50% reduction in tuberculosis incidence rate (less than 55 tuberculosis cases per 100 000 population) – No affected families facing catastrophic costs due to tuberculosis
Targets for 2035	95% reduction in tuberculosis deaths (compared with 2015) 90% reduction in tuberculosis incidence rate (less than 10 tuberculosis cases per 100 000 population) – No affected families facing catastrophic costs due to tuberculosis

Principles
1. Government stewardship and accountability, with monitoring and evaluation
2. Strong coalition with civil society organizations and communities
3. Protection and promotion of human rights, ethics and equity
4. Adaptation of the strategy and targets at country level, with global collaboration

Pillars and components

1. Integrated, patient-centred care and prevention
A. Early diagnosis of tuberculosis including universal drug-susceptibility testing, and systematic screening of contacts and high-risk groups
B. Treatment of all people with tuberculosis including drug-resistant tuberculosis, and patient support
C. Collaborative tuberculosis/HIV activities, and management of comorbidities
D. Preventive treatment of persons at high risk, and vaccination against tuberculosis

2. Bold policies and supportive systems
A. Political commitment with adequate resources for tuberculosis care and prevention
B. Engagement of communities, civil society organizations, and public and private care providers
C. Universal health coverage policy, and regulatory frameworks for case notification, vital registration, quality and rational use of medicines, and infection control
D. Social protection,poverty alleviation and actions on other determinants of tuberculosis

3. Intensified research and innovation
A. Discovery, development and rapid uptake of new tools, interventions and strategies
B. Research to optimize implementation and impact, and promote innovations

Fig. 14.1 Post-2015 global tuberculosis strategy framework

5. Extensive drug resistance (XDR): Resistance to any fluoroquinolone and at least one of three second-line injectable drugs (capreomycin, kanamycin, and amikacin), in addition to multidrug.

This process of resistance has been known since the development of the first antituberculous drug that was streptomycin, as a biological phenomenon of *Mycobacterium tuberculosis* [16]. Subsequently, with the development of new drugs such as thioacetazone and para-aminosalicylic acid in 1948 and isoniazid in 1952, it is known that the combination of antituberculous drugs prevents resistance; by that time, the treatments were given for 18 months. With the creation and use of rifampicin in 1957, shorter and more effective treatments were initiated, based on regimens containing this drug – rifampicin – and isoniazid. As of 1993 in resource-limited settings, the DOTS (directly observed treatment, short course) strategy was started as the standard TB treatment.

The foregoing is important to mention, because some of the known causes of the development of MDR-TB is attributed to the following:

1. Chaotic treatments: before the 1980s, many countries did not treat TB with standard treatment protocols and did not have patient tracking systems, which is worsened by the socioeconomic instability of some regions, which does not ensure a continuous treatment and with little adherence.

2. Amplifying effect of short-term treatments: when resistance to a drug occurs, paradoxically, the DOTS strategy can exacerbate the problem because when using the same treatment for short periods of time, a kind of resistant TB is generated to first-line treatments [17]. This mechanism is responsible for epidemics in countries where resistant TB is not properly diagnosed or treated [18].
3. Community transmission: current models of transmission indicate that in many countries, patients infected with MDR-TB were initially infected with an MDR-TB strain, instead of a bacterium that has slowly acquired resistance caused by inadequate or irregular treatment [19].
4. Facility-based transmission: this mechanism is important in the development of epidemics in patients above all HIV positive, as well as in health personnel, where in health centers frequented with patients receiving treatment for drug-sensitive TB, they become infected with MDR-TB [20].

Resistance to anti-TB drugs can occur in two ways:

1. Primary: occurs when the patient is infected by a strain of resistant mycobacteria, which can occur by spontaneous mutations without the pressure produced by the presence of anti-TB drugs [21, 22].
2. Acquired: occurs when this resistance occurs during the period in which the patient receives treatment with few active drugs, where the mycobacteria is able to mutate. These mutations have been measured and predicted [23].

It is important to clarify that the acquisition of resistance to anti-TB drugs does not confer changes in the virulence or transmission of *Mycobacterium tuberculosis*, although some exceptions have been described [24, 25].

The risk factors described for MDR-TB are the following [26, 27]:

1. Failure to respond to a first-line DOTS regimen (WHO Category I or II)
2. Relapse after a full course of treatment with a first-line regimen
3. Treatment after defaulting from treatment with a first-line regimen
4. Exposure to a known case of MDR-TB
5. Exposure to TB in institutions with high prevalence of MDR-TB, such as a prison or hospital
6. Living in areas or countries with high prevalence of MDR-TB
7. HIV co-infection

Diagnosis of MDR-TB

There is no difference in clinical presentation between patients with TB and MDR-TB. Both types of bacteria present the same symptoms which are fever, prolonged cough of more than 2–3 weeks, weight loss, night sweating, loss of appetite, and fatigue. If the disease progresses to the pulmonary level, chest pain and hemoptysis may occur, as well as other extrapulmonary manifestations such as lymphadenopathy (tuberculous lymphadenitis), altered mental status and meningism (central nervous system tuberculosis), pain and abdominal distension (peritoneal TB), etc. [28, 29]. Thus, there is no initial clinical clue that identifies the presence of an MDR-TB infection, except for patients with HIV who usually have a more advanced initial presentation when they have an infection due to this type of bacteria (MDR-TB).

Additionally both types of infection share the same diagnostic challenges such as there is a low diagnostic yield of the traditionally used diagnostic test, that is, the sputum smear, and it loses between 50% and 70% of active lung infections and this is more accentuated in patients with HIV [30]. This fact leads to the underdiagnosis of TB cases in poor countries, which only have this diagnostic method, and in any case, as the culture does not tell us about sensitivity to anti-HIV drugs. TB [31]

To determine the sensitivity to anti-TB drugs, it is usually required with standard means between 3 and 6 weeks, and taking into account from the moment that the sputum is taken, it can be between 8 and 16 weeks or more, taking into account the isolation of the germ and determination of sensitivity. In view of the above, a treatment with four drugs (usually isoniazid, ethambutol, rifampicin, and pyrazinamide) is initiated under the assumption that TB is treated with at least one effective drug, which also increases the potential for MDR development. TB

The WHO recommends the use of rapid drug sensitivity testing (DTS) for isoniazid and rifampicin, which requires 2 days; however, it has been estimated that 1 in 20 patients with MDR-TB is diagnosed using the systems and tools used [32].

The sensitivity tests to the anti-TB can be separated into two categories, to which we will refer briefly since many are in development and commercialization, not to mention that in many places with low resources, some of these tools are very expensive. In such way it has:

1. Phenotypic/culture-based tests (phenotypic/culture-based assays)
2. Genotypic tests/molecular tests (genotypic/molecular assays)

Phenotypic/Culture-Based Diagnostic Tests for Drug Susceptibility

These tests are based in the cultures results are the less expensive test and are the most frequently used and the choice to determine resistance to drugs. Its maximum disadvantage is the duration to obtain the results, which may require weeks or months.

Tests have been developed from crops, to obtain faster results such as:

(a) Nitrate reductase assay (NRA), in which it detects the reduction of nitrate to nitrite by mycobacteria, using colorimetric methods [33]
(b) Microscopic observation drug susceptibility (MODS) [34]
(c) Thin-layer agar (TLA)

These last two use an inoculation of the culture in a medium, with known concentrations of the drugs, in which they evaluate microscopically the bacterial growth [35]

These three methods are not expensive, they are not commercial tests, and they require between 5 and 18 days after having the crops [35].

There are commercial methods for the detection of TB and its resistance, which are rapid (results are obtained in less than 14 days), but they are expensive and are used in developed countries. For illustrative purposes, some of these will be mentioned: Epsilometer tests (E-tests), the BACTEC460 radiometric system (Becton Dickinson Diagnostic Instruments, Sparks, MD), and Mycobacteria Growth Indicator Tube (MGIT) 960 (Becton Dickinson Diagnostic Instruments, Sparks, MD), a fluorometric assay (Lemus 2004). Both the BACTEC460 and MGIT 960 systems.

Genotypic/Molecular Tests

These systems for the determination of *Mycobacterium tuberculosis* and its antibiotic sensitivity are based on the detection of specific genetic sequences both for the germ and to determine if there is specific resistance to drugs [36].

They use technology available from techniques derived from the polymerase chain reaction (PCR) to commercial one-step tests, which allows the detection and determination of resistance in a very short time, between 2 and 48 hours.

The two most important classes are line probe assays (LPAs) and nucleic acid amplification tests. The second generation of LPAs can detect resistance to fluoroquinolone, which allows the diagnosis [37].

Tuberculosis in Critical Care

Tuberculosis produces several conditions that can cause patients to be tributaries to critical care for reasons derived from the same infection or treatment, which causes respiratory failure, altered state of consciousness, or multiorgan failure.

The most frequent condition is respiratory failure in patients with active TB who present a high mortality, reported between 33% and 67% [38–40], taking into account that if the diagnosis is prolonged, mortality increases [41]. In addition, these patients may have diseases that worsen their condition such as bacterial pneumonias, COPD (chronic obstructive pulmonary disease), and malignancy, which may be present in about 72% of patients [42].

Other conditions for which these patients may require critical care are summarized in the following conditions and their causes [43]:

1. Massive hemoptysis due to Rasmussen aneurysm
2. Cardiogenic shock due to massive pericardial effusion
3. Known tuberculosis patient electively admitted to ICU with post-thoracic surgery
4. Liver failure due to drug reaction

5. Renal failure due to drug reaction (usually rifampicin)
6. Disseminated intravascular coagulation due to miliary TB
7. Pituitary apoplexy/stroke mimic due to cerebral tuberculoma
8. Airway obstruction due to laryngeal/retropharyngeal TB
9. Adrenal insufficiency with refractory hypotension or hyponatremia

All the above involve a challenge not only for the diagnosis but for the treatment of complications and the individualization of the treatment, especially if there is any renal or hepatic deterioration.

The use of corticosteroids in patients has been accepted in several international guidelines, in the following situations:

1. Miliary tuberculosis where the corticosteroids reduce the risk of death or disability [44, 45].
2. Tuberculous pericardial effusion, where corticosteroids reduce speed and risk of re-accumulation [45, 46].
3. Paradoxical reactions/immune reconstitution inflammatory syndrome, which is a clinical radiological reaction of worsening of pre-existing tuberculosis lesions or the development of new lesions, in patients who have received anti-TB drugs, in the absence of an explanation such as drug resistance, ineffective drug delivery, or a secondary diagnosis [47]. It occurs with an average of 26 days of treatment initiation [48], but may occur in the following months, especially in patients with low levels of rapidly recovering CD4 and HAART initiated within 2 months of diagnosis [49]. Montelukast and thalidomide have also been used in severe CNS TB paradoxical reactions unresponsive to corticosteroids [50].

Treatment

Regarding the treatment of MDR-TB, it is important to note that when compared to the standard treatment of TB, it has the following disadvantages:

1. It is more complex.
2. It implies the use of four or more drugs.
3. It has longer time, including 24 months.
4. It has low rates of healing.
5. It has more adverse effects.
6. It has a higher mortality [51–54].

Recently the WHO developed the "WHO treatment guidelines for multidrug- and rifampicin-resistant tuberculosis, 2018 update" [55], which summarizes the latest evidence available in the treatment of the MDR-TB.

For the usual treatment of TB, first-line drugs are used, such as ethambutol, isoniazid, and pyrazinamide, but they can also be used in the treatment of MDR-TB; it is important to emphasize that streptomycin is now considered a second-line substitute, when there is no proven resistance to amikacin.

There are two types of regimens in the treatment of MDR-TB:

1. *Prolonged regime (longer regimens)*, which is recommended in Section 2

   The duration of longer MDR-TB regimens
   Recommendation:

   2.1 In MDR/RR-TB patients on longer regimens, a total treatment duration of 18–20 months is suggested for most patients, and the duration may be modified according to the patient's response to therapy (conditional recommendation, very low certainty in the estimates of effect).
   2.2 In MDR/RR-TB patients on longer regimens, a treatment duration of 15 to 17 months after culture conversion is suggested for most patients, and the duration may be modified according to the patient's response to therapy (conditional recommendation, very low certainty in the estimates of effect).
   2.3 In MDR/RR-TB patients on longer regimens containing amikacin or streptomycin, an intensive phase of 6–7 months is suggested for most patients, and the duration may be reduced or increased according to the patient's.

2. *Short regimen*

   Section 3. The use of the standardized shorter MDR-TB regimen
   Recommendation:

   In MDR/RR-TB patients who have not been previously treated for more than one month with second-line medicines used in the shorter MDR regimen or in whom resistance to fluoroquinolones and second-line injectable agents has been excluded, a shorter MDR-TB regimen of 9–12 months may be used instead of the longer regimens (conditional recommendation; low certainty in the estimates of effect).

This regimen can be chosen when the patient does NOT present any of the following characteristics:

(a) Preference by the clinician and patient for a longer MDR-TB regimen
(b) Confirmed resistance or suspected ineffectiveness to a medicine in the shorter MDR-TB regimen (except isoniazid resistance)
(c) Exposure to one or more second-line medicines in the shorter MDR-TB regimen for >1 month (unless susceptibility to these 2nd line medicines is confirmed)
(d) Intolerance to medicines in the shorter MDR-TB regimen or risk of toxicity (e.g. drug-drug interactions)
(e) Pregnancy
(f) Disseminated, meningeal or central nervous system TB
(g) Any extrapulmonary disease in PLHIV
(h) One or more medicines in the shorter MDR-TB regimen not available

However, if the patient has any of these characteristics and/or there is a failure in the short regimen or there is no response, drug intolerance occurs or emerges from any of these exclusive characteristics; one must opt for an individualized regime of prolonged time.

The second-line anti-TB drugs (Fig. 14.2) are those drugs only available for the treatment of MDR-TB. The new classification divides it into three groups, for drugs with prolonged regimens:

Groups and steps	Medicine	Abrev.
Group A: Include all three medicines	Levofloxacin **OR**	Lfx
	Moxifloxacin	Mfx
	Bedaquine [2,3]	Bdq
	Linezolid [4]	Lzd
Group B: Add one or both medicines	Clofazimine	Cfz
	Cicloserine **OR**	Cs
	Terizidone	Trd
Group C: Add to complete the retimen and when medicines from Groups A and B cannot be used	Ethambutol	E
	Delamanid [3,5]	Dim
	Pyrazinamide [6]	Z
	Imipenem-cilastatina **OR**	Ipm-Cln
	Meropenem [7]	Mpm
	Amikacin	Am
	(OR Streptomycin) [8]	(S)
	Ethionamide **OR**	Eto
	Prothionamide [9]	Pto
	p-aminosalicylic acid [9]	PAS

1 This table is intended to guide the design of individualized, longer MDR-TB regimens (the composition of the recommended shorter MDR-TB regimen is largely standardized; see Section 3). Medicines in Group C are ranked by decreasing order of usual preference for use subject to other considerations. The 2018 IPD-MA for longer regimens included no patients on thioacetazone (T) and too few patients on gatifloxacin (Gfx) and high-dose isoniazid (Hh) for a meaningful analysis. No recommendation on perchlozone, interferon gamma or sutezolid was possible owing to the absence of final patient treatment outcome data from appropriate studies.
2 Evidence on the safety and effectiveness of Bdq beyond 6 months and below the age of 6 years was insufficient for review. Use of Bdq beyond these limits should follow best practices in "off-label" use.
3 Evidence on the concurrent use of Bdq and Dlm was insufficient for review.
4 Use of Lzd for at least 6 months was shown to increase effectiveness, although toxicity may limit use. The analysis suggested that using Lzd for the whole duration of treatment would optimize its effect (about 70% of patients on Lzd with data received it for more than 6 months and 30% for 18 months or the whole duration). No patient predictors for early cessation of Lzd could be inferred from the IPD sub-analysis.
5 Evidence on the safety and effectiveness of Dlm beyond 6 months and below the age of 3 years was insufficient for review. Use of Dlm beyond these limits should follow best practices in "off-label" use.
6 Z is only counted as an effective agent when DST results confirm susceptibility.
7 Every dose of Imp-Cln and Mpm is administered with clavulanic acid, which is only available in formulations combined with amoxicillin (Amx-Clv). Amx-Clv is not counted as an additional effective TB agent and should not be used without Imp-Cln or Mpm.
8 Am and S are only to be considered if DST results confirm susceptibility and high-quality audiometry monitoring for hearing loss can be ensured. S is to be considered only if Am cannot be used (unavailable or documented resistance) and if DST results confirm susceptibility (S resistance is not detectable with second line molecular line probe assays and phenotypic DST is required). Kanamycin (Km) and capreomycin (Cm) are no longer recommended for use in MDR-TB regimens.
9 These agents only showed effectivenessin regimens without Bdq, Lzd, Cfz or Dlm and are thus only proposed when other options to compose a regimen are not possible.

Fig. 14.2 Grouping of medicines recommended for use in longer MDR-TB regimens [1]

The WHO guidelines recommend for *monitoring response* to MDR-TB treatment:

Section 4. Monitoring patient response to MDR-TB treating using culture
Recommendation:

In MDR/RR-TB patients on longer regimens, the performance of sputum culture in addition to sputum smear microscopy is recommended to monitor treatment response (strong recommendation, moderate certainty in the estimates of test accuracy). It is desirable for sputum culture to be repeated at monthly intervals.

The WHO, recommends the following antibiotic doses for the treatment of MDR-TB (Figs. 14.3 and 14.4):

Surgery for MDR-TB

Surgery was a frequent treatment for tuberculosis; however, with the development of effective medications, its usefulness was limited to the treatment of complications such as pneumothorax, fistulas, massive hemoptysis, and empyemas. Its current application is in 5% of cases [56].

For MDR-TB, surgery became important again in terms of helping to reduce the bacillary load, in removing tissue with poor penetration of drugs, in the treatment of complications, and in possibly shortening treatment.

The patient must receive at least 2 months of treatment with anti-TB drugs before performing the surgery, understanding it as a coadjuvant therapy [57].

According to the criteria of Iseman et al. [58], published in 1990, there are three indications for surgery in MDR-TB, which are:

1. Drug resistance is extensive and there is a high failure of treatment with medications alone.
2. Disease is localized, allowing resection and sufficient lung function subsequently.
3. Effective drug therapy is available to treat residual disease.

Such surgeries have a mortality of less than 3% [58, 59], with the performance of lobectomies, segmentectomy, and cavernoplasties, as the case may be; with complications reported by 26%; with sputum smear negative a month after surgery in more than 80%; and in series reported in Romania, Seoul, Japan, and China [60–63].

Special Situations

There are some important scenarios to consider [64]:

1. Extrapulmonary MDR-TB: it is necessary to insist on obtaining samples for the diagnosis and sensitivity of MDR-TB:

    (a) Tuberculous lymphadenitis – prolonged treatment should be given as if it were a pulmonary MDR-TB; the time required is really unknown.

Dosing of medicines used in second-line MDR-TB regimens by weight band in patients older than 14 years

Group	Medicine	Weight-based daily dose	Formulation	30–35 kg	36–45 kg	46–55 kg	56–70 kg	>70 kg	Usual upper daily dose[b]	Comments
A	*Fluoroquinolones*									
	Levofloxacin	–,c	250 mg tab	3	3	4	4	4		
			500 mg tab	1.5	1.5	2	2	2	1.5 g	
			750 mg tab	1	1	1.5	1.5	1.5		
	Moxifloxacin	standard dose[c,d]	400 mg tab	1	1	1	1	1	400 mg	as used in the standardized shorter MDR-TB regimen
		high dose[c,d]	400 mg tab	1 or 1.5	1.5	1.5 or 2	2	2	800 mg	
	Bedaquiline	c	100 mg tab	\multicolumn 4 tabs od for first 2 weeks; then 2 tabs od M/W/F for 22 weeks					400 mg	
	Linezolid	c	600 mg tab	(<15 y)	(<15 y)	1	1	1	1.2 g	
B	Clofazimine	c	50 mg cap or tab	2	2	2	2	2	100 mg	
			100 mg cap or tab	1	1	1	1	1	100 mg	
	Cycloserine or terizidone	10–15 mg/kg	250 mg cap	2	2	3	3	3	1 g	
	Ethambutol	15–25 mg/kg	400 mg tab	2	2	3	3	3	–	
	Delamanid	–,c	50 mg tab	2 bd	2 bd	2 bd	2 bd	2 bd	200 mg	
	Pyrazinamide	20–30 mg/kg	400 mg tab	3	4	4	4	5	–	
			500 mg tab	2	3	3	3	4		
C	Imipenem–cilastatin	c	0.5 g + 0.5 g vial	\multicolumn 2 vials (1 g + 1 g) bd					–	To be used with clavulanic acid
	Meropenem	c	1 g vial (20 ml)	1 vial 3 times per day or 2 vials bd						To be used with clavulanic acid
	Amikacin	15–20 mg/kg	500 mg/2 ml vial[e]	2.5 ml	3 ml	3 to 4 ml	4 ml	4 ml	1 g	
	Streptomycin	12–18 mg/kg	1 g vial[e]	Calculate according to the dilution used					1 g	
	Ethionamide or prothionamide	15–20 mg/kg	250 mg tablet	2	2	3	3	4	1 g	Once daily dose advised but can start with 2 divided doses until tolerance improves
	p-aminosalicylic acid	8–12 g/day in 2–3 divided doses	PAS sodium salt (4 g) sachet	1 bd	1 bd	1 bd	1 bd	1 to 1.5 bd	12 g	Only to be used with carbapenems
			PAS acid (4 g) sachet	1 bd	1 bd	1 bd	1 bd	1 to 1.5 bd		
Other medicines[f]	Isoniazid	4–6 mg/kg (standard dose)[d]	300 mg tab	2/3	1	1	1	1		100 mg isoniazid tablet can facilitate the administration of certain dosages Pyridoxine given with isoniazid in patients at risk (such as those with HIV, malnutrition)
		10–15 mg/kg (high dose)[d]	300 mg tablet	1.5	1.5	2	2	2		
	Clavulanic acid[7]		125 mg tab[g]	1 bd	1 bd	1 bd	1 bd	1 bd		
	Kanamycin	15–20 mg/kg	500 mg/2 ml vial[e]	2 to 2.5 ml	2.5 to 3 ml	3 to 4 ml	4 ml	4 ml	1 g	M/W/F dosing of aminoglycosides at 25 mg/kg/day may limit toxicity and inconvenience when the injectable agents are used in longer MDR-TB regimens
	Capreomycin	15–20 mg/kg	500 mg/2 ml vial[e]	2.5 ml	3ml	3 to 4 ml	4 ml	4 ml	1 g	
	Gatifloxacin	c	400 mg tab	2	2	2	2	2	800 mg	Not used in <18 year olds (no quality assured product currently available)
	Thioacetazone	c	150 mg tab	1	1	1	1	1	–	Not used in <18 year olds (no quality assured product currently available)

(<15 y) = follow the separate dose schedule for patients younger than 15 years of age; bd = two times a day; cap = capsule; g = gram; im = intramuscular; iv = intravenous; kg = kilogram; ml = millilitre; mg = milligram; M/W/F = Monday, Wednesday, Friday; soln = solution; susp = suspension; tab = tablet

Fig. 14.3 Dosage by weight band for medicines used in MDR-TB regimens in adult

Footnotes

a   Dosages were established by the Guideline Development Group for the WHO treatment guidelines for rifampicin-and multidrug-resistant tuberculosis, 2018 update and the WHO Global task force on the pharmacokinetics and pharmacodynamics (PK/PD) of TB medicines and other experts. They are based on the most recent reviews and best practices in the treatment of MDR/RR-TB. For certain agents the dosages were informed by pharmacokinetic modelling results based on the principle of allometric scaling (Anderson BJ, Holford NH. Mechanism-based concepts of size and maturity in pharmacokinetics. Annu Rev Pharmacol Toxicol 2008;48:303–32). Due to the pharmacokinetic properties of certain medicines the doses proposed may exceed the mg/kg/day ranges shown here in order to achieve blood concentrations similar to target levels in an average adult patient. In patients <30 kg follow the schedule for <15-year olds unless otherwise indicated. If multiple dose options are given for one weight band select the lower or higher option depending on whether the patient is at the lower or higher limit of the body weight range. Dosing more closely to the target mg/kg/day should be aimed for, and is more feasible with oral or parenteral fluids and when solid forms of different dosages are available. Fractioning of tablets into halves or less should be avoided, if possible. Therapeutic drug monitoring is advised when the dose is at the upper and lower ends of the range to minimize the adverse therapeutic consequences of over-and under-exposure, respectively (especially for injectable agents, linezolid and fluoroquinolones).

     Clinicians may decide to exceed these values in particular cases to improve therapeutic effect.

b   No weight-based dosing is proposed.
c   Unless there is risk of toxicity, the high dose may be used if antimicrobial levels may be lowered because of pharmacokinetic interactions, malabsorption or other metabolic reasons or if the strain has low-level drug resistance.
e   Weight-based daily dose is for 6 or 7days/week administration (M/W/F scheduling may permit higher dosing). Volumes shown may differ by preparation. Streptomycin may be diluted in three different ways. For iv use, the volume may be increased.
f   In the 2018 WHO treatment guidelines, these agents are either no longer recommended (kanamycin, capreomycin), only recommended as a companion agent (amoxicillin/clavulanic acid) or not included because of lack of data from the latest analysis on longer MDR-TB regimens in adults (gatifloxacin, isoniazid and thioacetazone).
g   Only available in combination with amoxicillin as co-amoxyclav (e.g. 500 mg amoxicillin/125 mg clavulanic acid fixed dose combination). It is given with each dose of carbapenem, either as 125 mg bd or 125 mg 3 times daily.

     See the text of the guidelines for more details on the use of medicines.

Fig. 14.3 (continued)

Dosing of medicines used in second-line MDR-TB regimens by weight band in patients under 15 years[a]

Group	Medicine	Weight-based daily dose[b]	Formulation	5–6 kg	7–9 kg	10–15 kg	16–23 kg	24–30 kg	31–34 kg	>34 kg	Usual upper daily dose[b]	Comments
A	*Fluoroquinolones*											
	Levofloxacin	15–20 mg/kg	100 mg dt	1	1.5	2 or 3	3 or 4	(>14 y)	(>14 y)	(>14 y)	1.5 g	
			250 mg tab	0.5	0.5	1 or 1.5	1.5 or 2	2	3	(>14 y)	1.5 g	
	Moxifloxacin	10–15 mg/kg	100 mg dt	0.8	1.5	2	3	4	(>14 y)	(>14 y)	400 mg	Use 10 mg/kg in <6 months
			400 mg tab[c]	2 ml[c]	3 ml[c]	5 ml[c]	0.5 or 0.75	1	(>14 y)	(>14 y)	400 mg	Only in patients >5 years old (lower dose from 15–29 kg; higher dose from >29 kg)
	Bedaquiline		100 mg tab	-	-	-	2 tabs od for two weeks; then 1 tab od M/W/F for 22 weeks	4 tabs od for 2 weeks; then 2 tabs od M/W/F for 22 weeks				
	Linezolid	15 mg/kg od in <16 kg; 10–12 mg/kg od in >15 kg	20 mg/ml susp	4 ml	6 ml	8 ml	11 ml	14 ml	15 ml	20 ml[d]	600 mg	
			600 mg tab[c]	0.25	0.25	0.25	0.5	0.5	0.5	0.75[d]	600 mg	
B	Clofazimine	2–5 mg/kg	50 mg cap or tab	1 alt days	1 alt days	1 alt days	1	2	2	(>14 y)	100 mg	Give on alternate days if dose in mg/kg/day is too high
			100 mg cap or tab	M/W/F	M/W/F	1 alt days	1 alt days	1	(>14 y)	(>14 y)	100 mg	
	Cycloserine or terizidone	15–20 mg/kg	125 mg mini capsule (cycloserine)	1	1	2	3	4	(>14 y)	(>14 y)	1 g	
			250 mg cap[c]	4–5 ml[c]	5–6 ml[c]	7–10 ml[c]	2	2	2	(>14 y)	1 g	
	Ethambutol	15–25 mg/kg	100 mg dt	1	2	3	4	-	-	-		
			400 mg tab[c]	3 ml[c]	4 ml[c]	6 ml[c]	1	1 or 1.5	2	(>14 y)		
	Delamanid		50 mg tab	-	-	*	*	1 bd	1 bd	2 bd	200 mg	Not used in patients <15 years (use meropenem)
	Pyrazinamide	30–40 mg/kg	150 mg dt	1	2	3	4 or 5	-	-	(>14 y)		
			400 mg tab	0.5	0.75	1	1.5 or 2	2.5	3	(>14 y)		
			500 mg tab	0.5	0.5	0.75 or 1	1.5	2	2.5	(>14 y)		
	Imipenem-cilastatin		0.5 g + 0.5 g vial	-	-	Calculate according to the dilution used					200 mg	To be used with clavulanic acid
C	Meropenem	20–40 mg/kg iv every 8 hours	1 g vial (20 ml)	2 ml	4 ml	6 ml	8–9 ml	11 ml	(>14 y)	(>14 y)	1 g	
	Amikacin	15–20 mg/kg	500 mg/2 ml vial[f]	0.4 ml	0.6 ml	0.8 – 1.0 ml	1.2 – 1.5 ml	2.0 ml	(>14 y)	(>14 y)	1 g	Only to be used with carbapenems
	Streptomycin	20–40 mg/kg	1 g vial[f]	Calculate according to the dilution used					(>14 y)	(>14 y)	1 g	
	Ethionamide or prothionamide	15–20 mg/kg	125 mg (ethionamide)	1	1	2	-	4	4	(>14 y)	1 g	
			250 mg tab	0.5	0.5	1	2	2	2	(>14 y)	1 g	
	p-aminosalicylic acid	200–300 mg/kg in 2 divided doses	PAS acid (4 g) sachet	0.5–0.75 g bd	0.75–1 g bd	1–2 g bd	2–3 g bd	3–3.5 g bd	(>14 y)	(>14 y)		Full dose can be given once daily if tolerated
			PAS sodium salt (4 g) sachet	0.5–0.75 g bd	0.75–1 g bd	1–2 g bd	2–3 g bd	3–3.5 g bd	(>14 y)	(>14 y)		
			PAS sodium salt 60% (9.2 g) sachet	1.5 g bd	2–3 g bd	3–4 g bd	4 or 6 g bd	6 or 8 g bd	8–12 g bd	8–12 g bd		
Other medicines[e]	Isoniazid	15–20 mg/kg (high dose)	50 mg/5 ml soln	8–10 ml	15 ml	20 ml	-	-	-	-		300 mg isoniazid tablet can be used in patients >20 kg. Pyridoxine is always given with high-dose isoniazid in children (12.5 mg od in <5 y olds and 25 mg od in >4 y olds)
			100 mg tab	1	1.5	2	3	4	4	(>14 y)		
	Clavulanic acid[f]		250 mg amoxicillin/62.5 mg clavulanic acid/5 ml susp[f]	2 ml bd[h]	3 ml bd[h]	5 ml bd[h]	8 ml bd[h]	10 ml bd[h]	(>14 y)	(>14 y)		Only to be used with carbapenems
	Kanamycin	15–20 mg/kg	500 mg/2 ml vial[f]	0.4 ml	0.6 ml	0.8–1.0 ml	1.2–1.5 ml	2.0 ml	(>14 y)	(>14 y)	1 g	1 g vials (3 ml) also available
	Capreomycin	15–20 mg/kg	500 mg/2 ml vial[f]	0.4 ml	0.6 ml	0.8–1.0 ml	1.2–1.5 ml	2.0 ml	(>14 y)	(>14 y)	1 g	1 g vials (2 ml) also available
	Gatifloxacin		400 mg tab	-								Not used in <18 y olds (no quality assured product currently available)
	Thioacetazone		-									Not used in <18 y olds (no quality assured product currently available)

(>14 y) = follow the separate dose schedule for patients older than 14 years of age; alt = alternate; bd = two times a day; cap = capsule; dt = dispersible tablet; g = gram; im = intramuscular; iv = intravenous; kg = kilogram; ml = millilitre; mg = milligram; M/W/F = Monday, Wednesday, Friday; soln = solution; susp = suspension; tab = tablet

Fig. 14.4 Dosage by weight band for medicines used in MDR-TB regimens in children

Footnotes

a Dosages were established by the Guideline Development Group for the WHO treatment guidelines for rifampicin- and multidrug-resistant tuberculosis, 2018 update and the WHO Global taskforce on the pharmacokinetics and pharmacodynamics (PK/PD) of TB medicines and other experts. They are based on the most recent reviews and best practices in the treatment of MDR/RR-TB. For certain agents the dosages were informed by pharmacokinetic modelling results based on the principle of allometric scaling (Anderson BJ, Holford NH. Mechanism-based concepts of size and maturity in pharmacokinetics. Annu Rev Pharmacol Toxicol 2008;48:303–32). Due to the pharmacokinetic properties of certain medicines the doses proposed may exceed the mg/kg/day ranges shown here in order to achieve blood concentrations similar to target levels in an average adult patient. In patients >30kg follow the schedule for >14 year olds unless otherwise indicated. If multiple dose options are given for one weight band select the lower or higher option depending on whether the patient is at the lower or higher limit of the body weight range. Dosing more closely to the target mg/kg/day should be aimed for, and is more feasible with oral or parenteral fluids and when solid forms of different dosage are available. Fractioning of tablets into halves or less should be avoided if possible. Therapeutic drug monitoring is advised when the dose is at the upper and lower ends of the range to minimize the adverse therapeutic consequences of over- and under-exposure respectively (especially for injectable agents, linezolid and fluoroquinolones).

b Clinicians may decide to exceed these values in particular cases to improve therapeutic effect.

c Dissolving in 10ml of water may facilitate administration in patients in lower weight-bands and avoids fractioning solid formulations, although bioavailability is uncertain (use of dispersible tablets is preferred if available).

d In individuals >44 kg a dose of 600mg od is proposed.

e May be used in children 3–5 years of age. Giving half a 50mg adult tablet in these children does not result in the same blood levels observed in trials using the special 25mg paediatric tablet. Bioavailability may further be altered when the 50 mg tablet is split, crushed or dissolved.

f Weight-based daily dose is for 6 or 7 days/week administration (M/W/F scheduling may permit higher dosing). Volumes shown may differ by preparation. Streptomycin may be diluted in three different ways. Dosing closer to the upper limit of the mg/kg/day is more desirable. For iv use, the volume may be increased.

g In the 2018 WHO treatment guidelines, these agents are either no longer recommended (kanamycin, capreomycin), only recommended as a companion agent (amoxicillin/clavulanic acid) or not included because of lack of data from the latest analysis on longer MDR -TB regimens in adults (gatifloxacin, isoniazid and thioacetazone).

h Only available in combination with amoxicillin as co-amoxiclav. Only to be used with carbapenems, in which case they are given together, e.g. 125 mg bd or 125 mg 3 times daily in the 24–30 kg weight band.

See the text of the guidelines for more details on the use of medicines.

Fig. 14.4 (continued)

(b) Tuberculosis in the bone or spine – it should be suspected if bone collections or compromises persist or increase despite anti-TB treatment.

(c) Meningeal tuberculosis – it must be remembered that the diagnosis is difficult due to the low concentration of mycobacteria in the CSF; so it becomes a clinic challenge. And second-line drugs do not properly penetrate the blood-brain barrier.

2. Children: their infection usually occurs due to the transmission of a member of their household, so it is convenient to research the people around them. The treatment is the same as that of the adult, and usually the second-line drugs are well tolerated.

3. Pregnant women: many of the second-line drugs produce abnormalities in the product, so the women treated should be informed about it, although it is clear that the benefit outweighs the risks. The risk of malformations is greater in the first trimester, so that treatment can be deferred to the second trimester depending on the patient's clinical and social condition.

   Amikacin, streptomycin, prothionamide, and ethionamide are contraindicated in pregnancy. In addition, the Bedaquiline and delamanid have a scant evidence of safety in pregnancy and lactation; so the treatment must be individualized.

4. Confection with HIV: this group of patients has a high risk of having MDR-TB, with a greater spread and mortality. The use of ART improves survival in patients with HIV and MDR-TB, which should start in the first week after starting anti-TB drugs. This group of patients have a high incidence of adverse effects with second-line drugs [65].

Bibliography

1. WHO. Global Tuberculosis Report 2018. Available at: https://www.who.int/tb/publications/global_report/gtbr2018_main_text_28Feb2019.pdf?ua=1. Accessed 02 Apr 2019.
2. Donoghue HD. Paleomicrobiology of human tuberculosis. Microbiol Spectr. 2016;4(4):113–30.
3. Daniel TM. The history of tuberculosis. Respir Med. 2006;100:1862–70.
4. Smith DG, Waksman SA. Tuberculostatic and tuberculocidal action of streptomycin. J Bacteriol. 1947;54(1):67.
5. Frith J. History of tuberculosis. Part 1- phthisis, consumption and the white plague. J Mil Veterans Health. 2014;22:30–5.
6. Frith J. History of tuberculosis. Part 2- the sanatoria and the discoveries of the tubercle bacillus. J Mil Veterans Health. 2014;22:36–41.
7. Barberis I, Bragazzi NL, Martini LG. The history of tuberculosis: from the first historical records to the isolation of Koch's bacillus. J Prev Med Hyg. 2017;58:E9–12.
8. First unit: tuberculosis through the history. Available at: https://www.scribd.com/document/7556133/History-of-Tuberculosis. Accessed 19 May 2018.
9. Ringer PH. The evolution of the treatment of pulmonary tuberculosis. Chest. 1938;4:8–13.
10. Shampo MA, Rosenow EC. A history of tuberculosis on stamps. Chest. 2009;136:578–82.
11. Davies PDO. A little history of tuberculosis. Available at: http://www.evolve360.co.uk/Data/10/Docs/19/19Davies.pdf. Accessed 7 Oct 2018.
12. Bayer R, Castro KG. Tuberculosis elimination in the United States—the need for renewed action. N Engl J Med. 2017;377:1109–11.

13. WHO. The end TB strategy. Available at: https://www.who.int/tb/strategy/End_TB_Strategy. pdf?ua=1. Accessed 10 Apr 2019.
14. Smith I. Mycobacterium tuberculosis pathogenesis and molecular determinants of virulence. Clin Microbiol Rev. 2003;16:463–96.
15. World Health Organization (WHO). Definitions and reporting framework for tuberculosis—2013 revision. Geneva: World Health Organization; 2013.
16. Pyle M. Relative number of resistant tubercle bacilli in sputa of patients before and during treatment with streptomycin. Proc Staff Meet. Mayo Clinic. 1947;22:465–73.
17. Seung KJ, Gelmanova IE, Peremitin GG, Golubchikova VT, Pavlova VE, Sirotkina OB, Yanova GV, Strelis AK. The effect of initial drug resistance on treatment response and acquired drug resistance during standardized short-course chemotherapy for tuberculosis. Clin Infect Dis. 2004;39:1321–8.
18. Keshavjee S, Farmer PE. Tuberculosis, drug resistance, and the history of modern medicine. New Engl J Med. 2012;367:931–6.
19. Lin H, Shin S, Blaya JA, Zhang Z, Cegielski P, Contreras C, Asencios L, Bonilla C, Bayona J, Paciore CJ, et al. Assessing spatiotemporal patterns of multidrug-resistant and drug-sensitive tuberculosis in a South American setting. Epidemiol Infect. 2011;139:1784–93.
20. Gelmanova IY, Keshavjee S, Golubchikova VT, Berezina VI, Strelis AK, Yanova GV, Atwood S, Murray M. Barriers to successful tuberculosis treatment in Tomsk, Russian Federation: non-adherence, default and the acquisition of multidrug resistance. Bull World Health Organ. 2007;85:703–11.
21. David HL. Probability distribution of drug-resistant mutants in unselected populations of Mycobacterium tuberculosis. Appl Microbiol. 1970;20:810–4.
22. Gillespie SH. Evolution of drug resistance in Mycobacterium tuberculosis: clinical and molecular perspective. Antimicrob Agents Chemother. 2002;46:267–74.
23. Mlambo CK, et al. Genotypic diversity of extensively drug-resistant tuberculosis (XDR-TB) in South Africa. Int J Tuberc Lung Dis. 2008;12:99–104.
24. Gandhi NR, et al. Multidrug-resistant and extensively drug-resistant tuberculosis: a threat to global control of tuberculosis. Lancet. 2010;375:1830–43.
25. Zignol M, Gemert W, Falzon D. Surveillance of anti-tuberculosis drug resistance in the world: an updated analysis, 2007–2010. Bull World Health Organ. 2012;90(2):111–119D.
26. Chavez Pachas AM, Blank R, Fawzi Smith MC, Bayona J, Becerra M, Mitnick CD. Identifying early treatment failure on category I therapy for pulmonary tuberculosis in Lima Ciudad, Peru. Int J Tuberc Lung Dis. 2004;8:52–8.
27. Satti H, McLaughlin MM, Seung KJ, Becerra MC, Keshavjee S. High risk of drug-resistant tuberculosis when first-line therapy fails in a high HIV prevalence setting. Int J Tuberc Lung Dis. 2013;17:100–6.
28. Hoa NB, et al. National survey of tuberculosis prevalence in Viet Nam. Bull World Health Organ. 2010;88:273–80.
29. Lawn SD, Zumla AI. Tuberculosis. Lancet. 2011;378:57–72.
30. Magee MJ, et al. Prevalence of drug resistant tuberculosis among patients at high-risk for HIV attending outpatient clinics in Delhi, India. Southeast Asian J Trop Med Public Health. 2012;43:354–63.
31. Zhang Y, Yew WW. Mechanisms of drug resistance in Mycobacterium tuberculosis. Int J Tuberc Lung Dis. 2009;13:1320–30.
32. Caws M, Ha DT. Scale-up of diagnostics for multidrug resistant tuberculosis. Lancet Infect Dis. 2010;10:656–8.
33. Angeby KA, Klintz L, Hoffner SE. Rapid and inexpensive drug susceptibility testing of Mycobacterium tuberculosis with a nitrate reductase assay. J Clin Microbiol. 2002;40:553–5.
34. Moore DA, et al. Microscopic-observation drug-susceptibility assay for the diagnosis of TB. N Engl J Med. 2006;355:1539–50.
35. Minion J, Leung E, Menzies D, et al. Microscopic-observation drug susceptibility and thin layer agar assays for the detection of drug resistant tuberculosis: a systematic review and meta-analysis. Lancet Infect Dis. 2010;10:688–98.

36. Müller B, Borrell S, Rose G, et al. The heterogeneous evolution of multidrug-resistant Mycobacterium tuberculosis. Trends Genet. 2012;29:160. https://doi.org/10.1016/j.tig.2012.11.005.

37. Ajbani K, et al. Evaluation of genotype MTBDRsl assay to detect drug resistance associated with fluoroquinolones, aminoglycosides and ethambutol on clinical sediments. PLoS One. 2012;7(11):e49433.

38. Levy H, Kallenbach JM, Feldman C, Thorburn JR, Abramowitz JA. Acute respiratory failure in active tuberculosis. Crit Care Med. 1987;15:221–5.

39. Silva DR, Menegotto DM, Schulz LF, Gazzana MB, Dalcin PT. Mortality among patients with tuberculosis requiring intensive care: a retrospective cohort study. BMC Infect Dis. 2010;10:54.

40. Lin SM, Wang TY, Liu WT. Predictive factors for mortality among non-HIV-infected patients with pulmonary tuberculosis and respiratory failure. Int J Tuberc Lung Dis. 2009;13:335–40.

41. Zahar JR, Azoulay E, Klement E, De Lassence A, Lucet JC, Regnier B, Schlemmer B, Bedos JP. Delayed treatment contributes to mortality in ICU patients with severe active pulmonary tuberculosis and acute respiratory failure. Intensive Care Med. 2001;27:513–20.

42. Frame RN, Johnson MC, Eichenhorn MS, Bower GC, Popovich J. Active tuberculosis in the medical intensive care unit: a 15-year retrospective analysis. Crit Care Med. 1987;15:1012–4.

43. Hagan G, Nathani N. Clinical review: tuberculosis on the intensive care unit. Crit Care. 2013;17:240.

44. Thwaites G, Fisher M, Hemingway C, Scott G, Solomon T, Innes J. British Infection Society guidelines for the diagnosis and treatment of tuberculosis of the central nervous system in adults and children. J Infect. 2009;59:167–87.

45. National Institute for Health and Clinical Excellence. Tuberculosis: clinical diagnosis and management of tuberculosis, and measures for its prevention and control. http://guidance.nice.org.uk/CG117.

46. Strang JI, Kakaza HH, Gibson DG, Girling DJ, Nunn AJ, Fox W. Controlled trial of prednisolone as adjuvant in treatment of tuberculous constrictive pericarditis in Transkei. Lancet. 1987;19:1418–22.

47. Bloch S, Wickremasinghe M, Wright A, Rice A, Thompson M, Kon OM. Paradoxical reactions in non-HIV tuberculosis presenting as endobronchial obstruction. Eur Resp J. 2009;18:295–9.

48. Cheng SL, Wang HC, Yang PC. Paradoxical response during antituberculosis treatment in HIV negative patients with pulmonary tuberculosis. Int J Tuberc Lung Dis. 2007;11:1290–5.

49. Pozniak AL, Coyne KM, Miller RF, Lipman MC, Freedman AR, Omerod LP, Johnson MA, Collins S, Lucas SB. British HIV Association guidelines for the treatment of TB/HIV coinfection. HIV Med. 2011;12:517–24.

50. Schoeman JF, Fieggen G, Seller N, Mandelson M, Hartzenberg B. Intractable intracranial tuberculous infection responsive to thalidomide: report of four cases. J Child Neurol. 2006;21:301–8.

51. Mukherjee JS, Rich ML, Socci AR, et al. Programmes and principles in treatment of multidrug-resistant tuberculosis. Lancet. 2004;363(9407):474–81.

52. Orenstein EW, et al. Treatment outcomes among patients with multidrug-resistant tuberculosis: systematic review and meta-analysis. Lancet Infect Dis. 2009;9:153–61.

53. Rajbhandary SS, Marks SM, Bock NN. Costs of patients hospitalized for multidrug-resistant tuberculosis. Int J Tuberc Lung Dis. 2004;8:1012–6.

54. Bloss E, et al. Adverse events related to multidrug-resistant tuberculosis treatment, Latvia, 2000-2004. Int J Tuberc Lung Dis. 2010;14:275–81.

55. WHO. WHO treatment guidelines for multidrug- and rifampicin-resistant tuberculosis, 2018 update. Available at https://www.who.int/tb/areas-of-work/drug-resistant-tb/guideline-update2018/en/. Acceded 16 Apr 2019.

56. Ahuja SD, et al. Multidrug resistant pulmonary tuberculosis treatment regimens and patient outcomes: an individual patient data meta-analysis of 9,153 patients. PLoS Med. 2012;e1001300:9.

57. Kumar K, Abubjakar I. Clinical implications of the global multidrug-resistant tuberculosis epidemic. Clin Med. 2015;15(6):s37–42.
58. Iseman MD, Madsen L, Goble M, et al. Surgical intervention in the treatment of pulmonary disease caused by drug-resistant Mycobacterium tuberculosis. Am Rev Respir Dis. 1990;141:623–5.
59. Rizzi A, et al. Results of surgical management of tuberculosis: experience in 206 patients undergoing operation. Ann Thorac Surg. 1995;59:896–900.
60. Man MA, Nicolau D. Surgical treatment to increase the success rate of multidrug-resistant tuberculosis. Eur J Cardiothorac Surg. 2012;42:e9–12.
61. Sung SW, et al. Surgery increased the chance of cure in multi-drug resistant pulmonary tuberculosis. Eur J Cardiothorac Surg. 1999;16:187–93.
62. Shiraishi Y, Katsuragi N, Kita H, et al. Different morbidity after pneumonectomy: multidrug-resistant tuberculosis versus non-tuberculous mycobacterial infection. Interact Cardiovasc Thorac Surg. 2010;11:429–32.
63. Yew WW, Leung CC. Management of multidrug-resistant tuberculosis: update 2007. Respirology. 2008;13:21–46.
64. Seung KJ, Keshavjee S, Rich ML. Multidrug- resistant tuberculosis and extensively drug-resistant tuberculosis. Cold Spring Harb Perspect Med. 2015;5(9):a017863.
65. Seung KJ, Omatayo DB, Keshavjee S, Furin JJ, Farmer PE, Satti H. Early outcomes of MDR-TB treatment in a high HIV-prevalence setting in Southern Africa. PLoS One. 2009;4:e7186.

Chapter 15
Preparing the ICU for a Highly Infectious Disease

Alex Loarca Chávez, Jorge Hidalgo, and Adel Mohamed Yasin Alsisi

Introduction

Several pandemics have existed around the world, and only from influenza, there have been 10 pandemics in 300 years, reaching to cause millions of deaths, for example, the pandemic that lasts year turned a century (the pandemic of 1918) caused 50–100 millions of deaths [1]. During the H1N1 epidemic in 2009, according to data from the Center for Disease Control (CDC), there were 12, 469 deaths. However, there were 274, 304 hospitalizations, only in the United States. However another type of infectious diseases with higher lethality, have oversaturated the intensive care units (ICUs), therefore caused the definition of disaster; such is the case of the Ebola epidemic in 2014, which according to CDC data of 27,000 cases, 11,000 deaths have been reported [2].

Taking into account that in most countries, ICUs are maintained with an occupation close to or equal to 100%, small increases in the number of cases of infectious diseases that require admission to ICU can cause a disaster. According to the WHO is defined as unforeseen situations that represent serious and immediate threats to public health or any public health situation that endangers the life or health of a significant number of people and demands immediate action; since the responsiveness of the ICUs and their teams will be significantly reduced [3].

A. L. Chávez (✉)
Adult Intensive Care, Hospital Regional de Occidente, San Juan de Dios, Quetzaltenango, Guatemala

J. Hidalgo
Division of Critical Care, Karl Heusner Memorial Hospital, Belize City, Belize

A. M. Y. Alsisi
Prime Healthcare Group, LLC, Dubai, UAE
e-mail: dradel@primehospital.ae

© Springer Nature Switzerland AG 2020
J. Hidalgo, L. Woc-Colburn (eds.), *Highly Infectious Diseases in Critical Care*,
https://doi.org/10.1007/978-3-030-33803-9_15

Development of the Plan

The center of the management of the plan should be the leaders of the ICUs and related services and public health authorities, who have the responsibility to coordinate efforts and develop policies to contain infectious diseases and their consequences; allocate material and human resources; advise and disclose the information, protocols, and management guides, for the control and treatment of infections; direct the obtaining of data for investigations; and maintain the morale of the personnel, as well as job security of the same. In addition, the leaders of the units must provide information to the health authorities.

It is proposed the development of "crisis team," composed of the leaders of the sub-teams of interdisciplinary professionals responsible for the care of the patients of the ICU, either directly or indirectly: clinical management, infection control, education, social service, communication, moral support to the team, obtaining data, research, and administration to ensure that resources are available. The role of the critical care crisis team will be to coordinate the actions of the various leaders; to avoid duplication of efforts through the regular exchange of information, problems, and support; work together to devise creative solutions; and anticipate future needs (Fig. 15.1).

Response Capacity of Intensive Care Units

Some ICUs operate at or near 100% bed occupancy. In many countries, ICUs have a limited response capacity in case of a small increase in the number of patients requiring admission to these units [4].

Fig. 15.1 The crisis team is signed by clinical management, infection control, education, service social, communication, moral support to the team, obtaining data, research, and administration to ensure that resources are available

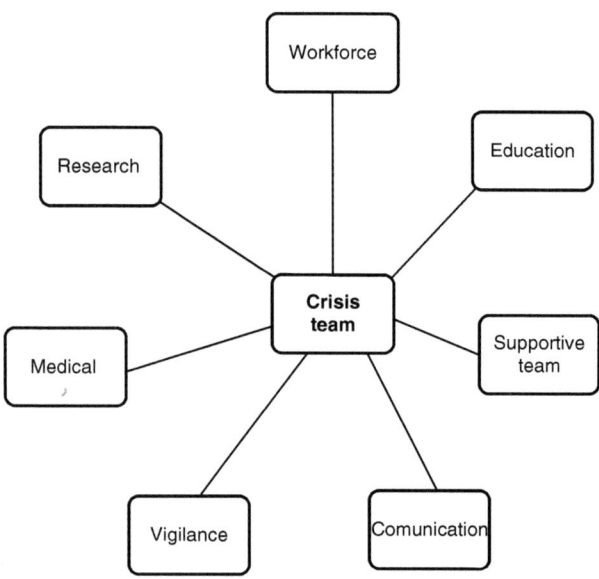

In addition, the ICU augmentation capacity, designed in most disaster planning, has been designed around mass casualty events with a large number of cases arriving in a period of a few hours. However, the prevalence rapidly decreases to over hours to days [5]. However, in infectious disease disasters, the increase in requirements of intensive care units usually lasts for several weeks, for example, during the H1N1 pandemic in 2009, patients required mechanical ventilation for 8 days, 25% for more than 16 days, only in Australia and New Zealand [6]. Besides, this type of epidemics is seasonal, and the time of occurrence of cases from 8 to 12 weeks may be prolonged [5].

Four factors can limit the response capacity concerning the expansion of ICU care:

- Staff availability
- Consumables and essential equipment such as mechanical fans
- Bed spaces
- Management and coordination systems [3]

Staff Availability

The availability of sufficient medical and paramedical personnel trained and experienced in the care of critical patients is the main factor that may or may not limit the ability to respond to a disaster. Therefore, during the epideiological alerte, vacations, ICU staff permits, changes in the nursing/patient relationship, and doctor/patient changes should be suspended, with mandatory extra hours. Personnel with previous experience in ICU, assigned to other services, can be reassigned to critical services during the alert. Besides, this person can be used in the care of critical patients in areas outside the ICU. Also, under no circumstances should attention be overlooked to health personnel who are working in the ICU, in terms of prevention of contagion of personnel, through vaccination, use of protective equipment, and hygiene measures. Psychological care and the needs of the staff, which for obvious reasons is prone to contagion and work fatigue, which will lead to inefficient work or work suspensions due to illness or, in the worse scenario, the hospitalization of health personnel [7].

Supplies and Equipment

The storage of medications, such as antivirals, is essential as a response strategy. Likewise, medications considered routine must have a significant amount for the response. The capacity of expansion of the ICU can be correctly anticipated, through prior planning and agreements with suppliers of supplies and equipment, for the immediate acquisition of the same for expansion. It is vital to take into account the supplies used for the protection of personnel, such as masks, gowns, diving suits, and hygiene materials, according to the cleaning protocol, which will be different depending on the level of infection that the epidemic in question may have, from infections such as diarrhea and even highly contagious infections like Ebola [8].

Availability of Spaces

In most countries, ICU bed occupancy is close to 100%, even without the pandemic. Which easily converts into infectious diseases disaster, to an increase of the cases of an infectious disease that due to the severity of the clinical picture, requires attention in ICU. Therefore, the creation of additional spaces, through the opening of previously closed spaces and conversion of other spaces in the ICU, such as intermediate care, anesthesia recovery rooms, coronary care units, areas of temporary emergency patient management, and even general care rooms, for which the response plan of each hospital must consider the mechanisms to convert these spaces into UCI spaces, taking into account the personnel that will attend those spaces and the necessary supplies. Without neglecting attention to the rest of patients who are already requiring ICUs, for other types of diseases, and ideally, the separation of these patients [5]. Figure 15.2 shows the impact that the infectious disaster can have on spaces in the ICU, which classifies the severity of the disaster concerning the increase in the percentage of saturation of the services [9].

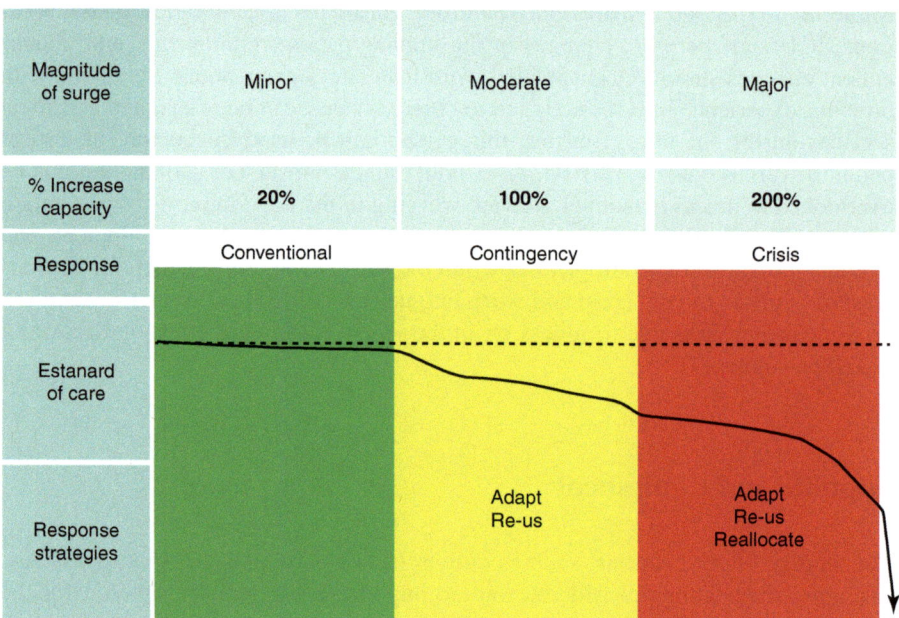

Fig. 15.2 The magnitude of crisis depends on the responsiveness of the systems, of the ability to maintain the balance between demand and response. According to the severity of the crisis will be the level of response

Management Systems

They are vital systems, which must respond in a scalable way, according to the pandemic. The management systems of the ICU should be understood within a response system of the hospital and by public health authorities [5]. The purpose of these systems is to establish avenues for communication and the elaboration of a disaster response plan. During the H1N1 pandemic in 2009, an infectious disaster response management system would have helped the planning and management of critical patient spaces in mechanical ventilation [5]. The management system must assemble the "crisis team," which, as already explained, is the interdisciplinary team that responds to the control of the infection.

Infection Control

The measures directed to the effective control of the infection are vital for the preparation and handling of the pandemic. The prevention of infections to health personnel and nosocomial infections to other hospitalized patients is of crucial importance, including the isolation of the first cases and the infection prevention measures, such as the use of gloves, gowns, caps, N95 masks, and face shield, according to the level of universal measures according to the bio-infectivity of the pandemic in question [7]. For which, the protection protocol must be individualized, as well as the disinfection of the equipment used with patients, beds, and all supplies [11].

Laboratory Capacity

The ability of the laboratory to develop and apply validated rapid diagnostic tests, such as PCR, represents a positive impact on the control of the pandemic, as it happened in the H1N1 pandemic of 2009. However, in critically ill patients, this type of tests has less sensitivity. The response capacity of the laboratory is easily overcome, due to the number of suspected cases that meet the definition of the case; therefore, the team of management systems should plan with the suppliers of the diagnostic tests, for a rapid response to the increase in demand in case of disaster [10].

Triage

During an infectious disease event that increases the number of admissions to the ICU, and therefore increases in the consumption of supplies, of the number of personnel in the ICU; To the extent that it exceeds the capacity of response of the same, it will be defined as a "disaster" of infectious diseases. Therefore, it will be mandatory to apply the *Triage*, which categorizes the type of patients that will be admitted

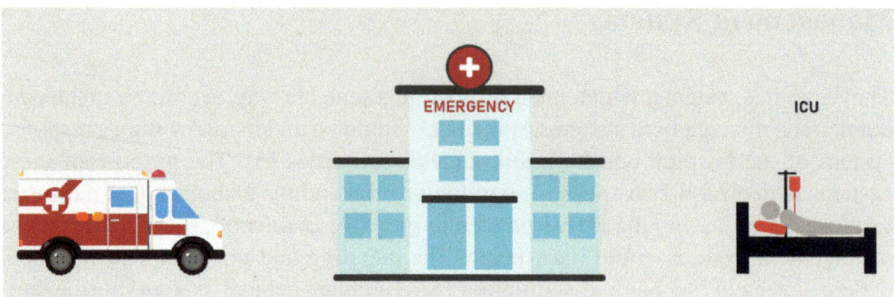

Fig. 15.3 The levels of triage are prehospital, emergency rooms, and the ICU

to the ICU services, as well as the services adapted for the care of critical patients during the disaster [9].

No significant alterations are observed in standards or processes of response to a crisis response where resource limitations cause significant alterations in standards and care processes to provide minimal critical care. In this context, the application of the triage that classifies which patient will receive this attention and who does not can reduce the number of losses and optimize the use of resources. The triage must be done at three levels: the first level is prehospital, the second is at the level of emergency rooms to prioritize or not the care of each patient, and the third involves the ICU, as shown in Fig. 15.3. It refers to the decision of the level of care needed by the patient within the hospital, to decide whether or not to enter the ICU. The following image exemplifies the above [9].

The decision flow process of the triadic triage, which involves the UCI, should be:

1. Inclusion criteria: refractory hypoxemia and persistent hypotension, among the most classic criteria.
2. The analysis of the exclusion criteria, because even if the patient meets inclusion criteria, if the patient has a low probability of survival or has comorbidities with a short period of life expectancy, he/she should be excluded.
3. Prioritization of attention; in the case of a disaster of infectious diseases, several patients at the same time may require their attention in the ICU, however, due to the oversaturation of the same, to give priority, according to the immediacy that the need, better prognosis and more significant benefit.
4. Daily reassessment, after admission, to establish discharge criteria or develop exclusion criteria during the stay.
5. Verification at 72 hours of the care that has been given to the patient, based on the objectives of the admission of each case, asking whether or not there is evidence of significant improvement [9, 12].

Conclusion

We will inevitably have future pandemics, many of which will require significant increases in the ICU's income, in addition to the devastating consequences of human losses as a result of infectious diseases; there is no doubt that we will never be sufficiently prepared. However, the planning of the response systems, simulations, and better organization of each unit will make us better prepared.

References

1. Osterholm MT. Preparing for the next pandemic. N Engl J Med. 2005;352:1839–42.
2. Gao HN, Lu HZ, Cao B, et al. Clinical findings in 111 cases of influenza A (H7N9) virus infection. N Engl J Med. 2013;368:2277–85.
3. World Health Organization, European Regional Office. Emergency preparedness & response program. EURO/EPR/90. Copenhagen: WHO, European Regional Office; 1990.
4. Devereaux AV, Dichter JR, Christian MD, et al. Definitive care for the critically ill during a disaster: a framework for allocation of scarce resources in mass critical care: from a task force for mass critical care summit meeting January 26–27 Chicago, IL. Chest. 2008;133(Suppl 5):51S–66S.
5. Hota S, Fried E, Burry L, et al. Preparing your intensive care unit for the second wave of H1N1 and future surges. Crit Care Med. 2010;38(Suppl 4):e110–9.
6. Webb SA, Pettila V, Seppelt I, et al. Critical care services and 2009 H1N1 influenza in Australia and New Zealand. N Engl J Med. 2009;361:1925–34.
7. Funk DJ, Siddiqui F, Wiebe K, et al. Practical lessons from the first outbreaks: clinical presentation, obstacles, and management strategies for severe pandemic (pH1N1) 2009 influenza pneumonitis. Crit Care Med. 2010;38(Suppl 4):e30–7.
8. Ver Infection prevention and control of epidemic- and pandemic-prone acute respiratory diseases in health care disponible en: http://www.who.int/csr/resources/publications/WHO_CD_EPR_2007_6/en/index.html.
9. Christian MD, et al. Triage care of the critically ill and injured during pandemics and disasters: chest consensus statement. Chest. 2014;146(4 Suppl):e61S–74S.
10. Iwasenko JM, Cretikos M, Paterson DL, et al. Enhanced diagnosis of pandemic (H1N1) 2009 influenza infection using molecular and serological testing in intensive care unit patients with suspected influenza. Clin Infect Dis. 2010;51:70–2.
11. Rutala WA, Weber DJ, et al. Guideline for disinfection and sterilization in healthcare facilities. 2008. Update: May 2019. Accessible version: https://www.cdc.gov/infectioncontrol/guidelines/disinfection/.
12. Cook D, Burns K, Finfer S, et al. Clinical research ethics for critically ill patients: a pandemic proposal. Crit Care Med. 2010;38(4 suppl):e138–42.

Chapter 16
Pandemic Declaration and Preparation

Michael J. Plotkowski

Pandemic Phase Descriptions

As defined by the World Health Organization:

Phase 1 No animal virus circulating among animals has been reported to cause infection in humans.

Phase 2 An animal virus circulating in domesticated or wild animals is known to have caused infection in humans and is therefore considered a specific potential pandemic threat.

Phase 3 An animal or human-animal virus has caused sporadic cases or small clusters of disease in people, but has not resulted in human-to-human transmission sufficient to sustain community-level outbreaks.

Phase 4 Human-to-human transmission of an animal or human-animal virus able to sustain community-level outbreaks has been verified.

Phase 5 The same identified virus has caused sustained community-level outbreaks in two or more countries in one WHO region.

Phase 6 In addition to the criteria defined in Phase 5, the same virus has caused sustained community-level outbreaks in at least one other country in another WHO region.

M. J. Plotkowski (✉)
Department of State, Foreign Service Medical Provider, U.S. Embassy Belmopan, Belmopan, Belize
e-mail: plotkowskimj@state.gov

© Springer Nature Switzerland AG 2020
J. Hidalgo, L. Woc-Colburn (eds.), *Highly Infectious Diseases in Critical Care*,
https://doi.org/10.1007/978-3-030-33803-9_16

Post-Peak Period Levels of the pandemic virus in most countries with adequate surveillance have dropped below peak levels.

Possible New Wave Level of pandemic virus activity in most countries with adequate surveillance rising again.

Post-Pandemic Period Levels of virus activity have returned to the levels seen for Phase 1/2 in most countries with adequate surveillance.[1]

As noted above, Phases 1–3 correlates with preparedness and surveillance, including capacity development and response planning activities. Phases 4–6 signal the need for response and mitigation efforts. Furthermore, periods after the first pandemic wave are elaborated to facilitate post-pandemic recovery activities.

Pandemic Preparation

Surveillance, Epidemiology, and Laboratory Activities – Better detection and monitoring of seasonal and emerging novel viruses are critical to assuring a rapid recognition and response to a pandemic.

Community Mitigation Measures – Incorporating actions and response measures people and communities can take to help slow the spread of a novel virus. Community mitigation measures may be used from the earliest stages of a pandemic, including the initial months when the most effective countermeasure – a vaccine against the new pandemic virus – might not yet be broadly available.

Medical Countermeasures: Diagnostic Devices, Vaccines, Therapeutics, and Respiratory Devices – Aggressive translation of applied research in diagnostics, therapeutics, and vaccines may yield breakthrough MCMs to mitigate the next pandemic. Building on existing systems for product logistics, as well as advances in technology and regulatory science, can increase access to and use of critical countermeasures to inform response activities.

Healthcare System Preparedness and Response Activities – Delivery system reform efforts of the past decade have made today's healthcare system dramatically different from 2005. The next 10 years will bring even more changes to delivery settings, provider types, reimbursement models, the sharing of electronic health information, referral patterns, business relationships, and expanded individual choice. Despite these changes, healthcare systems must be prepared to respond to a pandemic, recognizing that potentially large numbers of people with symptoms of the virus, as well as those concerned about the pandemic, will present for care. Systems must implement surge strategies, so people receive care that is appropriate to their level of need, thereby conserving higher levels of care for those who need them.

---

[1] https://www.who.int/csr/disease/swineflu/phase/en/

Communications and Public Outreach – Communication planning is integral to early and effective messaging when a pandemic threatens, establishes itself, and expands. Accurate, consistent, timely, and actionable communication is enhanced by the use of plain language and accessible formats. Testing messages and using appropriate channels and spokespeople will enhance our ability to deliver consistent and accurate information to multiple audiences.

Scientific Infrastructure and Preparedness – A robust scientific infrastructure underpins everything to prepare for, and respond to, pandemic and other emerging infectious diseases. Strong scientific foundations are needed to develop new vaccines and therapeutics and to determine how well other control efforts are working. Rigorous scientific methods applied during a pandemic response yield information to improve both ongoing and future responses.

Domestic and International Response Policy, Incident Management, and Global Partnerships and Capacity Building – Coordinate both domestic and international pandemic preparedness and response activities. This will include having clearly defined mechanisms for rapid exchange of information, data, reagents, and other resources needed domestically and globally, to prepare for and respond to a pandemic outbreak.[2]

Preparation with Limited Resources

The medical staff in the local healthcare facility with limited resources will be challenged to appropriately plan for and manage an epidemic, let alone a pandemic. In this case, we need to concentrate on the basics of preparation and planning.

Recognition of a communicable disease depends on surveillance – looking for evidence of infection.

Viral surveillance – determines what viral strains are circulating in the community. Collecting at the local level and contributing to a worldwide database in order to determine new viral recombinant. Without viral surveillance, early identification of the novel agent would be delayed.

Hand in hand with confirmation of the specific agent is disease surveillance. Disease surveillance entails collecting information on epidemiological and clinical features of specific disease caused by a viral illness. Important information to obtain are:

1. Estimated incubation period
2. Duration of illness
3. Level of infectivity
4. Case fatality and complication rate

---

[2] https://www.cdc.gov/flu/pandemic-resources/pdf/pan-flu-report-2017v2.pdf

5. Sensitivity to antibiotics/antivirals and development of clinical drug resistance
6. Changes in the viral signature/characteristics
7. Disease activity in a given location

Local health facilities should contribute to assisting organizations doing worldwide monitoring for new disease outbreaks by supplying specimens for analysis through existing surveillance programs.

Viral confirmation (PCR confirmation) is vital in disease management early in the course of a disease outbreak or early pandemic. PCR confirmation extrapolates specific diseases when encountering a cluster of signs and symptoms. PCR confirmation becomes less critical when in an outbreak with widespread disease and active cases; the local facility should have an excellent idea of what is causing the viral illness based on surveillance done early in the surveillance process. As an example, the www.cdc.gov/h1n1flu/casedef.htm provides the definition of Influenza-like illness (ILI): fever 100 °F or higher and cough/sore throat without other explanation. If these signs and symptoms are present, the condition meets criteria for possible ILI; the history of exposure or positive rapid testing for Influenza suggests suspected ILI, and positive PCR confirmation is specific for seasonal influenza or novel H1N1 influenza infection.

Health facilities should submit specimens to nationally designated organizations year-round for patients meeting surveillance case definition and other entry criteria after obtaining informed consent for participation. Review surveillance protocols regularly to assure the healthcare facility is collecting data on eligible patients and is familiar with the screening and collection protocols.

Review specimen handling protocols, shipping requirements. Perform a test run of a specimen, primarily if an international commercial carrier is being used to forward specimens to international labs. If the healthcare facility will have to forward specimens internationally to any lab as part of a study or for lab confirmation of infection, have shipping information available ahead of time. Proper labeling and packaging of specimens are critical to the safe and successful shipment of surveillance specimens. International transport requirements are available at www.transport.org. Check with commercial shippers to assure diagnostic samples will be accepted.

Use proper personal protective equipment when collecting potentially infectious materials: goggles, gloves, gowns, and N95 respirators that fit. Close exposure to droplets and aerosolized materials is always a probability when doing nasopharyngeal swabs for respiratory organism collection. Medical staffs performing such collections need to regularly review collection techniques and ideally have performed collections during training exercises. To ensure the best and most timely results, review before an outbreak situation to avoid delay and mismanaged samples.

Planning with Limited Resources

In planning for a pandemic medical response, healthcare providers need to engage in several levels of activities. Pandemic response preparation requires regular review of supplies and review of response protocols. Designation of tasks to specific staff and cross-training in the event of illness or staff absences is essential. Review and updates of inventories and protocols need to be performed at regular intervals as part of staff in-house training and orientation for all personnel. These components should be consistent throughout national healthcare facilities and include universal blood-borne precautions; droplet, contact, and respiratory precautions; PPE use and mask fit testing (if not previously performed); community prevention measures; and health facility triage for outpatients. Antiviral drugs, PPE, and other pandemic-related supplies should be well maintained, regularly inventoried, and readily available.

The seasonal flu vaccine is recommended for all; not only is it effective against the seasonal flu, but in the event of a viral pandemic, it may lessen the morbidity and mortality. Clinical differentiation between seasonal Influenza and other viral illness may be difficult, and reducing the incidence of seasonal flu in the community will decrease the necessity for such clinical dilemmas.

Each medical facility is unique in its staffing, resources, access to resources, and potential barriers to getting patients to medical care. The time to think about resources and barriers is now; identify them ahead of time. Determine how the facility will deal with high-risk patients and those who develop a worsening infection. If the number and severity of cases exceed your resources and training, a plan must be already established. Medical transfer capabilities and resources, as well as their alternatives, must be known and reliable. Medical resources in the community should be identified, and it is vital to establish a good working relationship and discuss preparations to manage a potential patient surge. Other considerations include establish what resources are in the community and whether there is any "surge capacity." During an outbreak, the anticipated hospital bed availability must be known.

Additionally, the healthcare facility must conserve a sufficient amount of medical supplies to maintain droplet isolation and general sanitation. Other important information to identify before an outbreak includes how many ventilators are in the local hospital and are the ICU facilities and training adequate to support an outbreak. Other questions to answer include the local facilities policy for hospitalization viral illness for minors and if parents are allowed to accompany them.

Local healthcare facilities must work through government and non-governmental health organizations to identify the ministry of health and other public health contacts in the community who can provide information on community outbreaks and national response. Additionally, the local healthcare facility must understand the local government's policies on isolation and quarantine, as well as the barriers to transferring patients to a higher level of care. The local health authorities must understand and comply with the particular criteria to make diagnosis, isolate, and quarantine patients.

All facility supervisors should discuss with personnel how to prioritize activities in the event of a pandemic. House calls, clinic hours, hospital visits, and dealing with telephone calls and other communications are the most prominent demands.

Conclusion

Planning and preparation at each level of patient care will augment the devastating effects of a pandemic. Surveillance is essential for detecting new viruses and will help specify and target alleviating countermeasures. Communication and coordination with governmental, non-governmental agencies, and the Ministry of Health can strengthen the response to a pandemic. Developing protocols and plans for the local health facility will ensure consistency and reliability in response to a pandemic. Additionally, practicing and reassessing protocols to reinforce good practices and adapt to changes is necessary to battle the effects of the pandemic.

Index

© Springer Nature Switzerland AG 2020
J. Hidalgo, L. Woc-Colburn (eds.), *Highly Infectious Diseases in Critical Care*,
https://doi.org/10.1007/978-3-030-33803-9